Language and Communication in Mental Retardation

Development, Processes, and Intervention

TOPICS IN APPLIED PSYCHOLINGUISTICS
Sheldon Rosenberg, Series Editor

Language and Communication in Mental Retardation

Development, Processes, and Intervention

Sheldon Rosenberg
University of Illinois at Chicago

Leonard Abbeduto
University of Wisconsin-Madison

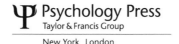
Ψ Psychology Press
Taylor & Francis Group

New York London

First Published by
Lawrence Erlbaum Associates, Inc., Publishers
365 Broadway
Hillsdale, New Jersey 07642

Transferred to Digital Printing 2009 by Psychology Press
270 Madison Avenue, New York NY 10016
27 Church Road, Hove, East Sussex BN3 2FA

Library of Congress Cataloging-in-Publication Data

Rosenberg, Sheldon.
Language and communication in mental retardation : Development,
processes, and intervention / Sheldon Rosenberg and Leonard
Abbeduto.
p.   cm. — (Topics in applied psycholinguistics)
Includes bibliographical references and index.
ISBN 0-8058-0302-5 (c) — ISBN 0-8058-0303-3 (p)
1. Communicative disorders in children. 2. Mentally handicapped
children—Language. I. Abbeduto, Leonard, 1954-   . II. Title.
III. Series.
RJ496.C67R68 1993
618.92 '8588—dc20   93-6806
                                                                CIP

Publisher's Note
The publisher has gone to great lengths to ensure the quality
of this reprint but points out that some imperfections in the
original may be apparent.

To Gordon Trevor and Clarke Sheldon with Grandpa's love

—S.R.

To Terry, Jackson, and Mack with all my love

—L.A.

Contents

Preface

This book is a volume in the series, *Topics in Applied Psycholinguistics* (Sheldon Rosenberg, Editor). The series is designed to make available critical, integrative reviews of research and theory in selected areas of applied psycholinguistics written at a level that will be useful to advanced undergraduate and first-year graduate students as primary or secondary texts in relevant courses in, for example, developmental psychology, cognitive psychology, linguistics, educational psychology, special education, and communication disorders. However, researchers, practitioners, and more advanced graduate students will also find the material useful for review or introductory purposes.

In this book, we present a critical, integrative review of research and theory on language and communication in persons with mental retardation. The basic assumption that guided our effort is that a characterization of linguistic knowledge, first-language acquisition, communicative knowledge, and the development of communicative competence in nondisabled persons is logically prior to the study of disorders of first-language acquisition. Therefore, we included in the book, especially with the needs of readers with a limited background in mind, introductory material on linguistic (chapter 2) and communicative (chapter 6) knowledge and development in nondisabled persons and additional background material as needed in the substantive chapters on language and communication in persons with mental retardation. Moreover, interested students and researchers will find throughout the book discussions of important theoretical issues in basic psycholinguistics (particularly as regards normal language acquisition) that are raised by the results of research on language and communication in persons with mental retardation.

The relevant substantive literature in mental retardation is organized along lines that are familiar in psycholinguistics. Thus, we treat phonological development in chapter 3, semantic development in chapter 4, morphosyntactic development in chapter 5, communicative development in chapter 7, and adult–child interactions in chapter 8. Work on language and communication intervention is reviewed in chapter 9. In our introduction (chapter 1), we discuss material on the nature of mental retardation and related work in cognitive development.

ACKNOWLEDGMENTS

We wish to acknowledge the assistance of members of the staff of the Department of Psychology at the University of Illinois at Chicago with the preparation of the final manuscript. We also wish to thank Glenis Benson, Catherine Short, and Jill Nuccio for comments on chapters. Finally, we are indebted to Judith Amsel, Vice President, Editorial at Lawrence Erlbaum Associates for her continuous support and encouragement during the preparation of the manuscript.

Leonard Abbeduto's work on this book was supported by grant No. RO1 HD24356 and grant No. P30 HD03352, both from the National Institute of Child Health and Human Development.

—Sheldon Rosenberg
—Leonard Abbeduto

1

Introduction

In this book, we describe and account for the linguistic and communicative capabilities of persons with mental retardation. As we understand it, *mental retardation* is a condition characterized by delayed (but not qualitatively different from normal) intellectual growth, as indexed by performance on a standardized test of intelligence. It is a condition, moreover, that appears early in life, tends to persist, has multiple causes, varies in severity, and has implications for the ability of an afflicted person to adjust to the demands of everyday independent living in a world of other people.

Given this picture of mental retardation and the common observation that intelligence includes both nonverbal and verbal components (Horn, 1976), we expect to find that language and communicative development in persons with mental retardation, as compared to chronological age (CA)-matched normal (non-retarded) persons, are characterized by: (a) later onset, (b) slower but not deviant development, (c) lower final level of achievement, and (d) variation in onset, rate of development, and final level of achievement. However, the reader will learn, as we did, that these expectations are not always supported by the available research literature. A lower final level of achievement, for example, is not an inevitable correlate of mental retardation. In other words, our examination of the research literature on language and communication in persons with mental retardation revealed a more complex relationship between mental retardation and development in these domains than one would have anticipated.

To illustrate this fact, we turn to a review of three studies of language functioning in persons with mental retardation. We then attempt to define mental retardation more fully.

1

SELECTED STUDIES

Dooley's 1976 PhD Dissertation

Dooley (1976) analyzed recorded samples of the spontaneous speech of two home-reared Down syndrome children, Timmy (IQ = 51, MA = 2;51, CA = 3;10 at time of testing) and Sharon (IQ = 44, MA = 2;11, CA = 5;2 at time of testing), at approximately 2-week intervals over a period of 12 months. (Age figures separated by a semicolon refer to years and months.) Down syndrome is a chromosomal disorder (in most cases, the cells of the affected individual contain three number 21 chromosomes instead of the normal two) that is associated with, among other things, mental retardation (Pisarchick, 1987). At the outset of the investigation, Timmy's CA was 3;9 and Sharon's was 5;1. Neither child displayed any hearing or speech-articulation problems that might have interfered with performance. The data analyzed by Dooley consisted of the first three (Sample I) and the last three (Sample II) sessions of the 12-month period. The specific measures he examined were computed from the children's analyzable single and multiword nonimitative utterances. An imitation was considered to be "a partial or complete repetition of any of the preceding five utterances of another speaker" (p. 23).

On a measure found to correlate positively with linguistic maturity in nondisabled preschoolers (Brown, 1973; Miller, 1981)—mean length of utterance (MLU)—both Timmy and Sharon were functioning at what is called Stage I of normal multiword syntactic development (Brown, 1973). Specifically, the MLUs of both children fell between 1 and 2 morphemes. Timmy's MLUs were 1.48 and 1.75 for Samples I and II, respectively; Sharon's were 1.84 and 1.73.

For readers with limited backgrounds in linguistics, the morpheme is the smallest linguistic unit that is assigned meaning in a language. Moreover, linguists distinguish between content morphemes (nouns, verbs, adjectives, and some adverbs) and grammatical morphemes (articles, prepositions, auxiliary *be*, modals such as *would* and *could*, tense markers on verbs, and pluralization markers on nouns). Thus, an utterance such as *John parked the car* consists of five morphemes: *John, park, -ed, the,* and *car*. In the main, grammatical morphemes serve to modulate and enrich the meanings of the basic sentence structures in a language (Brown, 1973) and play a fundamental role in sentence grammar (Radford, 1990a).

How do Timmy and Sharon's MLUs compare with those of nonmentally retarded children? Dooley compared their MLUs with that of Kathryn, a nondisabled child whose spontaneous speech had been studied by L. Bloom (1970). Kathryn's MLU at 1;9, when the first sample of her spontaneous speech was taken, was 1.32. Six weeks later it was 1.92, whereas 3 months later it was 2.83. Clearly, Kathryn made more progress in 6 weeks than Timmy and Sharon made in a year.

On the basis of data from nondisabled children reported by Miller (1981, pp. 26–27), it is possible to predict, within certain limits, the MLUs of children from their CAs and vice versa. According to these norms, at the outset of Dooley's study, Timmy's MLU should have fallen somewhere between 4.09 and 4.40, whereas Sharon's should have been somewhere between 5.63 and 6.00. Instead, as indicated, Timmy's MLU was 1.48 and Sharon's 1.84 in Sample I. Furthermore, in Sample II, Timmy's MLU increased to only 1.75, whereas Sharon's actually decreased somewhat to 1.73. In terms of Miller's norms, Timmy and Sharon's MLUs for Samples I and II combined were characteristic of nondisabled children whose CAs were 2;0 and 2;1, respectively. Therefore, according to their MLUs, both children (and Sharon to a greater extent than Timmy) appear to have developed language at an appreciably slower rate than their nonmentally retarded CA-matched counterparts. Moreover, it appears that their language development was also slow for their MAs.

During the early stages of normal language acquisition, there is an increase in the use of multiword utterances. Thus, another estimate of the rate of development of language employed by Dooley was the percentage of nonimitated spontaneous productions that were multiword utterances. On this measure, Sharon showed less change from Sample I (38%) to Sample II (41%) than did Timmy (37% to 48%). Dooley reported, however, that over a period of only 1 month (from CA 1;9), Kathryn's multiword utterances grew from 32% to 54%.

Expressive lexicon (vocabulary) size increased from Sample I to Sample II for both Timmy and Sharon, as did utterance diversity, which was somewhat similar to that of the utterances produced by 3 nondisabled children studied by Brown (1973), whose MLUs and CAs at the time ranged from 1.68 to 2.06 and 1;6 to 2;3, respectively.

The above measures, of course, do not identify the specific linguistic structures that are developing. We turn now to data that do.

During Stage I of language development, nondisabled children (Brown, 1973) make considerable progress in the mastery of the multiword syntactic structures that express semantic relations such as: (a) *nomination* (e.g., *It's a duck, Me doctor*), (b) *nonexistence* (e.g., *No knife, It gone*), (c) *agent–action* (e.g., *It spilled, The cat sleeping*), (d) *entity-locative* (e.g., *It's outside, They here*), and (e) *possessor-possession* (e.g., *My comb, Baby bed*). Dooley found that such structures and relations accounted for a substantial percentage of Timmy's and Sharon's multiword utterances in Samples I and II. Indeed, these examples, which look very much like the utterances produced by nondisabled children during Stage I, were actually produced by Sharon (Dooley, 1976, Appendix B.2). Similar examples can be found in Timmy's protocol. Timmy and Sharon both showed a substantial increase in the relative use of basic semantic relations from Sample I to Sample II, although Timmy's use of such relations increased to a greater extent than Sharon's. On this and other measures, then, Dooley's two Down Syndrome children with mental retardation differed in their rates of language development. Such differences, of course, are also characteristic of nondisabled children (Brown, 1973).

Dooley compared his subjects' performance on semantic relations with that of a younger nondisabled child, Kendall (Bowerman, 1973), for whom data were available at two different times (CA 1;10 and 1;11). He reported that "Kendall's growth in one month was approximately half the growth shown over a period of a year by Timmy and Sharon" (Dooley, 1976, p. 88). Moreover, it appears that Timmy and Sharon achieved a level of use of semantic relations not unlike that of the 3 younger (CAs 1;6, 2;3, and 2;3) nondisabled children studied by Brown (1973). Therefore, we have further evidence of delay in the mastery of these relations, although the delay is not as great as that suggested by the comparison with Kendall.

From an examination of cross-linguistic studies of early multiword utterances in nondisabled children, Bowerman (1975) proposed that, in the main, "word order corresponds to the dominant (or only) adult order" (p. 280). In other words, young nondisabled children appear to recognize early the significance of word-order constraints in the local language. Do children with mental retardation show similar sensitivity? The answer, based upon Rosenberg's (1982) analysis of the multiword utterances of Timmy and Sharon, is yes. According to Rosenberg, both children "appear to have been sensitive to word order constraints in expressing semantic relations in the earliest stage of combinatorial speech" (p. 340).

One of the most thoroughly investigated aspects of language development in English-speaking children is the mastery of grammatical morphemes, 14 of which were made famous by Brown (1973). These grammatical morphemes included the present progressive (-*ing*), the plural, the uncontractible copula (e.g., *Are they nice?*), the past regular (-*ed*), and the third person irregular (e.g., *He has* or *does*).

To a considerable extent, an examination of the linguistic and nonlinguistic environments of communication allows one to identify contexts that require a particular grammatical morpheme. Thus, if a person is asked the question "How did John get home last night?" we would find appropriate "He walked," but not "He walks," "He will walk," or "He walking." Brown (1973) employed 90% correct usage in obligatory contexts as a criterion of grammatical morpheme mastery.

In brief, what Brown and other developmental psycholinguists found regarding the 14 grammatical morphemes is a more or less invariant order of mastery among nondisabled children. What is more, on the average, the process of mastery begins late in Stage I. Given these findings, it was inevitable that Dooley would examine the progress of mastery of the 14 grammatical morphemes in Timmy and Sharon.

According to this investigator, these Stage I children "had not acquired productive usage of any of the 14 grammatical morphemes considered . . ."

(Dooley, 1976, p. 98). Timmy and Sharon's performance on the 14 grammatical morphemes was comparable to that of Brown's 3 younger nondisabled children at Stage I, who had also failed to acquire any of these morphemes. However, an examination of the percentage of correct usage in obligatory contexts for these morphemes did not suggest that they were mastering them in an order different from that of Brown's 3 nondisabled children.

Finally, Timmy and Sharon employed pronouns rather than nouns in the expression of a number of the basic semantic relations (e.g., agent–action), and a substantial proportion of their multiword utterances were syntactically unanalyzed routines or formulas (e.g., multiword utterances such as *thank you* and *say cheese* in which at least one of the words does not appear in combination with any other word or words).

Thus, like nondisabled children, Timmy and Sharon produced both pronouns and formulaic utterances; however, as Dooley pointed out, they also employed nouns to express, for example, the agent role in agent-action utterances and displayed productive use of a number of syntactic structures in their word combinations.

In summary, Dooley's subjects developed the same linguistic structures that nondisabled children develop, albeit at an appreciably slower rate. Moreover, the rate varied with the measure under investigation. In addition, like nondisabled children, Timmy and Sharon differed in the progress they made during Stage I of language acquisition. Finally, none of the findings suggested that the strategies Timmy and Sharon employed in mastering English differed from those employed by nondisabled children whose language development has been studied. In general, then, we found evidence of exceptional delay relative to CA and MA but no evidence of deviance in the language development of Dooley's 2 children with Down syndrome.

Rosenberg and Abbeduto's Research on the Linguistic Competence of Adults with Mild Mental Retardation

Rosenberg and Abbeduto's (1987) investigation differed in a number of respects from Dooley's:

1. Their subjects were adults (CAs 21 to 31) whose MAs were higher.
2. The subject sample was larger.
3. Although the factors responsible for (i.e., the etiologies of) their mental retardation were unknown, none of Rosenberg and Abbeduto's subjects appeared to be suffering from Down syndrome.
4. The data consisted of measures of linguistic competence—grammatical morpheme and complex sentence usage (percentage of total number of

sentences)—taken from the spontaneous conversations of triads of the subjects.

The focus of the analysis of grammatical morphemes in this study was the 14 items studied by Brown (1973). On average, Rosenberg and Abbeduto's subjects had reached Brown's criterion of 90% correct usage in obligatory contexts on all but three of these morphemes. Moreover, a significant positive correlation was found ''between mean percent correct usage in obligatory contexts and Brown's rank order of acquisition'' (p. 23) in nondisabled children. Thus, the errors made by the adults with mental retardation on the 14 grammatical morphemes, although quite limited in number, tended to occur on items that young nondisabled children (as well as Dooley's Down syndrome children) also found difficult. It is possible, therefore, that all such individuals acquire the 14 grammatical morphemes in a similar manner.

Mature complex sentence usage reflects a mastery of grammatical operations that allow one to combine simple sentences. Moreover, complex sentences are complex both syntactically and semantically. It is not surprising, then, that it takes nondisabled children a number of years to master such structures (Bowerman, 1979; Karmiloff-Smith, 1986).

Overall, the largest percentage of complex sentences produced by Rosenberg and Abbeduto's adults with mental retardation (31.1%) were those composed of three or more simple sentences. Moreover, 28% of their conversational turns contained one or more complex sentences. In addition, these investigators noted that their subjects produced instances of the majority of the complex sentence types in the English language.

The subjects in this study, then, displayed a relatively high level of (if not normal) mastery of complex sentence structures and 14 grammatical morphemes. This group of persons with mental retardation, therefore, may have evidenced little or no delay in language development or, if they were appreciably delayed, were eventually able to catch up to their nondisabled counterparts. In any event, it is clear that mental retardation is not a disorder that necessarily results in a lower than normal level of mastery of an individual's first language.

In brief, a group of individuals with mental retardation whose MAs were estimated in adulthood at between 8 and 13 years were able to master rather abstract features of language. In other words, their linguistic competence showed more consistency with their MAs than Dooley's (1976) subjects with Down syndrome. These same subjects, moreover, displayed appreciable mastery of some of the requirements of conversation (Abbeduto & Rosenberg, 1980), including: (a) the mechanics of turn taking, (b) the means for expressing and recognizing such communicative functions as assertations, questions, and directives, (c) topic introduction and maintenance procedures, and (d) the means for making and responding to requests for clarification and more information appropriately.

Curtiss' Case Studies

Curtiss (1988b; see also Curtiss, 1988a) reported on case studies of 3 children with mental retardation whose grammars appeared to be intact. Curtiss and her associates carried out detailed, in-depth studies of the children's linguistic (expressive and receptive) and nonlinguistic capabilities. The etiology of the mental retardation was known in only one of the three cases.

The first case Curtiss described was that of a child named Antony who was studied when he was between 6 and 7 years of age. Estimates of his IQ ran from 50 to 56. His MA was reported to be 2;9 when his CA was 5;6. Although he was reported to be developmentally delayed in a variety of areas (according to parental reports), he began speaking at CA 1;0. Curtiss found that Antony made grammatical errors that were typical for his CA. Moreover, his language was phonologically and syntactically well formed and morphologically elaborate. It also included complex sentence structures. Curtiss noted, however, that Antony was considerably deficient in the domain of semantics. This included incorrect word usage and deficiencies in the expression and comprehension of propositions (i.e., ideas) that led to communication failures, although there were areas of conversational communicative competence in which his behavior was appropriate. Thus, within the domain of language, Antony had developed a selective talent for the acquisition of phonology, morphology, and syntax (i.e., grammar).

On a variety of nonlinguistic cognitive tasks (e.g., attention span, drawing, play, classification, logical reasoning), his performance placed him at or below a level comparable to that achieved by nondisabled 2-year-old children. He performed above expectation, however, in one area—auditory verbal short-term memory.

The second case reported by Curtiss was that of a teenager named Marta (also known as Laura; see chapter 5). Estimates of her IQ varied from 41 to 48. Prior to CA 4 to 5 years, Marta was both nonlinguistically and linguistically delayed. Afterwards, however, language became her major area of development and, like Antony, she evidenced a high level of mastery of phonology, morphology, and syntax but a clearly less developed semantic and communicative competence. Furthermore, her overall nonlinguistic cognitive capabilities looked more like those of a preschooler than a teenager.

The third case reported by Curtiss was a 15-year-old boy named Rick who displayed a broad range of developmental difficulties during childhood. There was an indication, moreover, that he had suffered from anoxia (oxygen deprivation) at birth. For most of his years, he was a patient in a state hospital for severely retarded individuals. Although his performance on nonlinguistic cognitive tasks was that of a preschooler, he evidenced a mastery of phonology, morphology, and syntax similar to that of Antony and Marta. His pragmatic (i.e., communicative) competence was superior to that displayed by Antony and Marta, although his semantic abilities were reported to be poorly developed.

In brief, these are cases of exceptional grammatical knowledge combined with seriously retarded cognitive development and deficient semantic and, in two out of three cases, deficient communicative abilities. The findings for semantics are not surprising, given the fact that semantics includes aspects of cognition that are linguistically coded. As for the communicative deficiencies, it is clear that linguistic communication is strongly influenced by cognitive factors (Abbeduto & Rosenberg, 1987). Thus, cognitive deficits should impact on both semantic and communicative development.

Clearly, these cases suggest that, to a significant extent, language development in persons with mental retardation is not paced by prior cognitive development. We say more about the relationship between linguistic and cognitive development in subsequent chapters.

Summary

We have seen, then, that there are children with mental retardation who suffer from exceptional language delay, mentally retarded adults whose linguistic competence is essentially normal, and cases of exceptional language development in seriously mentally retarded children. The relationship between language and intelligence in persons with mental retardation is indeed more complex than one would have anticipated; therefore, we address this finding repeatedly in this book. It is remarkable, however, that none of the previous studies suggested that the process of language acquisition in (or the language acquired by) persons with mental retardation is different from what we find in normal language development.

THE NATURE OF MENTAL RETARDATION

Recent thinking on the nature of mental retardation is reflected in a book by Cartwright, Cartwright, and Ward (1984). According to the American Association on Mental Deficiency (AAMD), "Mental retardation refers to a significantly subaverage intellectual functioning resulting in or associated with impairments in adaptive behavior and manifested during the developmental period" (Grossman, 1983, p. 11; cited by Cartwright et al. 1984). Subaverage intellectual functioning falls below 68 on the Stanford-Binet Intelligence Test and below 70 on the Wechsler tests. Four levels of mental retardation are identified: mild, moderate, severe, and profound. Mild mental retardation begins at 53 on the Stanford-Binet and 56 on the Wechsler; moderate mental retardation ranges from 37 to 52 and 41 to 55, respectively, on these tests; severe mental retardation ranges from 20 to 36 on the Stanford-Binet and 26 to 40 on the Wechsler; profound mental retardation is 19 and below on the Stanford-Binet and 25 and below on the Wechsler. The developmental period referred to in the AAMD definition is prior to 18 years of age.

The definition of adaptive behavior emphasizes personal independence and social responsibility and includes communication skills (speech and language). However, some investigators (e.g., Zigler & Hodapp, 1986) questioned the validity of the adaptive behavior component of the AAMD definition of mental retardation, mainly on the grounds that there are nondisabled individuals with adaptive behavior problems and individuals with mental retardation who can adapt to the demands of everyday living. In other words, "social adaptation is not intrinsic to mental retardation" (Zigler & Hodapp, 1986, p. 11) and, therefore, should not be one of its defining features. These concerns notwithstanding, however, the high incidence of adaptive nonlinguistic and linguistic deficiencies among persons with mental retardation (Cartwright et al., 1984), particularly among lower level mentally retarded individuals, requires that researchers and practitioners in the field of mental retardation concern themselves with those aspects of development that impact on a person's capacity for independent community living.

To continue with the account in Cartwright et al. (1984), an alternative to the classification system that has been widely used in schools in the United States identifies three subgroups: (a) educable mentally retarded (EMR), (b) trainable mentally retarded (TMR), and (c) severely and profoundly impaired (SPI) mentally retarded persons. IQs in the first subgroup range from 50 or 55 to 75, in the second from 30 or 35 to 55, and in the third from 0 to 30. Thus, EMR persons are mainly mildly retarded and TMR persons mainly moderately retarded. However, the rationale for these distinctions is educational potential.

A number of other observations should be of interest to students of mental retardation. We summarize them here:

1. The incidence of mental retardation in the general population lies somewhere between 1 and 2%. The mildly retarded range covers 85 to 87% of the population of persons with mental retardation, and the moderate range includes 6 to 10%. Approximately 3.5% fall in the severe range, with 1.0% in the profound range.

2. The incidence of multiple handicaps among persons with mental retardation (e.g., blindness, deafness, motor paralysis) increases as one goes from mild to profound retardation. The incidence of brain damage and physical handicaps is highest among profoundly mentally retarded individuals.

3. Language and communication skills tend to decrease as one moves down the scale of mental retardation from mild to profound.

4. Proportionally fewer majority than minority group children are classified mildly mentally retarded.

5. More children from low-income families are classified mildly mentally retarded than are children from higher income families. Fewer females than males are classified mentally retarded.

Issues in the Characterization of Mental Retardation

Although the previous characterization of mental retardation enjoys considerable acceptance, it is not without its detractors. As we have already seen, one issue concerns whether to include individual differences in adaptive behavior in the definition of mental retardation. In addition, not everyone agrees on where normal intelligence leaves off and mental retardation begins. Note, for example, the differences in the IQ ranges based on the AAMD definition and the ranges associated with classification according to educational potential. Also, with a view toward prevention, workers in the field of mental retardation are looking increasingly toward classification in terms of etiology (i.e., cause).

According to Zigler and Hodapp's (1986) estimates, identifiable genetic and acquired insults account for less than half the population of persons with mental retardation. The remainder of the population does not evidence any clear-cut organic disturbances. Included in the former category are cases resulting from, for example, Down syndrome, metabolic disorders, infectious diseases, drugs, toxic agents, oxygen deprivation at birth, and head trauma. The nonorganic population includes individuals who have experienced extreme environmental deprivation, individuals from families with one or more cases of nonorganic mental retardation (the so-called familial group), and some for whom no cause can be discerned. Studies reviewed by Zigler and Hodapp suggest that ''organically retarded children are found about equally in all socioeconomic levels, whereas familial retarded children come predominantly from lower SES [socioeconomic status] families'' (p. 34), a finding supported by a recent large-scale longitudinal study of cognitive development in young mentally retarded and nondisabled children (Browman, Nichols, Shaughnessy, & Kennedy, 1987).

In the Browman et al. study, subjects were considered severely retarded if their IQs fell below 50, and mildly retarded if their IQs fell in the 50 to 69 range. Most highly related to severe retardation were such organic conditions as Down syndrome, cerebral palsy, and malformations of the central nervous system. Such was not the case for children with mild mental retardation. Central nervous system disorders were not the major factor here. Maternal education and SES were better predictors for the mildly retarded children. Moreover, the incidence of retardation in the families of the mildly retarded children was relatively high.

In the absence of a documented history of, for example, injuries, diseases, and genetic anomalies associated with mental retardation, investigators typically depend on standard neurological examinations for evidence of organic disturbance, which was essentially the procedure followed by Browman et al. (1987). Unfortunately, the standard neurological exam cannot detect many subtle forms of neurological dysfunction that are detectable by other methods. As a result, a number of observers (e.g., Huttenlocher, 1975; Jellinger, 1972) disputed the claim that familial (or cultural-familial as they are sometimes called) mentally retarded individuals tend to be free of neuropathology. It appears to be the case that: (a) the incidence of severe organic disorders and multiple handicaps among persons with mild mental retardation is low, (b) such individuals tend to come from low SES families, and (c) the incidence of mental retardation in the families of mildly retarded persons is relatively high. This pattern, however, does not characterize severe and profound mental retardation.

According to Zigler and his associates (1986), familial mentally retarded individuals, whose IQs tend to fall in the moderate to mild range of mental retardation, represent the lower end of the normal, bell-shaped distribution of intelligence. Furthermore, since their intellectual apparatus has not been damaged, it is expected that their cognitive development will be delayed but not deviant, with a final level of achievement lower than that of CA-matched, nondisabled individuals. Although there is evidence (Weisz & Zigler, 1979) that they go through the same stages of cognitive development as nondisabled individuals, organic mentally retarded persons may nonetheless display deviant cognitive processes. It is to be noted that Zigler and Hodapp (1986) do not claim that cognitive deviance is a necessary result of organicity. According to these investigators, too little is known to make such a claim. They do believe that on the average, when mentally retarded and nondisabled persons are matched on MA, the likelihood of differences on intellectual tasks is significantly greater for organic than for familial mentally retarded persons. This finding, of course, would indicate that IQ tests afford only a partial assessment of cognitive ability.

Piagetian theorists (e.g., Inhelder, 1968) subscribe to the view that, regardless of etiology, persons with mental retardation go through the same stages of development in the same order as intellectually normal children but at a rate and final level of achievement commensurate with their mental age (see Klein & Safford, 1977, for a review of research relevant to this view). Hence, according to Inhelder, development beyond the stage of concrete operations to a level where abstract reasoning is possible is rare among persons with mental retardation. On the other hand, Piagetians do not appear to believe that development in persons with organic mental retardation results in qualitatively different cognitive structures. According to Zigler and Hodapp (1986), this claim rests on the belief that developmental "sequences are logically ordered, that the environment promotes development of such sequences, and that the human nervous system may be preprogrammed to develop according to . . . specific stages" (p. 30).

For readers who are unfamiliar with Piaget's theory, we briefly point out its major claims. According to Piaget (e.g., Piaget & Inhelder, 1969, and the reviews in Flavell, 1985, and Kitano, 1987), cognitive development from birth onward is organized into four cumulative invariant stages or ways of thinking about and interacting with the world. Invariant means that all children go through the same stages in the same order, although there may be some variability from child to child in the rate of progression through the stages and in whether or not they achieve the highest stage possible (that of formal operations). Cumulative refers to the claim that, in large measure, the achievements of each successive stage are dependent upon a child's having achieved the previous stage. In brief, progress in cognitive development comes about as a result of the child's operating on the environment through the use of two complementary cognitive processes—*assimilation* and *accommodation*—within the constraints of his or her current stage-determined thinking style. Assimilation occurs when new environmental input is acted on in terms of already established cognitive structures; accommodation occurs when new environmental input leads to the modification of existing cognitive structures or the addition of new structures. The four stages are:

1. The *sensorimotor period* (birth to 2 years), which takes the child from reflex activity to the achievement of symbolic activity (the ability to mentally represent and manipulate objects and events in their absence, including the onset and early stages of language acquisition).
2. The *preoperational period* (2 to 6 years), when symbolic thinking is not constrained by principles of logic.
3. The *period of concrete operations* (7 to 11 years), when children develop the ability to go beyond the appearance of things or the information given to solve problems involving concrete objects and events.
4. The *period of formal operations* (from 12 on), when adolescents and adults become capable of abstract reasoning (e.g., in mathematics).

To return to our exposition, based on the extensive review by Weisz and Yeates (1981) of studies that employed Piagetian measures of cognitive functioning, it appears that nondisabled and familial retarded children matched on MA do not differ in their performance on a variety of other cognitive tasks. However, proportionally more studies showed differences between MA-matched, nondisabled subjects and subjects with mental retardation when the retarded group included organic children. Moreover, in research on profiles of IQ test performance (Groff & Linden, 1982), no differences were found between MA- or CA-matched, familial mentally retarded and nondisabled subjects.

The results of studies of information processing (memory, input organization, selective attention, discrimination learning, learning set, incidental learning, concept utilization and matching, hypothesis testing, and comprehension of humor) in MA-matched, nondisabled children and nonorganically impaired children with mental retardation, however, tell a different story. According to Weiss, Weisz, and Bromfield's (1986) review of research in this area, there is evidence of differences in favor of the nondisabled, MA-matched subjects (45% of the group comparisons showed such differences). In addition, the differences tended to increase as MA increased. However, performance deficits were not in evidence on the higher level information-processing tasks, such as concept utilization, concept matching, and hypothesis testing. There were noteworthy differences on some but not all memorial, discrimination, and attentional tasks. However, subjects' awareness of "the strategies they used in the various experiments" (p. 169) showed consistent differences favoring the nondisabled group.

Weiss et al. (1986) examined a number of alternative interpretations of the failure to confirm the earlier findings from the review by Weisz and Yeates (1981) of studies that employed Piagetian tasks, including: (a) artifacts of research design, (b) the possibility that information-processing tasks are more demanding and more artificial than Piagetian tasks, (c) differences in mode of processing (nonverbal vs. verbal) between Piagetian and information-processing tasks, (d) motivational factors, and (e) learned helplessness in the subjects with mental retardation, but concluded that none of them necessarily followed from the available data. It is possible, therefore, that MA-matched, familial and nondisabled children differ in certain cognitive information-processing abilities that are not captured by other tests of cognitive functioning. Indeed, in general, it is likely that matching groups on MA, or any given measure of cognitive maturity, is no guarantee that the groups do not differ on other measures of cognitive maturity.

Although these findings are problematic for developmental theorists such as Zigler and Piaget, they are not considered as such by proponents (e.g., Ellis & Cavalier, 1982) of an alternative view that mental retardation is fundamentally a disorder of specific cognitive processes.

Before proceeding, we need to alert the reader to a serious problem in the interpretation of significant differences in performance on cognitive tasks—or in the patterns of performance on the individual items of an intelligence test— between MA-matched, mentally retarded and nondisabled subjects (see also Baumeister, 1967). There is a tendency in the literature (e.g., Weiss et al., 1986) to assume that such differences signal qualitative differences between persons with mental retardation and nondisabled individuals in the processes that underlay cognitive development and performance, even though individuals in both groups appear to go through identical stages of cognitive development in the same order (Zigler & Hodapp, 1986). However, equality of MA does not necessarily mean equality of performance on all the items of an intelligence test. For example, one subject might be strong on Item A and weak on Item B, yet their overall performance might result in the same MA. Then, a subject's level of performance on a given item of an intelligence test or a given information-processing task tells us nothing about the processes that went into that performance. For example, some subjects may try to group the items in a memory task according to perceived patterns of similarity; others may not. In other words, claims concerning the processes that underlie performance on intelligence-test items and information-processing tasks must be supported by independent evidence (e.g., error analyses). In the case of the profile analysis of performance on the individual items of an intelligence test (or a battery of information-processing tasks), we want to know whether any of the profiles coincide with the order of acquisition of the abilities the items assess.

It appears, then, that neither standardized intelligence tests nor such tests combined with Piagetian or information-processing measures of cognitive development tell the whole story regarding the intellectual capacities, achievements, and processes of persons with mental retardation.

We also draw the reader's attention to a problem in the interpretation of the results of studies in which MA-matched persons with mental retardation and nondisabled subjects (or different subgroups of persons with mental retardation) are compared on their language performance. The problem in question has to do with how MA is assessed. The assessment can be based on a measure of verbal intelligence (e.g., a picture vocabulary test), a measure of nonverbal (performance) intelligence, or one that includes both a verbal and a nonverbal component. (Unfortunately, in some instances, the test of MA is not identified in an article.) The problem is that a test of verbal intelligence is also likely to assess aspects of linguistic knowledge (e.g., vocabulary, semantics, syntax). As a result, matching on verbal MA is likely to decrease differences that might exist in retarded and nondisabled subjects' linguistic knowledge. Thus, one who is primarily interested in the detection of differences in linguistic knowledge in MA-matched groups should equate the groups on a measure of performance MA (or, ideally, on a battery of nonlinguistic cognitive tasks) to avoid the problem that intelligence tests assess a limited number of nonlinguistic cognitive abilities). Of course, the nature of the test of MA should also be a factor in the interpretation of studies of nonlinguistic functions in which, for example, different subgroups of persons with mental retardation are matched on MA.

Traditional intelligence tests have frequently been criticized on the grounds that they assess only a narrow range of mental abilities (Sternberg, 1988b), and Piagetian assessments of cognitive development because they tend to underestimate children's cognitive capabilities (Smith, Sera, & Gattuso, 1988; Sternberg, 1988b). Sternberg (1988a, 1988b) offers an alternative to these measures that stresses the importance of three kinds of information-processing components: (a) *metacomponents*, (b) *performance components*, and (c) *knowledge acquisition components*. According to Sternberg, the first set of components "are higher order control processes used for executive planning, monitoring, and evaluation of one's performance in a task" (1988a, p. 269); the second "are lower order processes used to execute various strategies in a task performance" (1988a, p. 269); the third "are processes involved in learning new information and storing it in memory" (1988a, p. 269). This approach attempts to consider, moreover, what are major sources of individual differences in intellectual performance, namely, verbal, quantitative, learning, inductive reasoning, deductive reasoning, and spatial ability. In this view, what constitutes intelligence (in particular, intelligence in the service of everyday cognitive demands) is an integration of these abilities. Traditional intelligence tests were mainly designed to assess mental abilities related to school performance.

The use of traditional intelligence tests is further complicated by an age-old conflict between theorists who believe that intelligence at its core is a general trait that cuts across performance on a variety of tasks (e.g., Spearman, 1927) and theorists who favor the view that intelligence is a set of specific independent factors (e.g., Thurstone, 1938). In more recent years, some theorists have combined these views into a hierarchic representation of intelligence with broad, general abilities at the top and more specific abilities at the bottom (e.g., Cattell, 1971; Vernon, 1971; see also the discussions in Sternberg, 1988b, and Zigler & Hodapp, 1986).

Finally, we wish to illustrate the research of investigators (Ferrara, Brown, & Campione, 1986, p. 1088), who claim that the findings of intelligence testing can be supplemented by direct assessments of the amount of instruction needed to bring a subject to successful performance on a particular type of problem, to maintain the competence achieved, and to transfer it to similar and further removed situations. However, the main objective of this research has been to assess learning potential rather than the products of learning.

The subjects in two experiments by Ferrara et al. (1986) were nondisabled third to fifth graders (CAs in the 8 to 10 range) in the IQ range of average to high. In brief, these investigators found a negative correlation between IQ and the amount of instruction needed for performance on cognitive measures during original learning. Transfer flexibility, furthermore, showed a similar relationship to IQ. Then, there was evidence of learning and transfer improvements associated with increased CA. The authors, moreover, pointed out that "even after children are equated on original learning, transfer differences related to age and IQ are significant, and they increase as the need for flexibility in applying the acquired rules increases" (p. 1096). Finally, Ferrara et al. indicated that findings similar to these have been reported for subjects with mental retardation (e.g., Campione, Brown, Ferrara, Jones, & Steinberg, 1985). However, they also indicated that "the lower the ability level, the less the modification of the original learning conditions required to induce disruption. Whereas average- and high-IQ children solve maintenance and near transfer tests easily, retarded students need assistance even on maintenance items" (p. 1096).

These experiments are part of a large-scale program of research on the cognitive information-processing capabilities of mildly mentally retarded persons (Brown, Bransford, Ferrara, & Campione, 1983; Campione, Brown, & Ferrara, 1982) that focused on the knowledge base of intellectual performance, strategies, metacognition (knowledge of cognition), executive control of cognitive activities, and speed of processing. These authors found that persons with mental retardation are less likely than nondisabled subjects to use what they know, to make spontaneous use of trained strategies, and to transfer them to new situations. They also noted that persons with mental retardation require specific training in the use of available cognitive strategies. The findings they summarize, in other words, stress the importance of metacognitive ability and executive control in cognitive performance and are thus related to Sternberg's (1988a, 1988b) view of intelligence.

SUMMARY

In this chapter, we saw evidence that the relationship between language and intelligence is a complex one. Language and cognition can develop at strikingly different rates in different persons with mental retardation and the final level of language competence achieved may exceed that of cognitive development.

We also encountered differing views concerning the nature of mental retardation and the role of etiological factors in mental retardation. A particularly influential view is that derived from Piaget's theory of cognitive development. However, we also described proposals of researchers who favor an information-processing approach to cognitive development and functioning, and pointed out some problems in the assessment of intellectual status. We also discussed some issues in the interpretation of studies in which persons with mental retardation are matched with nondisabled persons on standardized intelligence tests, Piagetian tasks, information-processing tasks, or some combination of such measures, and alerted the reader to a problem in the interpretation of studies in which groups are matched on verbal MA.

2

Linguistic Background and Language Development in Nondisabled Persons

In the first section of this chapter, we introduce a number of basic concepts (traditional and recent) in linguistics. In addition, we review some of the developments in linguistic theory that have influenced research on language acquisition and performance, with special emphasis on the contributions of Chomsky (e.g., 1965, 1981, 1986, 1988; see also the reviews of his work in Cook, 1988, Haegeman, 1991, Sells, 1985, and the introductory linguistics text by Fromkin & Rodman, 1988).

In the second section, we review some major trends of research and theory in the study of language development in nondisabled children. This prepares the reader for comparisons made throughout the book between persons with mental retardation and nondisabled individuals in the domains of language development and language functioning, and the attempts to explain the phenomena encountered in these populations.

LINGUISTIC BACKGROUND

Linguists have taught us that the sentences of a language are organized on a number of levels simultaneously, and that the levels are arranged hierarchically. At the top of this hierarchy is the sentence as a whole (symbolized S) which consists of, at the next lowest level, a noun phrase (NP) and a verb phrase (VP). The VP consists of a verb (V) in the intransitive case (e.g., *John complained*) or a V and another NP in the transitive case (e.g., *The boy hit the ball*). A third type of VP in English contains adjectives (e.g., *The man is old*), a fourth type predicate nouns (e.g., *The man is a teacher*), and a fifth type prepositional phrases (e.g., *The book is on the table*).

A NP can consist of a single noun (N), such as *men*, a determiner (DET) and a N (e.g., *The men*), any number of adjectives (ADJs) and a N (e.g., *The nice old men*), or a N followed by a whole S (e.g., *The children liked the idea that we could buy a sailboat*). There are a number of rules, known as *recursions*, that allow the grammar to combine sentences ad infinitum. One rule governs relative clause constructions (e.g., *The man who lives next door married my sister*). Another makes it possible to string together any number of sentences through the use of coordinating conjunctions (e.g., *and, or*). Then, simple sentences can be elaborated through the addition of certain types of phrases and other constituents (e.g., *The boy dusted the books on the shelf; The old king ruled wisely*), which also contributes to the vast productive potential of a language.

At the next level of linguistic structure, phrases are broken down into their word constituents (e.g., *The + dogs + chased + the + cat*) and then, at the next level, words are broken down into their *morphemes* (e.g., *The + dog + s + chase + ed + the + cat*). Morphemes are the minimal meaningful units in a grammar and consist of a very large class of content items (e.g., nouns and verbs), a small class of function words (e.g., articles, prepositions, conjunctions), and *bound* morphemes or inflections such as the past tense marker on regular verbs (*-ed*) and the pluralization marker on certain nouns in English (e.g., *-s*). Thus, some words consist of a rule-governed combination of morphemes. Other examples of morpheme combinations in English (*boyish, quietly, vicarage, alcoholic, exwife*) represent *derivational morphology*, which involves adding meaning to a word and often changing its grammatical form as well, through the addition of certain types of morphemes (e.g., *quiet + ly = quietly*).

Morphemes honor rules of the sound or *phonological* system of a language that specify permissible combinations of sound types or classes called *phonemes* (e.g., consonants and vowels). Therefore, the immediate constituents—the next lowest level in the sentence hierarchy—of morpheme strings are strings of phonemes (e.g., *B + o + b + l + e + f + t*, etc.), which can be further broken down into a description of the articulatory gestures that produce them or the physical signal the ear receives in the process of speech-sound recognition (the so-called *phonetic* level of a sentence).

Included in the phonological representation of a sentence are such *prosodic* phenomena as phrase and sentence pitch (intonation) and word stress, which can play an important role in signaling meaning. For example, a rising intonation in an English sentence (such as *John kissed Mary*) rather than the usual falling intonation can convert it from an assertion to a question. Then, the topic of an English sentence in communication—the given or old information it conveys—is frequently unstressed or receives less stress than the comment or new information it expresses, which is frequently the most heavily stressed constituent. Contrast, for example, *JOHN kissed Mary* with *John kissed MARY*, where *John* receives the heaviest stress in the first rendition and *Mary* in the second.

The hierarchically organized structure we have been describing through the morphological level is frequently referred to as the *surface structure* of a sentence. However, there is another level of linguistic structure that many linguists (e.g., Chomsky, 1965; Jacobs & Rosenbaum, 1968) would include in the description of a sentence—*deep structure*. The notion of deep structure was motivated primarily by the observation that surface structures imperfectly signal the meaning of a sentence, mainly because of the abstract nature of such grammatical relations or functions as *subject* and *direct object*. For example, the surface structure of the sentence *The police stopped drinking at the club* does not allow the grammar to specify who was doing the drinking, the police or some other group of individuals. The sentence, in other words, is ambiguous. On one reading, the police are doing the drinking; on the second reading, others are doing the drinking.

Take as another example the case of the sentence pair *John is eager to please* and *John is easy to please*. The reader will readily note that although these sentences have virtually identical surface structures, the *John* of the first sentence is subject of the underlying (or deep) sentence *John pleases someone*, whereas the *John* of the second sentence is object of the verb in the underlying sentence *Someone pleases John*.

Deep structure is also the level at which certain constituents that are missing from the surface structure are identified. For example, in English, the surface structure *John is fond of Mary but dislikes Sarah* is understood to mean *John is fond of Mary but (the same) John dislikes Sarah*. (For purposes of exposition, these representations of deep and surface structure are simplified versions of the structures in question.)

In brief, deep structure is the level at which linguistic information essential to semantic interpretation not contained in the surface structure of a sentence is represented. However, having drawn the distinction between deep and surface structures, it became necessary to posit a grammatical device for relating the two; That was *transformations* (e.g., Chomsky, 1965). In the simplest cases, transformational rules add to, delete, and permute (rearrange) information in the deep structure on the way to the surface structure. For example, the sentences *The dog chased the cat* and *The cat was chased by the dog* are derived from two separate deep structures that have a NP AUX (auxiliary) VP structure in common. In the case of the active construction *The dog chased the cat*, a transformational rule has deleted the auxiliary constituent, whereas in the case of the passive construction *The cat was chased by the dog*, a transformation has resulted in a rearrangement of the subject and object NPs, the addition of the preposition *by*, and selection of the appropriate form of the AUX *be* (Jacobs & Rosenbaum, 1968). Such rules, it should be stressed, are formal grammatical devices and not attempts to describe how sentences are actually produced by language users.

Transformations also figure in the derivation of surface structures that contain two or more simple sentences. For example, the identical NP deletion transformation plus a transformation that deletes *for* applied to the deep string (roughly) *The doctor prepared for the doctor to examine the boy* results in the surface string *The doctor prepared to examine the boy* (Jacobs & Rosenbaum, 1968).

On the basis of this distinction between deep and surface structures and other considerations, Chomsky developed a model of mature linguistic competence (1965) that, along with an earlier model (1957), was the inspiration for much of the research on language development and mature language performance for approximately two decades. In its most popular version, the model posited a grammar with three basic components; (a) a *syntactic component*, (b) a *semantic component*, and (c) a *phonological component*. The syntactic component was subdivided into a surface-structure component and a deep-structure component, with the two related through the operation of a transformational component. The surface structure of a sentence was the input to the phonological component, which functioned to supply a representation of the sentence at the level of speech sounds. The deep-structure component was itself subdivided into a *categorial component* and a *lexicon* and contained linguistic information essential to semantic interpretation (which was the responsibility of the semantic component). The categorial subcomponent listed the phrase structure rules for generating deep-structure sentences, and they took the form of *rewrite rules*, a partial set being:

$$S \rightarrow NP\ AUX\ VP$$
$$NP \rightarrow (DET)\ N\ (S)$$
$$VP \rightarrow V\ (NP).$$

A given arrow means, simply, that the symbol on the left can be rewritten as, or consists of, the symbol or symbols on the right. The symbols in parentheses refer to constituents that are optional; a NP, for example, can consist of a N, a DET and a N, or a N and another S. Also, in some constructions, an AUX appears in the surface structure of a sentence (e.g., *Tornadoes can destroy towns*), whereas in others it is not represented in the surface structure (e.g., *Tornadoes destroy towns*). The relationships in question are also depicted in the following simplified deep-structure tree diagram for the sentence *Tornadoes can destroy towns.*

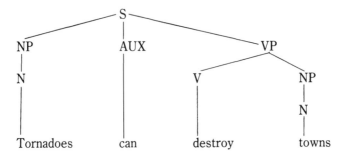

Grammatical functions are defined in terms of phrase-structure configurations in the deep structure. For example, the subject of a sentence is the NP immediately dominated by S in the deep structure (*Tornadoes* in the previous example), whereas the direct object is the NP immediately dominated by VP (*towns*). However, the surface-structure location of the deep-structure subject does not necessarily correspond to its standard location in the deep structure. This applies similarly for the deep-structure direct object. Contrast, for example, *Tornadoes destroy towns* with *Towns are destroyed by tornadoes*. Despite the differences between these surface structures (one an active and the other a passive construction), each is derived from a deep structure in which the subject is the NP *Tornadoes*, which is immediately dominated by S, and the direct object is the NP *towns*, which is immediately dominated by VP. Their surface-structure differences are due to the application of different transformations.

The reader should note that grammatical functions are not to be confused with such semantic roles as *agent* (the doer of an action) and *recipient* (the person affected by the action). For example, whereas *Jane* is deep structure grammatical subject in the sentences *Jane washed her car* and *Jane underwent an operation*, Jane is the agent of an action in the first sentence but the recipient in the second sentence. Moreover, in English, as in many other languages, the subject of a sentence is not necessarily its *topic* (given information); it could be its *comment* (new information), as when the heaviest stress is placed upon the first noun in the sentence *JOHN sliced the salami*.

Each word of the lexicon of the deep-structure component of a grammar is associated with a list of features that simultaneously distinguish it from and relate it to other words of the language. *Honesty*, for example, is a common, abstract, mass noun, whereas *John* is a proper, concrete, human, count noun. Moreover, in the examples given, some features can subcategorize their nouns to prevent certain ungrammatical structures. Proper nouns serving as the head of a NP do not normally take articles (e.g., *Tom likes carrots* but not *The Tom likes carrots*), and so on. Furthermore, some of these features restrict the types of words that can appear in the same phrase or sentence, and thus prevent the creation of semantically anomalous sentences. Hence, *Tornadoes destroy towns* but not *Towns destroy tornadoes; Professors admire hard-working students* but not *Sincerity admires hard-working students*. The verb *admires*, for example, requires a living, animate, human, adult as subject.

Chomsky's theory underwent extensive revision to account for these observations:

1. On the basis of rather limited input, normal human beings acquire an incredibly rich system of linguistic knowledge.
2. Although any given linguistic input a child might encounter is consistent with any number of different grammars, the child ends up with the correct grammar for his or her native language.

At the center of Chomsky's latest account of grammatical competence, known as *Government and Binding or Principles and Parameters Theory*, is the concept of *Universal Grammar* (Chomsky, 1981, 1986, 1988, and the reviews in Cook, 1988, Haegeman, 1991, and Sells, 1985). This is a system of innate linguistic principles and parameters (features that vary across languages but within a narrow range) that guide the acquisition of language. What is fundamental to this account, as Cook (1988) pointed out, is that "knowledge of language comes down to variations in a small number of properties" (p. 1), thus greatly reducing the child's task in acquiring a language. Universal Grammar, therefore, is a hypothesis about the initial state of the child's linguistic knowledge. Hence, language acquisition boils down to "learning how these principles apply to a particular language and which value is appropriate for each parameter" (p. 2).

In brief, Universal Grammar plus the linguistic input to which a child is exposed serve to instantiate the principles in question in the local language and to set the value of each of the parameters for that language as well, resulting in what Chomsky (e.g., 1981) called a *core grammar*. However, Chomsky also posited a periphery of language, consisting of linguistic phenomena acquired outside of Universal Grammar that might involve, for example, properties that play a role in conversational communication.

Perhaps the most important principle of Universal Grammar is that of *structure dependence* (see the discussion of linguistic universals in Comrie, 1981, 1988, Hawkins, 1988, and Cook, 1988). According to this principle, the syntactic structures of language are not dependent on the linear order of the words in a sentence but on the abstract syntactic categories of the words and structural relationships within a sentence. For example, as we have already seen, the subject of S in English is a NP that bears a particular relationship to S; the direct object is a NP that bears a specific relationship to a different constituent, VP. Also, subject-of-S is a relationship that takes in the entire sentence, whereas direct-object-of-VP is a relationship that involves only the VP or predicate. Thus, the relationship between subject and verb and direct object and verb are fundamentally different. This asymmetry involving subject and predicate, moreover, is considered to be a universal property of human languages that serves as additional evidence for the operation of the principle of structure dependence (e.g., Chomsky, 1988). Finally, as we pointed out earlier, subject-of-S is not to be equated with the semantic role *agent* or the pragmatic function *topic* in English. Like direct object, it is a structural syntactic phenomenon.

As indicated, human languages display not only similarities but differences as well. Those differences that are part of their core grammars are handled by the concept of parameters, which are features of Universal Grammar that can take on a narrow range of innately determined values. Among other things, the process of language acquisition involves selecting the value of each parameter that is consistent with the local language. For example, in acquiring French, the parameters receive one pattern of settings, and in acquiring English, another pattern. All the parameters in question have not been identified, but a few have been characterized in some detail. One of these is the so-called *pro-drop parameter*; another is the *head parameter*. The latter, as Cook (1988) indicated, describes how the constituents of sentences are ordered. The former concerns whether or not a language licenses subjectless sentences (Cook, 1988; Hyams, 1986). Thus, in acquiring Italian, which is a pro-drop language, children discover that subjectless declarative sentences are well formed. In Italian, one can say, for example, *parla (speaks)*, meaning *he speaks*, whereas English requires an explicit subject (*he speaks*) (Cook, 1988, p. 40). Hence, children acquiring English must discover that sentences other than the imperative (e.g., *Take me home*) require an overt subject.

The languages of the world vary in terms of whether the heads of phrases (e.g., the preposition in a prepositional phrase, the N in a NP) appear first or on the left side of phrases (as in English; e.g., *on the table*) or last or on the right side of phrases (as in Japanese; e.g., *Japan in*). (Examples are from Cook, 1988, p. 9.) In acquiring English, the head parameter is set on the left; in the case of Japanese, it is set on the right.

According to *Government and Binding Theory*, a grammar consists of: (a) a lexicon, with a greatly expanded role in determining the syntactic-categorical structure of sentences, (b) a deep structure (d-structure) component, (c) a small transformational component concerned with the movement of constituents from d-structure to (d) surface structure (s-structure) component, (e) a Phonetic Form (PF) component that represents s-structure at the level of sound, and (f) a Logical Form (LF) component that represents the contribution of syntactic structure to meaning. Because of its importance, we describe the lexical component of the grammar in greater detail.

First of all, a word in the lexicon (Chomsky, 1986, pp. 86–92) is represented as an abstract phonological form. Its associated semantic properties are then listed, including those that determine the semantic properties of the words (e.g., nouns and verbs) with which it can be combined in phrases and sentences. For example, *kick* can be combined with a noun—an object in the semantic role of recipient of an action (e.g., *Bill*). Moreover, the lexical entry for *kick* will also specify that the semantic role of its subject is that of agent. Finally, specification of the semantic selectional properties of a word results in the specification of its syntactic categorical properties (Chomsky, 1981, p. 86). For example, *kick*, a V, takes a NP complement (e.g., Bill). Here is a convention for expressing these facts.

hit, V, [_____ NP] <Agent, Recipient>

In short, the semantic selectional properties of lexical items can be said to project onto the syntactic structure of the sentence and, therefore, to integrate semantic and syntactic knowledge. This claim is summarized in Chomsky's latest theory as the *projection principle* (e.g., Chomsky, 1986; Cook, 1988). This principle is considered to be a universal property of the child's innate linguistic knowledge that greatly reduces (or possibly eliminates) the need for separate specification of phrase-structure rules in the description of grammatical competence because they can be expressed as projections from the lexicon.

An important implication of this characterization is that language acquisition is largely a matter of the child's discovering (a) the semantic-syntactic properties of words under the guidance of such universal language principles as the projection principle and structure dependence, and (b) how the parametric variations of universal grammar are set in the local language. It also suggests that the semantic and syntactic properties of words should be the focus of our attempts to understand language-performance processes (i.e., language production and language comprehension).

There is much more to the linguistic concepts and theoretical claims that we have reviewed. Moreover, principles and parameters theory contains a number of subtheories that we have not described. However, we need not devote more space to such matters at this point. Additional concepts and theoretical material pertaining to language structure are introduced to the reader as needed throughout the book.

LANGUAGE DEVELOPMENT
IN NONDISABLED PERSONS

Language acquisition appears to begin with the phenomenon of infant speech-sound perception. This refers to the ability of infants as young as 1 month of age to discriminate among many of the phonemes in the languages of the world (including some that are not part of the sound system of their native language) and to fail to discriminate variants of the same phoneme, evidently on the basis of particular sensitivities of the auditory system (e.g., Eimas, 1974; Eimas, Sigueland, Jusczyk, & Vigorito, 1971; Kuhl & Miller, 1975; Kuhl & Padden, 1982; Trehub, 1976; and the reviews of Aslin, Pisoni, & Jusczyk, 1983, Sachs, 1989, and Werker, 1989).

The next important developmental phenomenon is babbling. At approximately 6 months of age, children from different language communities begin to produce meaningless vocalizations within which different types of consonants, vowels, and sequences of consonants and vowels can be detected. Later in the babbling period, the child's vocalizations begin to resemble phenomena in the sound system of the local language (de Boysson-Bardies, Halle, Sagart, & Durand, 1989). There is evidence that aspects of babbling constrain the sound structure of later meaningful speech (Matthei, 1989). In addition, babbling contains intonation patterns that eventually start to resemble those of the local language. Major articles in this area, in addition to those already cited, are those of de Boysson-

Bardies, Sagart, and Bacri (1981), Oller and Eilers (1982), Oller, Weiman, Doyle, and Ross (1976), Smith (1982), and Smith and Oller (1981). (See also the reviews by Smith, 1988, and Stark, 1986.)

At approximately 12 months of age, children enter a stage of language development in which they produce mostly one-word, monosyllabic, consonant–vowel combinations that appear to express, initially, already established concepts and semantic relations involving concrete objects and events in the immediate environment (e.g., see the reviews of Carroll, 1986, Fromkin & Rodman, 1988, Pease, Gleason, & Pan, 1989, Smith & Locke, 1988, and Nelson's classic 1973 study of the development of the first 50 words). Such words appear to serve a variety of functions—for example, requesting, greeting, labeling, and expressing actions, states, possession, and location (Greenfield & Smith, 1976; Griffiths' 1986 review). During this stage, children typically comprehend more words than they produce (e.g., Benedict, 1979).

Between about 18 and 24 months, children begin to combine words into sentences in a systematic fashion that reflects a beginning mastery of syntax in language production (see the review in Tager-Flusberg, 1989). However, there is some evidence that the onset of sensitivity to syntax in comprehension antedates the onset in production (Golinkoff & Hirsh-Pasek, 1987, cited in Tager-Flusberg, 1989, p. 144). Furthermore, according to Slobin (1982), cross-linguistic studies reveal an early sensitivity to both word order and grammatical inflections, depending on their significance in the structure of the local language.

There is considerable controversy over the question of the nature of children's early syntactic structures, with some psycholinguists proposing that they are semantically based and derived from the child's prelinguistic general cognitive and/or pragmatic achievements (e.g., Bowerman, 1982; Snow, 1986), and others proposing that they reflect an early mastery of abstract grammatical categories (e.g., noun, verb) and relations (e.g., subject) under the guidance of the innate specifically linguistic principles and parameters of Universal Grammar (e.g., Hyams, 1986). On the semantic view, according to Hyams:

> early grammars map underlying semantic categories, for example, *agent, action, entity, attribute*, etc., directly onto a linear position in a surface expression. These grammars do not contain the syntactic categories, relations, or rules which define the adult system. Hierarchical structure is also assumed to be absent. (p. 128)

On the basis of her examination of data from studies of children acquiring English, Italian, Polish, and Hebrew, Hyams argued "that very young children do have knowledge of basic syntactic categories and relations" (p. 134). There is evidence, for example, that the process of setting the pro-drop parameter (i.e., of determining whether or not one's native language licenses subjectless sentences) begins with the earliest multiword utterances of Italian- and English-speaking children. In the following and in chapter 5, we cite additional evidence consistent with Hyams' claim regarding early syntactic categories and relations.

Early word combinations display a number of other interesting characteristics (Brown, 1973; Tager-Flusberg, 1989):

1. They are *telegraphic*; that is, they consist mainly of uninflected content words (nouns, verbs, and adjectives). In other words, the grammatical morphemes tend to be missing.

2. As Bowerman (1975) and others pointed out, for the most part, the order of words in early combinatorial speech "corresponds to the dominant (or only) adult order" (p. 280).

3. Early word combinations express a small set of semantic relations (e.g., agent–action, action–object, entity–location, possessor–possession, entity–attribute) that are thought by some (e.g., Brown, 1973) to reflect the conceptual achievements of Piaget's sensorimotor period of intellectual growth (see our discussion of Piaget's theory in chapter 1 and following).

These are all features of what Brown (1973) termed Stage I of combinatorial speech, when a child's MLU is approximately 1.75. The process of mastering the grammatical morphemes that were largely missing during this stage begins when children's MLUs are in the neighborhood of 2.25 (Brown's Stage II). Such morphemes (e.g., present progressive *-ing, and, in, on,* plural *-s*, third person present tense of regular verbs as in She talk*s*) are said to modulate the meanings within simple sentences. Moreover, although the acquisition process for grammatical morphemes begins early, it takes several years to complete and, according to Brown's findings, is influenced by a combination of syntactic and semantic complexity. Brown's research, confirmed by other investigators, revealed a range of individual differences in the rate of acquisition of the 14 grammatical morphemes he studied but an invariant order of mastery. However, there is some evidence (Brown, 1973) that spontaneous speech samples date the mastery of these morphemes earlier than do controlled observation procedures (Berko, 1958).

When children reach an MLU of 2.75, they begin Stage III of syntactic development (Brown, 1973) and the mastery of simple sentence modality, that is, negatives, questions, and imperatives. For example, on the basis of her review of the literature, Tager-Flusberg concluded "that the development of negation reflects a complex interaction of syntactic, semantic, and input factors that may combine in different ways for different children learning various languages in the early stages" (1989, p. 151).

Another later developing construction in preschoolers is the passive (e.g., *The cat was chased by the dog*), which is used infrequently. This construction focuses the attention of the listener on the object rather than the subject of a sentence. Tager-Flusberg's (1989) review of research in this area revealed, among other things, that:

1. Truncated passives (e.g., *The lawn was mowed*) are used much more often than full passives by younger children.

2. Animate subjects (e.g., *dog, boy*) are much more common in full than in truncated passives, whereas inanimate subjects (e.g., *hammer, lamp*) are much more common in truncated than in full passives.

3. Irreversible passives (e.g., *The book was dropped by the boy*) are comprehended earlier than reversible passives (e.g., *The girl was pushed by the boy*).

4. Passives with action verbs are comprehended earlier than passives with nonaction verbs.

Between 2½ and 3 years of age, children begin to master sentence-combining operations, including sentence conjunction (coordinating—e.g., *and, but*; subordinating—e.g., *because, before, after*) and sentence embedding (e.g., see L. Bloom, Lahey, Hood, Lifter, & Fiess, 1980; L. Bloom, Rispoli, Gartner, & Hafitz, 1989; Limber, 1973, 1976; Miller, 1981; Rosenberg & Abbeduto, 1987; and the reviews in Bowerman, 1979, and Tager-Flusberg, 1989). Subordination includes, among other constructions, object noun-phrase complements (e.g., *I think I can fix it*), indirect or embedded *wh-* questions (*Whoever took my hat must return it; John gave me what I wanted*), and relative clauses (e.g., *The man who lives next door married my sister*). However, the process of mastering sentence-combining operations continues for several years.

We turn now to a discussion of the process of language acquisition in normal individuals. Theories of how language is acquired by nondisabled persons are not only important from the standpoint of the basic science of psycholinguistics, but are also relevant to the task of trying to describe, explain, and ameliorate the problems of language-disordered individuals. For example, if one believes that certain nonlinguistic cognitive abilities are a prerequisite for the onset of language acquisition, he or she is likely to favor a language-training program for nonverbal severely retarded persons who have not acquired these abilities that begins with an attempt to facilitate the acquisition of the abilities (e.g., Kahn, 1975).

THEORIES OF LANGUAGE ACQUISITION

Three views of the language acquisition process in nonmentally retarded persons have dominated work in this area: (a) the innateness hypothesis, (b) the cognition-first hypothesis, and (c) the motherese hypothesis. We describe and discuss each of these theories here.

Innateness

Human natural languages are rich, complex, and highly organized systems of abstract knowledge with properties that are unique to these systems of knowledge (e.g., structure dependence). Also, there is no limit to the number and variety of utterances their users can generate. Yet, informal observation suggests that normal children of the world, across a wide range of IQ (from approximately 70 to well over 150) and regardless of the level of sophistication of their culture (from the most primitive to the most civilized industrial culture), are able to acquire any such language in a relatively short period of time, without special training, on the basis of a limited sample of linguistic input, and with little or no negative feedback concerning errors, during a period when much knowledge of lesser complexity cannot be acquired. Moreover, children are universally able to zero in on just the grammar of the local language, even though the linguistic input they receive is consistent with a very large number of different grammars (e.g., Berman, 1986; Chomsky, 1986). This state of affairs has led many to propose that children must have some built-in constraints on language acquisition that are specifically linguistic in nature. According to Chomsky and others (e.g., Lightfoot, 1991), these constraints are captured by the principles and parameters of Universal Grammar.

In this view (Chomsky, 1980; see also Curtiss, 1988a), knowledge of language, in a broad sense, consists of distinct but interacting components or modules, specifically:

1. A grammatical component, which includes syntactic, morphological, phonological, and certain semantic categories and rules.
2. A conceptual component, which includes, for example, knowledge of objects and relations in the world.
3. A pragmatic component, which includes rules for the use of grammatical and conceptual competence in communication.

According to Chomsky, as important as communication may be, it is not the only or necessarily the chief function of our grammatical-conceptual competence. This issue is discussed in a recent book by Bickerton (1990), who pointed out that language is an enormously powerful representational system at the service of our cognitive information-processing capabilities. In this capacity, it allows us to create abstract concepts, transmit such concepts, formulate logical arguments, represent imaginary objects and events, and so forth.

The grammatical component of language computes form–meaning relations (e.g., sentences) and is considered to be the output of the operation of the innate specifically linguistic–biological component in language acquisition (i.e., the principles and parameters of Universal Grammar). The conceptual system may be involved in a variety of nonlinguistic cognitive activities (e.g., visual information processing, problem solving, imagination, nonverbal learning), and the pragmatic component may be recruited in, for example, social interaction. Moreover, language (and other human endowments) "can flourish, or can be restricted and suppressed, depending on the conditions provided for their growth" (Chomsky, 1990, p. 634) and the child's memory and attention capacities. However, the major factor in language acquisition is still the child's innate language-acquisition system.

If the components of our knowledge of language are truly modular, we should expect to find evidence of independent operation in adulthood and development (Chomsky, 1980). Marshall (1990) recently reviewed evidence that these domains can be selectively impaired in adulthood by damage to the brain in certain areas. For example, grammatical competence might be impaired although the other components remain intact. Moreover, according to Marshall, there is evidence (Zangwill, 1969) that severity of grammatical impairment is not necessarily related to the extent of any intellectual impairment in patients with focal brain damage. In addition, selective impairment in the conceptual domain appears possible in the absence of a general deterioration in intellectual functions. Linguistic–conceptual impairment is found in cases of diffuse brain damage, pragmatic impairment is evidently "most common and extensive in patients with right-hemisphere damage" (Marshall, 1990, p. viii), and left-hemisphere lesions are typically found in cases of grammatical impairment associated with brain damage.

Is there also evidence of selective impairment in components of language competence in cases of developmental disability? On the basis of available evidence (e.g., Curtiss, 1988a; Gopnik, 1990, 1992; Yamada, 1990), the answer is yes.

Other observations considered relevant to the innateness view are listed here. We also elaborate on some of the previously mentioned claims:

1. The languages of the world share many properties—for example, structure dependence, grammatical relations, and categories such as vowel, noun, verb, sentence (Comrie, 1981, 1988; Crystal, 1987, pp. 84–85; Hawkins, 1988; Pinker, 1987, pp. 406–408). In addition, the differences between languages appear to vary within limits having to do with, for example, how grammatical relations are expressed, the order of phrase and sentence constituents, whether subjectless declarative sentences are possible, and possible phonemes and phoneme combinations. Such similarities are considered, by proponents of the innateness hypothesis, to be a reflection of human beings' common biological propensity for language.

2. There appears to be no logical necessity for languages to be structured as they are. Therefore, they are set apart biologically from systems of knowledge acquired through the operation of general purpose, nonlinguistic, cognitive information-processing capabilities. Of course, we can artificially create differ-

ently structured languages that would be learnable through explicit instruction, but "these would not be human languages" (Chomsky, 1988, p. 26), and they would not be learned as human beings acquire natural languages, with apparently little or no conscious awareness.

3. Language performance (speech production and speech comprehension), including that of children during the period of language acquisition, is constrained by a variety of factors other than grammatical competence, including, for example, conceptual ability, real-world knowledge, personality, motivation, culture, and communicative competence (Carroll, 1986; Foss & Hakes, 1978; Gleason, 1989). Moreover, language communities (and homes within a given language community) can differ in the linguistic input they provide and the manner in which they provide linguistic input for young children (Snow, 1986).

Given these observations, it is not surprising that children differ to some extent in the rate at which they acquire language, the types of utterances they produce, and the manner in which they produce them (Bates, Bretherton, & Snyder, 1988, and Goldfield & Snow, 1989, reviewed the research on individual differences in language acquisition). However, some investigators have proposed that certain differences signal individual differences in the process of language acquisition (e.g., Bretherton, McNew, Snyder, & Bates, 1983; Nelson, 1975; Peters, 1983). Peters, for example, distinguished between gestalt and analytic language learners. In brief, Peters claims that the former begin with large routinized or formulaic utterances and then proceed to discover their underlying syntax, whereas the latter begin with single-word utterances and build up an understanding of the syntax of larger constructions, component by component. However, it is important to note that, although some children may use one strategy more often than the other, most children appear to utilize both strategies (Bretherton et al., 1983; Nelson, 1981) during language acquisition. Some observations of Peters (1977, 1983) suggest that the choice of one strategy over the other in a given child is frequently determined by context. The analytic strategy was generally employed in referential contexts (e.g., picture naming), the gestalt strategy in social contexts (e.g., playing with brother). Thus, it remains to be established whether these strategies signal differences in underlying language-acquisition strategies (Carroll, 1986; see also the methodological issues raised by Pine & Lievin, 1990, and the treatment of individual differences within the concept of Universal Grammar by McDaniel, Cairns, & Hsu, 1990/1991). In Chomsky's (1980, 1986) view, great individual differences are possible in the use of language, including its creative use, many of which are associated with cognitive capabilities and powerful social and other environmental factors.

Regardless of the ultimate status of such differences, one has to deal with the fact that children from different language communities go through a number of similar, if not identical, stages on the journey toward mastery of adult language (Tager-Flusberg, 1989), and different children in a given language community end up with essentially the same linguistic system. In the innateness view, such similarities are the result, by and large, of innate specifically linguistic constraints on the form that languages can take and, thus, the language-acquisition process.

4. Hyams (1986) reported that the earliest two-word utterances of children reflect a significant understanding (unconscious, of course) of the abstract grammatical relation subject-of-sentence. Other investigators (e.g., P. Bloom, 1990) reported finding evidence of abstract grammatical categories and relations in children's early combinatorial speech as well. Thus, there are aspects of children's linguistic achievements that are underdetermined by—indeed, far in excess of (Wexler, 1991)—the linguistic input and are thus likely to reflect preexperiential linguistic biases that they bring to the task of language acquisition.

5. Human language as we know it is species specific; that is, no other species of animal has evolved or has been successfully taught a language system with all of the characteristics of human language (e.g., Petitto, 1988). For example, on the basis of her review of attempts to teach American Sign Language (ASL) to primates, Petitto concluded, consistent with Chomsky's view, that "Language represents a species-specific distinct domain of knowledge, separate from other forms of knowledge. . . . aspects of human language (in particular, syntax) could simply not be trained, regardless of the intelligence of the organism" (pp. 189–190). Human children, on the other hand, seem unable to avoid acquiring language.

6. Studies of brain functions in brain-damaged and nonbrain-damaged adults and children and brain-surgical patients (e.g., see the reviews in Carroll, 1986, Hahn, 1987, and Witelson, 1988) led to the discovery of centers in the human brain which control language functions. From birth onward, in right-handed individuals and to a lesser extent in left handers, anatomically identifiable areas in the left hemisphere appear to control speech production, syntax, and phonemic decoding. Areas in the right hemisphere, on the other hand, show a bias for holistic-integrative processing that is largely visual in nature (e.g., shape, color, and spatial perception) but also involves musical and other stimuli.

Some research has suggested that language is controlled by the left hemisphere through the mechanism of a bias for any type of analytic sequential processing (Witelson, 1988). However, more recent evidence suggests that the language areas of the brain are specialized for linguistic processing. Poizner, Klima, and Bellugi (1987) showed that language, regardless of modality (auditory–vocal language vs. the visual–manual language of deaf signers) is a left-hemisphere function. What would ordinarily be a right-hemisphere function—the spatial relationships of ASL—has come under the control of the left hemisphere in deaf users of ASL, as is clear from Poizner et al.'s research with brain-injured deaf users of ASL. Although "ASL tends to transmit structural information in a simultaneously layered fashion rather than in temporally sequential fashion" (p. 107), speakers of ASL are left-hemisphere dominant for language. In brief, there appears to be a neurological separation of visuospatial gestures used linguistically and such gestures used nonlinguistically. Thus, the type of processing thought to characterize left-hemisphere functioning, (i.e., sequential–motor and general symbolic processing) cannot be the source of the left-hemisphere specialization for language. Also, it is clear that "auditory experience is not necessary for the development of hemispheric specialization" (p. 191). Thus, it is possible "that the left cerebral hemisphere in humans may have an innate predisposition for the central components of language independent of language modality" (p. 212).

Further evidence for a dissociation of left-hemisphere language processing from nonlinguistic sequential processing is presented in chapter 5 where we discuss the research by Yamada (1990) with a person with mental retardation whose grammatical achievements far outdistance her nonlinguistic cognitive abilities.

Caplan's (1988) observations regarding the biological basis for language are also relevant here. According to Caplan, recent research in aphasia indicated:

> . . . that sociological and environmental factors play no role in the determination of the neural basis for language. There is no indication that processing components are differentially localized in languages with different structures. . . . These findings apply both to the localization and to the lateralization of language functions and strongly suggest that internal organic factors, possibly entirely genetic, determine the location of processing subcomponents of the language system within a specified area of the human brain. (pp. 248–249)

Caplan concluded, "Data presently available regarding the biological basis for language is . . . in keeping with a strong nativist [innatist] position regarding the physical mechanisms underlying human language capacities" (p. 253).

7. From our brief review of milestones of language development, it should be clear that right from the beginning language competence and language performance are highly structured. The types of errors young children make indicate that they are sensitive to language-significant features of the linguistic input and are not distracted by features that tell them nothing about the local language or language generally, such as correlated variations in loudness and voice quality. Also, many possible types of linguistic errors do not occur; for example, verb tense markers are not attached to inappropriate words (Hyams, 1986). Why is the child not distracted by certain correlated features of the linguistic input? Why do many possible types of linguistic errors fail to occur? Because, according to the innateness view, the child approaches the task of language acquisition with certain genetically determined expectations concerning the nature of language.

8. Across a wide range of conditions associated with disorders of first-language acquisiton—from such conditions as profound deafness to mental retardation caused by genetic anomaly—there are striking similarities among

language-disordered children, and between language-disordered and nonlanguage-disordered children, in the language acquired (in a given language community) and in the stages of language acquisition (Rosenberg, 1984). According to Rosenberg, this finding "suggests that there are strong specifically linguistic biological constraints on first-language acquisition that limit significantly the manner in which a wide variety of insults can affect language competence and its development" (p. 228). For example, Bellugi (1988) showed that despite the differences that exist between spoken language and the signed language of deaf persons, these groups have evolved languages with similar linguistic structures that develop in similar stages.

9. If there is a strong, innate, specifically linguistic component in language acquisition, then, to an appreciable extent, language should develop independently of nonlinguistic cognitive development. Consistent with this view would be cases of seriously mentally retarded individuals whose language development is normal or essentially normal (Curtiss, 1988b; Sabo, Bellugi, & Vaid, 1986; see also Yamada, 1990, and the reviews in Cromer, 1988, 1991). In addition, there are cases in the literature of seriously language-impaired children whose performance on standardized tests of nonlinguistic intelligence falls within the normal range (Leonard, 1982, 1987; see also Gopnik, 1990, 1992). Moreover, studies of the correlation between stage of nonlinguistic cognitive development and stage of language development reported inconsistent findings (e.g., Miller, Chapman, Branston, & Reichle, 1980). Also, research on adults with mild mental retardation (Rosenberg & Abbeduto, 1987) revealed that such individuals display a mastery of complex abstract syntax that differs little from that of nondisabled adults. Indeed, as we pointed out earlier, there is evidence that children begin to master abstract syntax with the appearance of their first productive two-word utterances (Hyams, 1986). Furthermore, normal sensorimotor growth is not necessary for language acquisition, as is clear from studies of individuals with severe motor disorders who were nonetheless able to master their native language (e.g., Fourcin, 1975). Language acquisition, moreover, requires the application of principles (e.g., structure dependence) that appear to be unique to linguistic knowledge (Chomsky, 1988).

In another vein, according to Abbeduto and Rosenberg (1987), there is a strong cognitive component in communicative (pragmatic) competence (e.g., perspective taking, inference making, topic maintenance; see also the material in chapter 6). At the same time, there is evidence that grammar can develop independently of pragmatic competence. For example, infantile autism is a disorder that is characterized by, among other things, a profound delay and possible deviance in pragmatic development (Fay & Mermelstein, 1982). Yet, such children evidence phonological and syntactic development at a rate that is clearly in excess of their rate of pragmatic development (1982). Blank, Gessner, and Esposito (1979) described the case of a nonautistic child whose pragmatic development was severely deficient but whose development in other areas (e.g., syntax) was normal or nearly normal. Then, recall the differential rates of development of pragmatics and/or semantics versus phonology, morphology, and syntax in the children with mental retardation studied by Curtiss (1988b).

Relevant also to the issue of the independence of language and cognition are some observations concerning first- (L1) and second- (L2) language acquisition. There is some recent evidence that, despite their superior cognitive capabilities, adults and adolescents are not as adept as children at acquiring either a first or a second language (Johnson & Newport, 1989; Newport & Supalla, 1987, cited in Johnson & Newport, 1989). In brief, this work suggests that, given the conditions of the studies, there is a critical period for ease of first- and second-language acquisition that cannot be attributed solely to such factors as general cognitive abilities, motivation, input, or attitude.

The innateness view does not hold that linguistic and nonlinguistic cognitive development are completely independent, only that the major factor in language acquisition is the child's innate, specifically linguistic language-acquisition system. In particular, the lexical-semantic and pragmatic components of language, by their very nature, require a certain level of general cognitive maturity for their development and utilization (Abbeduto & Rosenberg, 1987). There is also evidence that aspects of language development shape certain cognitive-semantic achievements (Blank, 1974, 1975; Bowerman, 1982, 1988; Cromer, 1988, 1991), for example, that children are first led to appreciate certain cognitive-semantic categories and relations because of their prior coding in the local language.

Cognition First

This view is most often associated with Piaget (e.g., Piaget, 1980, Piaget & Inhelder, 1969, Sinclair, 1975, and the reviews in Rice, 1983, and Yamada, 1990), who claimed that language is one of a number of achievements of sensorimotor development. In this view, language is made possible by the development of the *symbolic function*, which is considered to be in operation when a child has available mental "representations by which he can evoke persons or objects in their absence" (Piaget & Inhelder, 1969, p. 3). The basis for this is the achievement of *object permanence* (the understanding that objects do not cease to exist when they are no longer in view). Symbolic function, which develops by the end of the sensorimotor stage of cognitive development (1½ to 2 years of age), is evidenced by *deferred imitation* (imitation in the absence of the original model), *symbolic play* (pretending), *drawing* (graphic imagery), and "verbal evocation of events that are not occurring at the time" (Piaget & Inhelder, 1969, p. 54). In addition, according to Piaget (1980, Piaget & Inhelder, 1969) language and other types of representational thinking are linked by deferred imitation.

According to this point of view, sensorimotor intelligence is necessary but not sufficient for language acquisition. A language model is required and children must recognize that language as a symbol system has some special features, although those special features are not thought to violate the constraints of prior nonlinguistic cognitive knowledge and processing capabilities. Also, nonlinguistic cognitive development is thought to constrain language acquisition at all stages of such acquisition, although "left open is the possibility that language development influences the development of *formal operations*, that is, the development of logical thinking and abstract thought in general" (Rosenberg, 1984, p. 202). Finally, this view explicitly denies the existence of an innate specifically linguistic component in language acquisition.

Thus, in Piaget's view, the mechanisms of language acquisition are the same as those of nonlinguistic cognitive development; therefore, at each stage of acquisition, the complexity and abstractness of a child's language should not exceed that of his or her nonlinguistic cognitive achievements. For example, children who have not yet acquired the requisite nonlinguistic knowledge should not have mastered the linguistic means of expressing that knowledge, whereas children who display the knowledge in question may or may not have also mastered the linguistic means of expressing it. That is, if we were to assess a child's acquisition of the requisite nonlinguistic knowledge in question at the point when he or she has just completed acquisition of that knowledge but has not yet had an opportunity to apply it to the mastery of the linguistic means of expressing it, we would record a lag in the acquisition of the linguistic means in question relative to the acquisition of the requisite nonlinguistic knowledge. However, the cognition-first view, as it currently stands, would not countenance an exceptional lag between the nonlinguistic and linguistic achievements.

The cognition-first view has generated much research and theoretical literature (see Rice, 1983, and Yamada, 1990, for reviews of this and related views). A good example of recent thinking in this area is the research of Gopnik & Meltzoff (1986; see also Gopnik & Meltzoff, 1987). In an examination of relevant literature (see also Cromer, 1988, 1991), these investigators pointed out that general measures of cognitive development (e.g., stage of sensorimotor intelligence) are not strongly related to general measures of language development such as MLU and age of language onset (e.g., Corrigan, 1978; Miller et al., 1980). Therefore, they set out to evaluate a "specificity hypothesis," namely, that specific lexical-semantic achievements (e.g., the appropriate and consistent use of disappearance words like *gone* and success/failure words like *did it*) are related to specific cognitive achievements (respectively, object permanence and means–ends understanding) that are not necessarily related to each other. Presumably, young children's ability to discover the meaning of an unfamiliar word in their linguistic environment will be facilitated by the prior achievement of the conceptual foundation for that meaning (e.g., object permanence) at a nonlinguistic level.

In the first of two studies by these researchers, word use and cognitive status were assessed in a cross-sectional investigation with a sample of 18-month-old children. Three levels of each of the cognitive variables were identified. As the level of mastery of object permanence increased, the percentage of subjects using disappearance words increased, but the percentage of subjects using success–failure words did not. Although not as regular, a positive relationship resulted between the level of means–ends understanding and the percentage of subjects using success–failure words but not the percentage of subjects using disappearance words. The reader should note that, even at the highest level of object permanence and means–ends understanding, there were a number of subjects who did not use the related words as well as some subjects using the words who had not reached the highest level on the cognitive dimensions. This indicates that the cognition-language relationship in question (the direction of which cannot be assessed in this cross-sectional study) is an imperfect one.

A second study by Gopnik and Meltzoff employed a longitudinal design to track the relationship in question over time and identify its direction. The children's ages at the beginning of the study ranged from 13 to 20 months. In this study, the authors assessed two levels of mastery of the object permanence and means–ends tasks.

The findings of interest are summarized here:

1. Seventeen of the 19 children solved the lower level object-permanence task before they evidenced acquisition of a disappearance word; 18 solved the lower level means–ends task before they acquired a success–failure word.

2. The time between solution of the higher level cognitive tasks and the acquisition of a related word was shorter than the time between solution of the lower level cognitive tasks and the acquisition of a related word.

3. Only 8 children solved the higher level object permanence task "before they acquired a disappearance word, while two children reversed this order, and nine children acquired the word and solved the task in the very same session" (Gopnik & Meltzoff, 1986, p. 1049). Similar tends were noted for the means–ends and success–failure relations.

4. The findings just described could not be accounted for in terms of the CAs of the children.

5. The highest correlations were between the age of solution of the higher level object-permanence task and the age of acquisition of disappearance words ($r = .70$) and between the age of solution of the higher level means–ends task and the age of acquisition of success–failure words ($r = .95$). The other correlations (e.g., the correlation between means–ends and disappearance words) were low and, for the most part, statistically nonsignificant. Thus, cognition-language (language-cognition) relations were found to be stronger than relations within the cognitive or semantic domains.

6. As in their first study, CA did not appear to be a factor in the relations that were observed between the cognitive and linguistic variables.

Thus, in the main, the lower level mastery of object permanence and means-ends understanding predated the appearance of related lexical-semantic achievements, a finding which suggests that there may be some minimal cognitive requirements for the establishment of certain lexical-semantic connections. Of course, given that these are correlational studies, it is always possible that some third variable, not yet identified, is responsible for the results. Moreover, the authors pointed out that the findings for the higher level cognitive tasks raised the possibility of a variety of cognition-language constraints, encompassing cognitive constraints on language acquisition, linguistic constraints on cognitive achievements, as well as the possibility of a close interaction between the two. In addition, studies (see Johnston, 1985, for a review) suggested that words other than those examined in the present studies may evidence different patterns of relations with nonlinguistic cognitive development. Also, the observation that, for some children, high-level cognitive achievements follow lexical acquisition is consistent with other evidence that, for certain concepts, the fact that they are coded in a language can help shape a child's appreciation and mastery of those concepts at a nonlinguistic level (Blank, 1974, 1975; Bowerman, 1978, 1982, 1988; Deutsch, 1979). Finally, the overall pattern of findings in these studies is thought to be more consistent with a specificity hypothesis regarding the relation between cognition and language than with one that is based on the classical Piagetian view of general cognitive stage (or substage) constraints on language acquisition.

The primary concern of studies such as those of Gopnik and Meltzoff (1986, 1987) is the impact of specific nonlinguistic cognitive achievements on the semantic aspects of lexical acquisition. Moreover, they address only the conceptual content of words and not their semantic relational (predicate argument) potentialities (e.g., agent–action–recipient). Clearly, lexical acquisition involves, in addition to these semantic factors, discovering how to represent the sound of a word, how to pronounce it, its morphological structure, and its syntactic potentialities or restrictions in phrasal, sentential, clausal, and discourse environments. Thus, those who claim that nonlinguistic cognitive achievements facilitate acquisition of the formal aspects of subsequent lexical acquisition must provide a mechanism or mechanisms for such facilitation. Unfortunately, this remains a persistent limitation of the cognition-first hypothesis, mainly because languages display formal features (e.g., structure dependency, syntactic categories) that are unique to the linguistic mode of cognition.

In a critical review of the cognition-first hypothesis, Cromer (1988; see also Cromer, 1991) indicated that the fact that early word combinations express semantic relations made possible by prior sensorimotor growth does not account for the acquisition of the formal grammatical means of expressing them. However, we add that although sensorimotor achievements might be helpful in identifying the semantic relational contents of basic sentence structures, this is clearly not the only route, because there are cases of individuals with, for example, severe motor problems beginning early in life (C. Brown, 1970; Fourcin, 1975) who are able to achieve mature linguistic, including semantic, competence.

An attempt by Johnston (1985) to account for the formal properties of language, including syntax, in cognitive terms emphasized the role of "biologically conditioned," nonlinguistic, cognitive "organizing capacities . . . that depend upon aspects of memory and attention . . . as well as properties of the sensory apparatus" (p. 986). Also, Johnston considered that children approach language acquisition "with the potential for creating intellectual structures of increasing complexity, flexibility, generality, and coordination" (p. 986; see also Slobin's, 1985, treatment of cognitive operating principles in language acquisition).

With respect to this last claim, an innateness theorist might point out that, according to Hyams' (1986) research on the development of the pro-drop parameter, the complexity of young children's linguistic knowledge is far in excess of that of their nonlinguistic achievements. Hence, it is possible that children are born with certain expectations about the nature of human language, certain information-processing capabilities that are unique to language, or both. Moreover, the achievement of this level of complexity does not depend on either a high-level or average general intellectual capacity, for, as Curtiss (1988b) and others have shown, there are cases of seriously mentally retarded individuals whose language competence exceeds their nonlinguistic cognitive ability.

The concern at issue here is expressed succinctly by Maratsos (1988), with a bit of irony, in the course of a critical treatment of the topic of linguistic universals in language acquisition. Maratsos stated:

> nativists are right on one count: Languages are enormously complex. If children
> do derive linguistic formulations from general data-processing procedures, or from
> such procedures combined with a few linguistically specific analytic biases or algorithms, very high general intelligence is called for in this type of task. (p. 147)

Thus, it must be the case that to an appreciable extent, as we indicated earlier, language develops independently of nonlinguistic cognitive achievements.

We turn now to some additional points regarding Piagetian and derivative views of the relationship between cognitive and language development. The innateness view that we presented earlier articulates a representation of mature linguistic competence that has evolved over a period of more than three decades, from (roughly) Chomsky, 1957, to Chomsky, 1988. The cognition-first view, on the other hand, has not aligned itself with a systematic integrated and well-motivated view of mature linguistic knowledge. Claims concerning cognition-language relations can only be fully evaluated with reference to such a view of mature linguistic competence. Unfortunately, the situation is further complicated by problems in the assessment of the achievements in the stages and substages of cognitive development Piagetian theory identifies (Bates & Snyder,

1987). Then, the stage concept so central to Piaget's theory of cognitive development has itself come under severe criticism in recent years (Brainerd, 1978; Fodor, 1980; and the review in Gelman & Baillargeon, 1983).

Three additional observations are appropriate here:

1. No cognitive account of the phenomenon of infant speech-sound perception has been forthcoming and although, as the reader will recall, an auditory sensory account is consistent with the available evidence, it should be recognized that only human beings have exploited this capacity linguistically.
2. To complement the universals of speech-sound perception, there are, as we mentioned earlier, universals of early speech-sound production that are best accounted for in terms of the maturation of innate vocal capacities.
3. Levy (1988) and Perez-Pereira (1991) provided evidence of formal morphosyntactic acquisition independent of meaning. If the cognition-first hypothesis is correct, one should expect to find a close relationship between form and meaning.

Motherese

Linguistic input is a fundamental factor in the language-acquisition process. Otherwise, it would be impossible to account for the fact that children acquire the particular language to which they are exposed. The innateness view attempts to identify the particular linguistic input responsible for instantiating innate principles of universal grammar in the local language (e.g., how the projection principle and structure dependence are realized) and setting the values of the innate parameters (Lightfoot, 1991). According to the cognition-first hypothesis, the linguistic environment must supply a model for the language-learning child to emulate if he or she is to master the local language through the operation of universal, general purpose, nonlinguistic cognitive capabilities such as those specified by Piagetian or information-processing theory. According to the motherese hypothesis, through the linguistic input they provide (in interaction with their young language-learning children) and the manner in which they provide it, mothers (and other caregivers) teach their children the local language or at least help to facilitate aspects of language acquisition.

Although the motherese hypothesis is a social-interaction-oriented view of language acquisition, it does not rule out an innate capacity for language acquisition as a factor in language development. The majority of its proponents, however, appear to prefer an account of the process of language acquisition that stresses the role of general purpose learning mechanisms (see Hoff-Ginsburg, 1985, 1990; Hoff-Ginsberg & Shatz, 1982; Snow & Ferguson, 1977; and the review of the literature on child-directed speech by Snow, 1986).

The motherese hypothesis derives from the observation that mothers modify their speech to their young language-learning children, hence the term motherese or baby talk. In comparison with their speech to older children and adults, mothers' speech to young children includes, among other features, the following: It is slower, shorter, and more grammatical. Moreover, it contains fewer pauses and false starts and more repetitions, is articulated more carefully, displays exaggerated intonation, employs some different lexical items, and tends to refer to the "here and now." However, according to Snow (1986; see also Brown, 1977), such modifications—which are thought to be simplifications by proponents of the motherese hypothesis—do not represent a conscious attempt on the part of mothers to teach the language; rather, they are a side-effect of their attempts to communicate with their young children. As a result, such adjustments are thought to facilitate not only phonological, syntactic, and morphological development, but semantic and pragmatic (e.g., conversational) development as well.

It is important to note that such adjustments, although common to a number of languages, are not universal (Harkness, 1977; Ochs & Schieffelin, 1984; Pye, 1986; Schieffelin, 1979, 1986). Mothers in some societies may attempt to direct their children's language development with input and activities that do not characterize motherese (e.g., Schieffelin, 1979). Nevertheless, it is clear that neither the adjustments of motherese nor the efforts to direct children's language development are a universal requirement of language acquisition. Additionally, there appears to be no evidence that children from societies with varying practices regarding child-directed speech develop language at different rates.

A study by Pye (1986) is illustrative of the comparative work on parental linguistic input. This investigator observed adult speakers of Quiché (a Mayan language spoken in a region of Guatemala) addressing their young children and found evidence of the use of a special register or style that overlapped to only a limited extent the one familiar to observers of motherese. He also reported evidence that, by and large, Quiché Mayan speech to children is not a simplification. He suggested, moreover, that the adjustments the Guatemalan parents make reflect features of the language in question and cultural beliefs and practices. In a cross-linguistic study of prosodic features of parental speech to preverbal infants in six languages, Fernald, Taeschner, Dunn, Papousek, de Boysson-Bardies, and Fukui (1989), found both similarities and language-specific features. However, Grieser and Kuhl (1988) reported finding some evidence of universal prosodic features in motherese, although we have no way of knowing whether such cues are used by infants (Pinker, 1989). Fernald speculated that the prosodic features of mothers' preverbal child-directed speech may serve as cues to the communicative functions of mothers' speech. Gleitman, Gleitman, Landau, & Wanner (1988), among others, suggested that such features may help in the segmentation of child-directed speech into linguistic units. Cooper and Aslin (1990) recently reported that infants show an early auditory preference for the exaggerated prosody of adult speech, but here, also, we have no way of knowing what role, if any, such a preference might play in language acquisition.

It appears then, from the cross-linguistic research on child-directed speech, that there is flexibility in at least the surface features of the linguistic input required for language acquisition and in the manner in which that input is presented. This, along with other observations presented earlier, argues for a strong role for the linguistic biases that proponents of the innateness hypothesis believe children bring to the task of language acquisition.

Of course, the role of linguistic input in language acquisition is not a trivial one, as is clear from the findings of research on children who have suffered extreme linguistic deprivation as the result of profound deafness (Quigley & King, 1982) and other forms of environmental deprivation (Curtiss, 1979, 1980). However, even in cases of serious linguistic deprivation (Sachs, Bard, & Johnson, 1981), considerable language development is possible. Moreover, Feldman, Goldin-Meadow, and Gleitman (1978) and Goldin-Meadow and Feldman (1977; see also Goldin-Meadow, 1982, and Goldin-Meadow & Mylander, 1990a, 1990b) reported finding instances of the spontaneous development of communicative gestures with language-like properties in young prelingually deaf children in the absence of visual–manual input.

Numerous studies have attempted to identify the impact of motherese (and other features of child-directed speech) on language acquisition using correlational analyses. Details aside, in a typical study, correlations are computed between aspects of mothers' child-directed speech at Time 1 and aspects of their children's speech at Time 2, while investigators attempt to control for relations with child CA and child-linguistic maturity at Time 1. In this design, the assumption is that any effects of maternal input (positive or negative) on the child variables will result in statistically significant correlations between the Time 1 mother and Time 2 child measures.

Unfortunately, such a design does not rule out the possibility that the relationship between maternal input and child language has aspects that are bidirectional or that some combination of factors is operating, depending on the child's CA or linguistic maturity or the particular linguistic measures that are being investigated (Smolak, 1987; Yoder & Kaiser, 1989). In addition, with correlational analyses there is always the possibility that a given statistically significant correlation is spurious, that is, due to some third variable that covaries with one or the other or both of the variables that are involved in the correlation.

Other problems that have plagued the research on maternal linguistic input (Schwartz & Camarata, 1985; see also the introduction in Barnes, Gutfreund, Satterly, & Wells, 1983) include:

1. Small numbers of subjects.
2. Limited samples of utterances.
3. Unknown or limited reliability of measures.

4. Lack of or unknown consistency of maternal and/or child behavior across observation sessions.

5. Too many statistical analyses for the number of subjects, which increases the likelihood of statistically significant correlations due to chance.

6. Lack of independence of the different maternal and child linguistic measures.

7. Bias of the particular measures chosen for analysis.

8. Disagreements over how to best measure child language growth (e.g., most investigators have chosen to use measures of frequency of occurrence of the linguistic variables, but there is no linguistic or other reason to expect frequency to be the crucial or only dimension of linguistic input relevant to language acquisition).

9. Confounding of syntactic with semantic or pragmatic aspects of maternal or child speech.

10. Bias associated with the conditions of observation (e.g., representativeness, naturalness, presence or absence of an observer in the home, environmental context).

11. Possible nonlinearity of various correlations.

12. The recent observation that children may make use of speech that is not addressed to them in acquiring some aspects of grammar (Oshima-Takane, 1988).

13. The exclusive reliance on child production measures.

These and other shortcomings created profound problems of interpretation of research findings in this area (see Scarborough & Wyckoff, 1986, for a methodological critique and a failure to confirm findings of earlier studies). Moreover, the problems were compounded by the fact that proponents of the motherese hypothesis have not proposed an explicit learning theory to account for presumed effects of maternal input (Pinker, 1988) or a consistent account of the mature linguistic competence toward which young children are moving. However, the interested reader will find some suggestions regarding possible learning mechanisms in Hoff-Ginsberg (1985), Kemler Nelson, Hirsh-Pasek, Jusczyk, and Wright Cassidy (1989), and Snow (1986). The following comments by Lightfoot (1991) illustrate the concerns raised by proponents of the innateness view regarding the claims of the motherese hypothesis:

1. We cannot tell what the child registers (i.e., identifies) in the linguistic input.

2. The hypothesis in question does not specify how the child induces, from the input provided, the appropriate language-specific grammatical principles, in particular, how the child ends up with such a rich system of knowledge with

an infinite output on the basis of positive evidence alone (essentially, little in the way of negative feedback—corrections—for errors: more about this later).

3. ". . . if the child registers only the simplified and well-formed sentences of motherese, the problem of language learning would be more difficult because the child's information would be more limited" (p. 18).

4. Correlational studies indicate that there is only a limited relationship between aspects of the speech directed to children and aspects of children's emerging grammar.

5. Motherese, as a set of adjustments, is not universal, within or across cultures. Yet, children do not appear to be inconvenienced by this with regard to their language acquisition.

We discuss briefly a small sample of the studies in this area. Newport, Gleitman, and Gleitman (1977) reported finding no relation between maternal input and children's acquisition of presumed universal aspects of syntax but did find a relation with aspects of syntax considered language specific. Findings consistent with these observations were reported by Gleitman, Newport, and Gleitman (1984) on the basis of a reanalysis of data from Newport et al. (1977). Gleitman et al. (1984) argued "that the effects of maternal speech are significantly modulated by biases of the child learner about how to store and manipulate incoming information, and about allowable structures and contents of a language" (p. 44).

Furrow and Nelson (1986) offered a rejoinder to Gleitman et al. (1984) in which they do not deny the possibility of internal biases in the child's approach to language acquisition. They believe, however, that the motherese literature has provided some suggestions concerning "what an effective teaching language might be" (p. 175):

1. Caregivers "would use language within contexts that are readily interpretable by the child on other grounds" (p. 175).
2. An effective teaching language "would adjust the length of utterances to the current ability of the child to integrate linguistic information" (p. 175).
3. This language "would be sensitive to the child's understanding, and would expand and recast utterances as needed to facilitate that understanding. Exact repetitions would not be helpful" (p. 176).

How such suggestions are to be implemented is still to be specified. More importantly, whether such suggestions actually follow from the available literature is still a matter of considerable debate.

Given the limitations of the studies of naturally occurring motherese, some investigators have turned to artificial experimental procedures to assess effects of linguistic input on language acquisition. Representative work in this area includes that of Nelson, Carskaddon, and Bonvillian (1973), Nelson (1977), Nelson, Denninger, Bonvillian, Kaplan, and Baker (1984), and Shatz, Hoff-Ginsberg, and MacIver (1989).

For example, Nelson et al. (1973) reported finding, among other things, a positive effect of sentence recasts by adults on measures of syntactic development in nursery school children. The recasts involved following children's complete sentences with new but related linguistic information that referred "to the same event or basic meaning . . . in a different form, such as a question in response to a child's affirmative statement" (p. 498), for example, *Is that Daddy's car?* in response to *Daddy car*.

Unfortunately, a number of problems complicate the interpretation of the research findings in this area (a possible exception is the study by Shatz et al., 1989). For one thing, if adult input is filtered through the child's current expectations concerning language structure and linguistic information-processing biases (which seems a strong possibility), then without information on these biases, results of training studies are difficult if not impossible to interpret. For example, a failure to find an effect of a given input may have resulted because that input is generally not effective or because it was presented at the wrong time vis-à-vis the child's biases. Then, a positive effect might be only temporary unless the input articulates with the child's current biases. Additionally, in most studies, long-term effects of an intervention and generalization of an intervention beyond the experimental setting are not assessed. Also, some effects of input may not appear for some time, may not appear in the measures of child language development employed in a given study, or crucially, might be at a level of abstraction that is far removed from the surface forms that are observed in experiments. Moreover, one would also have to account for any individual differences that might be observed in the effects of a given input in children at comparable levels of linguistic maturity. Finally, a given positive finding may indicate only that it is possible to produce an effect artificially, not that such input is necessary to language acquisition.

An issue that has been treated in the context of research on child-directed speech is whether caregivers respond with negative (i.e., corrective) feedback to young children's departures from the grammar of the adult language (e.g., Bohannon & Stanowicz, 1988; Brown & Hanlon, 1970; Demetras, Post, & Snow, 1986; Hirsh-Pasek, Treiman, & Schneiderman, 1984; Penner, 1987). Such feedback might take the form of direct signals of ungrammaticality (e.g., "That's not right," "Don't say it that way") or direct comparisons of incorrect with correct utterances (e.g., "Don't say *Daddy car*; say *Daddy's car*").

Proponents of the innateness hypothesis (e.g., Pinker, 1984, 1988; Wexler & Culicover, 1980) claimed that children do not receive negative feedback on their ungrammatical utterances, although Chomsky (1981) made provision for a possible contribution of indirect negative evidence to language acquisition. Specifically, repeated failures to encounter certain possible (from the standpoint of Universal Grammar) utterance types in linguistic input may lead the child to conclude that such types are not licensed in the local language. However, the innateness hypothesis contends that children acquire grammar mainly from positive instances; because much of the grammar of particular languages is not revealed in the structure of heard utterances, it must be induced with the assistance of innately determined linguistic biases of the language learner.

One source of evidence proponents of the innateness hypothesis cite in favor of the no negative evidence view is the informal observation that much of what young children say is grammatical in the local language right from the beginning when they have received limited feedback from the environment. Second, there is the related observation that even abstract principles of Universal Grammar such as structure dependence are in evidence in children's earliest multiword utterances (Hyams, 1986, and the critical discussion of negative evidence in Cook, 1988, and Morgan & Travis, 1989). A third source of evidence in favor of the no negative evidence view derives from the results of a study by Brown and Hanlon (1970) of parents' reactions to a sample of grammatical and ungrammatical children's ($N = 3$) utterances. Brown and Hanlon found that parents corrected their children's semantic but not their grammatical mistakes. In addition, the findings suggested that the parents were also able to comprehend their children's ungrammatical sentences.

Other investigators, however, reported evidence of possible indirect negative feedback in parents' responses to their children's mistakes (Bohannon & Stanowicz, 1988; Demetras et al., 1986; Hirsh-Pasek et al., 1984; Penner, 1987). We discuss here the study by Bohannon and Stanowicz (1988), which attempted to correct certain shortcomings in the other investigations. However, they did not address the facts that much of language structure is not represented in the surface form of the utterances children hear, or that natural languages are highly integrated; as a result, mastering one linguistic rule may assist in the discovery or instantiation of a related linguistic rule. Thus, we see again the problems that can arise when investigators approach the tasks of describing and accounting for language acquisition without a characterization of mature linguistic knowledge that reflects the breadth and depth of linguistic phenomena natural languages display.

Bohannon and Stanowicz (1988) analyzed two sets of data, one consisting of conversations between adult nonparents and a single child (CA = 2;8) and the other consisting of conversations between parents and their children (mean CA = 2;3). Three types of errors were coded: (a) syntactic (e.g., word order), (b) semantic (incorrect lexical items), and (c) phonological (incorrect pronunciations). The errors of a given type in a given sentence, moreover, were coded as single or multiple. The adult responses consisted of four types of repetitions of their children's preceding utterances: (a) exact repetitions, (b) contracted repetitions (elements of the child's utterance missing; e.g., Child: "That is a duke"; Adult: "A duke"), (c) recasts (meaning preserving with replacements;

e.g., "That be monkey" repeated as "That is a monkey"), and (d) expanded repetitions (addition of new information to major elements of the child's utterance; e.g., Child: "Monkey climbing"; Adult: "The monkey is climbing to the top of the tree"). Two other adult responses were coded: (a) requests for clarification, and (b) questions that did not repeat major elements of the child's preceding utterance.

Unfortunately, this scoring procedure is not exhaustive and, more importantly, is indiscriminate with respect to the specific type of ill-formed utterance produced by the child (e.g., overgeneralizations, omissions; Bowerman, 1987). Also, it does not take into account the child's level of understanding of the grammar underlying well-formed productions. A child's understanding of a grammatical rule would be considered less than perfect if his or her speech also contained utterances that violate the structure of the well-formed utterances. Such a factor might conceivably mediate the possible effectiveness of parental feedback.

Coding reliability for a sample of transcripts (two independent coders) was reported to range from 71% to 100% but was not tested for significance (an all too common occurrence in the literature, unfortunately). As for the results, semantic errors were infrequent in the children's speech, although parents (but not nonparents) tended to correct them overtly. According to the authors, the finding for nonparents may have reflected the fact that the child's mother was present during the sessions with nonparents.

Other findings confirmed earlier observations (e.g., Hirsh-Pasek et al., 1984) that presumed indirect measures of negative feedback do not discriminate between grammatical and ungrammatical utterances 100% of the time, although the authors still believe that such feedback is adequate to assist learning.

Exact repetitions were more common after well-formed utterances, whereas presumed negative feedback was more common after ill-formed utterances. However, more often than not, the children's language errors were not followed by any adult feedback and the presumed negative feedback followed well-formed speech approximately 14% of the time. Then, whereas adults tended to request clarification of children's syntactic and phonological errors relatively more often than they requested clarification of their well-formed utterances (21.1%, 16.7%, and 7.8%, respectively), the differences were not all-or-none and the percentages of requests for clarification of ill-formed utterances totalled only 37.8%.

What is the child to make of such inconsistencies? Even if the findings were all-or-none in favor of the presumed indirect negative feedback, there would still be the problem of determining whether such feedback actually facilitates language acquisition for all children for all aspects of linguistic competence, and if so, what the specific mechanisms of facilitation are. Indeed, even when the feedback contrasts a child's error with the correct utterance, we still must determine whether it actually facilitates language acquisition and, if it does, what the mechanism of facilitation is.

Interested readers should consult the original article for additional findings and discussion relevant to claims that language acquisition is shaped largely by the linguistic environment, the critical article by Gordon (1990), and the response by Bohannon, MacWhinney, and Snow (1990). Recent applications of associative-learning proposals to language acquisition can be found in the work of MacWhinney and his associates (e.g., MacWhinney, 1989; MacWhinney & Leinbach, 1991; MacWhinney, Leinbach, Taraban, & McDonald, 1989). Pinker (1991) found evidence for the operation of both rule-governed and associative factors in the acquisition of the past tense of verbs.

At present, the view that language acquisition is largely the result of shaping by the linguistic environment continues to be challenged by such considerations as the following (see also Fodor & Pylyshyn, 1988):

1. It is not clear that the type of negative feedback discussed by Bohannon et al. (1990) is necessary for language acquisition.
2. How is it possible, on the learning view, for persons with serious cognitive (e.g., conceptual, learning and memory, problem-solving) deficits (e.g., Yamada, 1990) to achieve mastery of complex, abstract, morphosyntactic structures?
3. How is it possible, on the learning view, for a child whose main language model is language disordered to acquire language normally, as shown by Sachs, Bard, and Johnson (1981; see also the work with language-deprived deaf children reviewed by Goldin-Meadow & Mylander, 1990a)?
4. Why, if the learning view is correct, does human language take the form it does?
5. How would a learning view account for observations concerning the organization of language in the brains of hearing and hearing-impaired persons?
6. If some form of corrective feedback for ungrammatical utterances is necessary for language acquisition, how does one account for the mature linguistic competence of an adult who was prevented from learning to talk by paralysis (Fourcin, 1975)?
7. How would the learning view account for cases of what appear to be an inherited, specific language disability involving the acquisition of grammatical morphology in persons who are not mentally retarded (Gopnik, 1990, 1992)?

Regardless of the outcome of the debate between proponents of the innateness and cognitive-learning views of language acquisition, a number of aspects of language competence are likely candidates for an explanation in terms of general learning mechanisms:

1. Content lexical form-meaning pairings in a given language are arbitrary. There are tens of thousands of them in a society like our own that have to be learned, which is why vocabulary tests have always played an important role in the assessment of intelligence.

2. Associative factors appear to play a crucial role in the acquisition of the past tense of irregular verbs (Pinker, 1991).

3. Many formulaic expressions ("Hi there") appear to be acquired by rote (Peters, 1983).

4. Some aspects of a given language are very likely historical accidents of experience rather than a reflection of the operation of principles of Universal Grammar (Chomsky, 1986).

5. Rather than being determined by the grammar, many pairings of social-communicative functions with linguistic expressions are arbitrary in a given language—for example, politeness conventions—and may therefore be learned in an associative fashion.

SUMMARY

In this chapter, we reviewed a number of basic concepts in linguistics and introduced the reader to Chomsky's theoretical efforts. As we pointed out, sentences are organized on a number of levels simultaneously, including the levels of the phrase, word, morpheme, phoneme, and phonetic segment. However, certain observations concerning language have led many linguists to distinguish between the surface and deep structures of a sentence. Linguistic information essential to the semantic interpretation of a sentence, which is not contained in its surface structure, is represented in its deep structure. The rules that operate on the deep structure of a sentence to convert it into a surface structure have been termed transformations.

We then discussed two versions of Chomsky's theory of grammar and their basic components. The recent version posits a Universal Grammar—the initial state of a child's innately determined linguistic knowledge—where principles and parameters (permissible variation across languages) act to constrain both the language-acquisition process and the resulting grammatical knowledge or competence. Of particular importance are the universal principle of structure dependence and the universal projection principle. We illustrated the notion of a parameter with reference to the pro-drop and head parameters and described ways in which certain aspects of the meaning of a word can constrain the syntax of the phrase and sentence structures in which it can appear.

Next, we turned our attention to a brief discussion of some of the highlights of language acquisition in nondisabled children. Included were the phenomena of infant speech-sound perception, babbling, one-word utterances, early combinatorial speech, grammatical morphemes, sentence modality, and complex sentences.

We ended the chapter with a detailed discussion of the three major theoretical accounts of language acquisition: (a) the innateness hypothesis, (b) the cognition-first view, and (c) the motherese hypothesis. According to the innateness hypothesis, the facts of language acquisition and mature linguistic competence require the existence of a strong, innate, specifically linguistic component in language acquisition. The cognition-first account, attributed to Piaget, posits that language acquisition is determined primarily by prior nonlinguistic cognitive achievements, whereas the motherese hypothesis stresses the role of parental linguistic input in the language-acquisition process.

3

Phonological Development

In this chapter, we review work on the development of the sound system of English in persons with mental retardation and contrast it with development in nondisabled individuals. We begin our exposition with a brief treatment of physical and linguistic aspects of speech sounds, followed by an overview of speech-sound development in nondisabled persons. More detailed treatments of these topics can be found in Fromkin and Rodman (1988), Menn (1989), and the chapters on phonological development in Fletcher and Garman (1986).

PHYSICAL AND LINGUISTIC ASPECTS OF SPEECH SOUNDS

The science of speech sounds is called *phonetics*. Speech sounds can be described in terms of: (a) how they are produced by the human articulatory apparatus, which involves the larynx, pharynx, mouth and nose (vocal tract), and the lips, tongue, teeth, and lower jaw, and (b) how they are perceived by the human auditory system. For example, if vibration of the vocal cords is involved (entirely or partially) in the production of a speech sound, it is said to be *voiced*. Speech sounds that do not require vocal-cord vibration are called *unvoiced* or *voiceless*. Such sounds (e.g., the [s] in *s*oap) are made possible by the friction-produced turbulence in the stream of air that passes through the mouth in the speech-articulation process. Other factors in speech-sound production include the shape of the mouth and the location of the tip of the tongue on the roof of the mouth.

The major classes of speech sounds (or *phonemes*, indicated by enclosing a symbol within / /) are called *vowels, consonants, glides,* and *liquids.* Menn (1989, p. 60) listed 14 vowel classes in American English, including, for example, the following:

- /i/ as in b*ea*d.
- /ej/ as in b*ai*t.
- /a/ as in t*o*t.
- /uw/ as in b*oo*t.

The chief physical characteristics of vowels are vocal-cord vibration and an essentially unobstructed passage of air through the vocal tract.

Consonant production involves constriction of the vocal tract. In phonology, this includes what are called *stops* (e.g., /p/ as in *p*ill, /k/ as in *k*eep or *c*ool, and /b/ as in *b*ill), *fricatives* (e.g., /f/ as in *f*ie, /θ/ as in *th*igh, and /ʒ/ as in sei-*z*ure), and *nasal consonants* (e.g., /m/ as in ra*m*, and /n/ as in ra*n*). The stops, moreover, include a subclass called *affricates* (/tʃ/ as in *ch*ill, and /dʒ/ as in *J*ill). Also, some consonants are voiced (e.g., /b/, /d/, and /g/) and some are unvoiced (e.g., /p/, /t/, and /k/).

The glides, or *semivowels* as they are sometimes called, are /j/ as in *y*et and /w/ as in *w*et; the liquids include /r/ as in *r*ed and /l/ as in *l*ed. Some constriction of the vocal tract is involved in the production of glides but not as much as in the production of liquids. The greatest amount of constriction occurs in the production of consonants. (Most of these examples come from Menn, 1989, p. 60.)

A phoneme represents a class of speech sounds that are similar in certain respects and different in others, which native speakers nevertheless treat as identical. Thus, the *p* sounds in *pot* and *spot* are said to be variants of the same phoneme (/p/, called *phones.* Some physically similar but not identical sounds are considered to be variants of different phonemes when they contrast in what is called a *minimal pair* of words. Thus, for example, the word *thigh* is kept distinct from the word *thy* in English in spite of some similarity in the pronunciation of the initial *th* sound in the words. The *th* in *thigh* is voiceless whereas the *th* in *thy* is voiced. Phonetic features that distinguish one phoneme from another are called *distinctive features* (Fromkin & Rodman, 1988, p. 73).

In the main, morphemes and words consist of combinations of speech sounds. Children, therefore, must master not only the basic phonological units of their native language but also its rules for phoneme combination (called *phonotactics*) as well. The sound system of a language is also enriched by such so-called *prosodic* features as stress and pitch, which can play important roles in signaling meaning. For example, the words *green* and *house* become *greenhouse* when the stress is placed on *green,* and *green house* when the two words are not differentially stressed or when the stress is placed on *house.* Pitch can function to convert an assertion like *John is nice* into the question *John is nice?*

by converting the falling intonation at the end of the sentence into a rising intonation.

The languages of the world display similarities and differences in the set of
phonemes they include, although a limited number of different phonemes are
employed in the known human languages. Furthermore, all languages combine
their phonemes in a limited number of ways to produce morphemes and words.
In the main, phonemes are meaningless. Distinctive features also figure in
speech-sound universals. According to Menn, "A primary object of linguistic
research is to describe the precise minimal set of features sufficient to characterize all language sounds in a way that will bring out phonological patterns op-
timally. . . ." (1989, p. 64, footnote 1). Thus, the phonological differences
between the languages of the world are of a limited number and variety, some
of which may lend themselves to treatment in terms of Chomsky's (e.g., 1986)
concept of universal parameters of variation among human natural languages
(see also the treatment of phonological universals in Locke, 1983).

SPEECH-SOUND DEVELOPMENT
IN NONRETARDED INDIVIDUALS

Presumably, phonological development builds on the capacity of infants as young
as 1 month of age "to discriminate most of the speech contrasts used phonologically by the world's languages" (MacKain, 1988, p. 52). Human beings
eventually lose this capacity but evidently not permanently (Werker, 1989). It
is likely the result of "a general auditory mechanism shared by all mammals"
(MacKain, 1988, p. 52), although no other mammals have exploited it as human
beings have for linguistic purposes. Thus, human infants approach the task of
mastering the phonology of the local language equipped with certain "expectations" concerning the phonological structure of human languages that are subsequently confirmed or modified by the phonological properties of their native
language. The role of early speech-sound recognition abilities in later phonological development has been addressed by Locke (1986, 1988).

Based on a critical review of research on vocal development in infancy, Stark
(1986, pp. 156–162), identified five overlapping stages prior to the production
of a child's first words:

1. Stage I (0 to 8 weeks) is characterized by reflex crying and the production of vegetative sounds (e.g., burping). Reflex crying is described as being
"predominantly vowel-like" (p. 156).

2. Stage II (8 to 20 weeks) is dominated by cooing (comfort sounds) and
laughter. The sounds of cooing are thought to be "vowel-like, but in fact they
contain brief consonantal elements also" (p. 157).

3. Vocal play characterizes Stage III (16 to 30 weeks), according to Stark. The chief features of this stage are that "longer series of segments are produced than in the cooing stage and . . . prolonged vowel- or consonant-like steady states" (p. 158) occur. However, the order of appearance of speech-sound segments produced during this stage can vary from infant to infant.

4. Stage IV runs from 25 to 50 weeks and is termed *reduplicated babbling*. This involves "the production of series of consonant-vowel syllables in which the consonant is the same in every syllable" (p. 160). An example would be *dada*. Such series, however, are frequently initiated by a brief vowel. According to Stark, infants do not use reduplicated babbling to communicate with adults; rather, it appears to serve as self-stimulation. "Towards the end of this stage, however, [it does appear in] ritual imitation games with adults" (p. 161).

5. The final stage prior to the onset of word production, Stage V, is labeled *nonreduplicated babbling*. It varies appreciably in its duration across infants and is characterized within individual children by a varied production of consonant-vowel and consonant-vowel-consonant syllable series, with consonant and/or vowel segments varying from syllable to syllable. Some sound types not found in reduplicated babbling are added to the child's repertoire of speech sounds during this stage. Moreover, various stress and intonation patterns may appear late in this stage.

As we pointed out earlier, late in the babbling period, children's vocalizations begin to resemble aspects of the sound system of their native language (de Boysson-Bardies et al., 1989). Furthermore, late in this period, some vocalizations appear to serve a conversational function (Menn, 1989, p. 73). Additionally, as Menn indicated in her review, "Early speech develops gradually out of babbling and typically coexists with it for several months at least" (p. 73). In other words, children's early word productions, including those that they have been observed to invent, appear to be constrained by features of the sound system that is operating by the end of the babbling period.

Finally, after an examination of the literature on the anatomical and neurophysiological underpinnings of early vocalizations, Stark (1986) concluded, "In spite of individual differences, the progression [from reflex sounds to first words] may have certain aspects which are universal" (p. 171) and, therefore, possibly genetic in origin. Genetic factors are also implicated in the finding that similarities in the difficulty of articulating certain sounds were greater for identical twins than for matched nonidentical twins (Locke & Mather, 1989). However, Stark also stressed the importance of auditory learning (in speech production and speech perception) and cognitive-social development (in spoken communication) during the period from reflex sounds to first words.

An implication of Stark's analysis of early speech-sound development is that the universal features of babbling are the result (largely) of the maturation of the articulatory system. However, recent research with deaf infants exposed to sign language from birth indicates, "Both manual and vocal babbling contain units and combinations of units that are organized in accordance with the phonetic and syllabic properties of human language. Thus, the form and organization of babbling is tied to the abstract linguistic structure of language" (Petitto & Marentette, 1991, p. 1494). Hence, striking differences in environmental input and mode of expression do not result in different underlying phonology. Needless to say, such findings make a strong case for the operation of innate specifically linguistic constraints in phonological development.

The period from late babbling to early word acquisition has been addressed by Vihman, Ferguson, and Elbert (1986; see also Locke & Pearson, 1990, and the reviews in Menyuk, Menn, & Silber, 1986, Smith, 1988, and Vihman & Miller, 1988) in a 7-month study of nonretarded children that began when they were approximately 9 months of age. Speech data were collected in free-play sessions at frequent intervals and subjected to a phonetic analysis using the International Phonetic Alphabet of human speech sounds supplemented by procedures designed for child speech transcription. Consistent with the results of other studies, these investigators found evidence of considerable individual differences among their subjects, although there were some relatively uniform trends as well, and some tendency towards increasing uniformity of speech sounds from subject to subject with increasing linguistic maturity.

These investigators also suggested that some speech sounds "are somehow biologically 'given,' or physiologically basic, in speech production" (Vihman et al., 1986, p. 31). However, they also presented evidence that other factors (e.g., features of the local language, auditory acuity, individual differences in phonological preferences, and cognitive strategies) also play a role in phonological development.

We turn now to a brief description of phonological processing strategies that have been observed in nonretarded children's speech data from a number of different languages.

In the period from 1½ to 4 years of age—from roughly a 50-word vocabulary to multiword utterances of varying complexity—children's phonological capabilities vis-à-vis the local language develop substantially (Ingram, 1986). Prior to attaining mastery of the sound system, however, they make numerous phonological errors that display considerable systematicity. Such errors have been referred to as *phonological processes* (Stampe, 1969, as cited in Ingram, 1986). According to Ingram, "Stampe sees these processes as consisting of a universal set of hierarchically ordered procedures used by children to simplify speech. They are universal to the extent that every child is born with the facility to simplify speech in a consistent fashion" (Ingram, 1986, pp. 223–224). However, Ingram warns the reader that the study of phonological processes must be supplemented with a consideration of the wide range of individual differences among children in their phonological productions.

Ingram (1986) described a number of the general phonological processes that have been observed in children acquiring a variety of different languages, including: (a) *substitution processes* (e.g., [du's] for *goose*, [wedi] for *ready*, and [apo] for *apple*), (b) *assimilatory processes* (e.g., [bip] for *bib* and [bit] for *bird*), and (c) *syllable structure processes* (e.g., [pe] for *play* and [ten] for *train*). These examples of syllable structure processes are called *cluster reduction*, which occurs when "a consonant cluster is reduced to a single consonant" (p. 229). Assimilation occurs when one sound segment in a word is assimilated to another sound segment in the same word. These examples of assimilation follow the simplifying rule that "Consonants tend to be voiced when preceding a vowel and devoiced [voiceless] at the end of a syllable" (p. 227). Thus, because the consonant that precedes the vowel in *bib* is voiced, the final voiced consonant [b] is changed to the unvoiced consonant [p].

It should be pointed out that phonological development in nonretarded children is by no means complete by 4 years of age; on the average, it continues for a number of years more. Moreover, from both a linguistic and a psycholinguistic standpoint, it involves more than our brief review suggests. For example, speech-sound errors characteristic of phonological processes can exist side by side with correct pronunciations of the same words or words containing the same phonological segments or clusters, which suggests that these processes not only simplify the acquisition process but speech articulation performance as well (Ingram, 1986).

PHONOLOGICAL DEVELOPMENT IN PERSONS WITH MENTAL RETARDATION

Speech-articulation problems have long characterized mentally retarded persons as a population, especially lower IQ, Down-syndrome, and other organically impaired retarded persons (see the reviews of earlier work in Ingram, 1976, Rosenberg, 1982, and Schlanger, 1973). We begin this section with a discussion of studies that have examined the prelinguistic (premeaningful) vocal behavior of retarded infants and children and then turn to research on older retarded persons.

The subjects in a study by Dodd (1972) were Down-syndrome and nonretarded infants in the age range 9 to 13 months, half male and half female in each group. All subjects came from middle-class, English-speaking homes. Performance on the Bayley Scales of Infant Development revealed differences in favor of the nonretarded group in cognitive and motor development, but no differences between the groups were found when they were compared on such variables as number and variety of consonants and vowels produced. Thus, despite the fact that the two groups differed in mental and motor development, they did not differ in the vocal behavior that was assessed, which led Dodd to suggest that babbling may develop independently of intelligence and motor development.

Smith and Oller (1981) examined more interesting aspects of babbling (e.g., age of onset of reduplicated babbling) than had Dodd in a longitudinal (birth through the second year) study of infants with Down syndrome and nonretarded infants. Thus, Smith and Oller's groups differed in mental age. However, the children with Down syndrome were all participating in "an intensive educational program," which may have had some influence on their phonological development. Recordings of the subjects' vocalizations were made every 3 months and a modified version of the International Phonetic Alphabet was used to transcribe their "relative speech-like" vocalizations.

The two groups did not differ in age of onset of reduplicated babbling (means of 8.4 months and 7.9 months for the Down-syndrome and nondisabled infants, respectively). The investigators also studied the development of consonant articulation with respect to three primary places of articulation, *labial* (e.g., *p*), *alveolar* (e.g., *d*), and *velar* (e.g., *ng*), which involve, respectively, adjustments of the lips and tongue, the placement of the tip of the tongue in the area behind the upper front teeth, and the raising of the back of the tongue to the soft palate at the back of the mouth (Fromkin & Rodman, 1988). On these measures, Smith and Oller (1981) found "a strong similarity of the developmental patterns of consonant production . . . by the normally developing and the Down's syndrome infants" (p. 49). A similar trend was noted when they looked at the development of vowel quality in their subjects.

Thus, Smith and Oller's (1981) findings were consistent with those of Dodd (1972) and reinforce the view that prelinguistic phonological development does not depend on intellectual status. The findings of these studies are also interesting because, on the average, language development from the one-word stage onward is delayed in Down-syndrome persons (e.g., Mahoney, Glover, & Finger, 1981; Miller, 1987, 1988; Smith & von Tetzchner, 1986). Of course, it is always possible that measures other than those employed by Dodd and by Smith and Oller might produce differences between Down-syndrome and nondisabled infants.

Oller and Seibert (1988) reported the results of a study of *canonical babbling* in prelinguistic retarded and nondisabled persons. According to these investigators, canonical babbling (e.g., "mamama") "represents the earliest production of syllables that could function in real words" (p. 370). In nondisabled infants, this stage is typically reached by 10 months of age (Oller, 1980; Stark, 1980). The subjects with mental retardation in this investigation were from a full-time cognitive, motor, and linguistic stimulation program in the CA range of 17 to 62 months ($M = 39$) and developmental age range of 5 to 42 months ($M = 17$). The hearing status of some of the subjects was unknown, however. None of the subjects displayed referential speech and, with respect to etiology, 5 were classified etiology unknown and 8 as Down-syndrome persons; the remainder were mainly organically impaired. The authors sampled the retarded children's vocalizations at various times as well as those of a control group of nondisabled infants at 5 and 6 months of age and between 11 and 13 months of age.

Most of the children with mental retardation evidenced canonical babbling, although there was considerable variability in its occurrence relative to the number of utterances they produced (the canonical babbling ratio). This raises the question of whether retarded persons in the age range of Oller and Seibert's nondisabled persons would show a similar trend. However, the canonical babbling ratio in the nondisabled sample was statistically greater than that in the group of retarded children, even though a number of the retarded children had a relatively high canonical babbling ratio. Neither CA nor developmental age appeared to predict the rate of canonical babbling in the sample of children with mental retardation. As for etiology, the only trend observed was for the Down-syndrome children, whose canonical babbling ratios fell "within the range of the nondisabled 11 to 13 month olds" (Oller & Seibert, 1988, p. 373). Unfortunately, this tells us nothing about the age of onset of canonical babbling in Down-syndrome as compared to non-Down-syndrome children. However, Smith and Oller (1981) indicated that CA-matched, nondisabled and Down-syndrome infants did not differ in age of onset of reduplicated babbling, and canonical babbling is a common form of reduplicated babbling. Thus, it is likely that the age of onset of canonical babbling in persons with Down syndrome is similar to that in nondisabled persons. However, why their relative use of canonical babbling at a later age should be similar to that of younger, nondisabled persons is not possible to determine on the basis of the available research. It would also be necessary to determine whether individual differences in the canonical babbling ratio predict individual differences in the onset and early acquisition of meaningful vocabulary.

PHONOLOGICAL DEVELOPMENT
IN LINGUISTICALLY ADVANCED PERSONS
WITH MENTAL RETARDATION

Dodd (1976) examined the phonological errors that severely retarded (home-reared and residential) Down-syndrome, severely retarded non-Down-syndrome, and nondisabled children produced on two tasks: (a) elicited picture naming, and (b) elicited lexical imitation. The groups were matched on Stanford-Binet MA (means between 3;0 and 4;0) and social background and were reported to be free of sensory, gross motor, and neurological deficits that might impair performance. The average CA in the nondisabled group was approximately 3;7 whereas in the groups of retarded subjects it was about 10;8. No information was provided on etiology for the group of non-Down-syndrome retarded children but, given their low IQ level, it is likely that the group contained a number of subjects whose retardation was the result of an organic condition (Cartwright et al., 1984; Zigler & Hodapp, 1986).

Analysis of phonetic transcriptions of the subjects' responses centered on three types of systematic phonological errors; *cluster reduction* (e.g., *poon* for *spoon*), (b) *consonant harmony* (e.g., cases in which only certain consonants are allowed in a word, for instance, *lellow* for *yellow*, the rule being that the only consonants allowed in a word are /l,r, j,w/), and (c) *simplification of the phonological system* (e.g., deletion of initial unstressed syllables, for instance, *brella* for *umbrella*). The children with Down syndrome produced more errors and a greater variety of error types than the other two groups, which did not differ from each other. However, in the absence of an estimate of overall linguistic maturity (e.g., MLU) for Dodd's subjects, it is impossible to determine whether the phonological performance of her Down-syndrome and non-Down-syndrome retarded children was consistent with their grammatical development. It evidently lagged behind their nonlinguistic cognitive status as assessed psychometrically. It will be recalled that there was some evidence of a lag in language acquisition relative to MA in Dooley's (1976) children with Down syndrome. Dooley, however, did not assess the phonological status of his subjects.

A fuller assessment of the phonological skills of a group of children with Down syndrome reared at home was provided by Stoel-Gammon (1980) on the basis of samples of continuous spontaneous speech recorded over a 4-week period. The children's CAs and MLUs ranged from 3;10 to 6;3 and 1.22 to 2.06, respectively, and they were classified as mildly mentally retarded persons. They displayed no complicating visual, auditory, or neurological problems, and they were participating in preschool programs. The speech samples were transcribed using the International Phonetic Alphabet modified for use with children and, because over 90% of the children's speech errors involved consonants, the analysis focused on this category of phonemes.

According to Stoel-Gammon, "although they made many pronunciation errors, the subjects were capable of producing nearly all the phonemes of English" (1980, p. 46). Moreover, the patterns of errors within words precluded an explanation in terms of oral structure abnormalities. Stoel-Gammon also studied the phonological processes underlying the children's errors and found the errors to be "systematically related to the adult forms in regular and predictable ways" (p. 46). Furthermore, Stoel-Gammon noted a strong tendency for her subjects' phonological skills to be consistent with, if not superior to, those reported in the literature for younger, nondisabled children with similar MLUs (Ingram, 1976). Finally, an analysis of individual differences among her subjects revealed processes identical to those reported in the literature on phonological development in nondisabled children (Ingram, 1976). Thus, phonological development kept pace with grammatical development in these mildly retarded Down-syndrome children, even though their language development in both domains was evidently delayed. Moreover, there was no evidence of linguistic deviance in their phonological behavior.

Down-syndrome children's use of phonological processes was examined in two other studies. One of them (Bleile, 1982) found evidence of the use of a strategy that had previously been observed in nondisabled children but not in children with Down syndrome (Stoel-Gammon, 1980). Bleile tested a single male person with down syndrome who was 4 years old at the start of the study. His MLU at 4 years of age was 1.25; his MA at 4;1 was 2;6 on the McCarthy scale.

Smith and Stoel-Gammon (1983) reported the results of a longitudinal study of stop consonant production in children with Down syndrome (observed from CA 3 to 6 years of age) and nondisabled children (observed from CA 18 to 36 months of age). The subjects were being reared at home. Hearing was described as normal in all subjects but no information was provided on MA, IQ, or MLU. However, there was evidently a rough, informal attempt to match the two groups on stage of language acquisition, taking into account the slower rate of linguistic development in children with Down-syndrome postbabbling.

Similar patterns of errors characterized the two groups; for example, both groups made more errors in producing the stop consonants in final position than in initial position in a word, the majority of errors in both groups were voicing errors, and there was some tendency in both groups to omit final consonants. Over the period of observation in each group, an examination of the use of four different phonological processes revealed less mature productions and a slower rate of improvement among the children with Down syndrome but "no major qualitative differences between the normal and the Down-syndrome children" (p. 117). There was also a trend toward an increase in the difference between the nondisabled and the Down-syndrome children over time in the maturity of their phonological productions.

Phonological process use by a group of non-Down-syndrome persons with mental retardation was the topic of an investigation by Prater (1982). The subjects were moderately retarded (no IQs provided) males with normal hearing in the CA range 3;0 to 6;3 "who did not evidence retardation associated with a clinical syndrome" (p. 400). Their MLUs, which ranged from 1.01 to 1.41, placed them in Brown's (1973) early Stage I of combinatorial speech. According to Miller's (1981, p. 26) norms for nondisabled children, this range of MLUs is associated with a CA range from 1;7 to 1;11. Each child's utterances were sampled at his school in a single session and scored independently by two judges. The analysis centered on the phonological processes of consonant assimilation and reduplication.

Consonant assimilation did not appear to serve primarily a simplifying function in the phonological development of Prater's subjects. More often than not, the children with mental retardation used consonant assimilation on phonological segments and clusters that they could correctly articulate, suggesting that consonant assimilation can serve a performance-simplifying function rather than, or in addition to, a facilitating function in original learning. However, wide individual differences were observed in the use of this process. According to

Prater, these findings are consistent with observations in the literature on phonological development in nondisabled children.

With respect to reduplication, Prater found that, among other things, this process was used almost exclusively with multisyllabic words. Moreover, all of these instances of reduplication "contained target consonants and consonant clusters that were not in the phonetic repertoires of the children" (1982, p. 403). According to Prater, these findings indicated that reduplication was "used by the children to generate multisyllabic words containing phonetic targets that the children could not produce" (p. 403).

For the phonological processes under investigation, there was generally no evidence of linguistic or developmental deviance in Prater's non-Down-syndrome retarded persons, who were functioning in the earliest stage of grammatical development, although their language development, including phonology, lagged behind what would be expected on the basis of their CAs.

Klink, Gerstman, Raphael, Schlanger, and Newsome (1986) provided data on a wide range of phonological process usage in mildly mentally retarded (IQs 50 to 75; test not specified), language-disordered (nonretarded), and normally developing children matched on mean MLU (3.6, 3.7, and 4.1, respectively). The mean IQs of the groups were 65, 100, and 114, respectively, and the mean CAs 5;0, 4;0, and 3;6, respectively. Thus, the groups were not matched on cognitive maturity. The subjects were enrolled in preschools and were from lower-middle-class homes. No information on etiology was provided for the children with mental retardation. Given their IQs, however, it is not likely that the group of children with mental retardation contained many subjects with identifiable organic disturbances.

Phonological process usage was evaluated using a test that allows assessment of 16 different error types. Subjects differed in the frequency with which they utilized the various phonological processes, although the patterns of process usage across the three groups were similar. The retarded and the nonretarded language-disordered groups did not differ in their overall use of the various processes. Both groups, however, used the processes significantly more frequently than did the normally developing children. Unfortunately, the analysis did not show instances in which subjects made errors on items they might have been able to articulate correctly at other times. When such errors occur frequently, the error by itself may not constitute a valid assessment of the subjects' phonological competence.

Group comparisons on each individual phonological process revealed only one statistically significant difference between the mentally retarded and nonretarded language-disordered children. However, the retarded and language-disordered groups each differed significantly from the normally developing controls on 10 processes, 8 of them the same. Thus, the problems (competence and/or performance) the high-level mentally retarded children in this study had in the domain of phonology were not unique to mental retardation but were also found in nonretarded language-delayed children. Moreover, both the retarded and the nonretarded language-disordered children were relatively more at risk for phonological problems than for grammatical problems because they were matched with the normally developing children on mean MLU.

Why phonological development did not keep pace with grammatical development in Klink et al.'s (1986) retarded and nonretarded language-disordered persons is not clear. However, the fact that these two groups displayed comparable phonological performance and both differed from MLU-matched normally developing children suggests that the nonlinguistic cognitive status of the children with mild mental retardation was not the major factor in their phonological delay. A specifically linguistic explanation seems more likely. Furthermore, an explanation that assigns major weight to nonlinguistic cognitive factors is also weakened by the results of Curtiss' (1988b) study of exceptional language development in children with mental retardation. In addition to the findings we discussed in chapter 1, Curtiss reported that Antony, Marta, and Rick's language was phonologically well formed. Phonological deficit, therefore, is not a necessary concomitant of mental retardation.

For the average nondisabled child, phonological development is complete or nearly complete by 8½ years of age (Reich, 1986, p. 57). There is evidence, however, that phonological errors (phonological processes) persist into adulthood, at least in the case of the moderately and severely retarded persons studied by Moran, Money, and Leonard (1984). The subjects in this investigation had spent most of their lives in institutions. Needless to say, phonological processing in adults with mental retardation is a topic that requires additional research.

SUMMARY AND DISCUSSION

Our brief linguistic introduction focused on a number of key concepts and phenomena in phonology. In broad outline, phonological development in nondisabled persons begins with the phenomenon of infant speech-sound perception, which is attributed to a universal acoustic capacity that humans appear to share with some other species but that only humans have exploited for linguistic purposes. Moreover, sometime during the second half of the first year of life, this capacity combines with a uniquely human (modality-independent) bias toward the use of phonological processes or strategies that serve to simplify early phonological acquisition and performance and possibly early lexical development as well. The end result of these largely task-specific (i.e., language-acquisition-oriented) biases and maturational changes is certain universal properties of the phonologies of human languages and phonological development. However, because children vary in, for example, their rate of phonological development, the order in which they identify the phonemes and phoneme combinations of the local language, and their use of phonological processes, nonlinguistic cognitive and social factors, and peculiarities of the local language may also play a role in phonological development.

This picture also characterizes phonological development among the persons with mental retardation of varying etiology and IQ level who have been studied thus far. Indeed, for retarded persons whose vocalizations have been studied during the prelinguistic stage of phonological development, specifically Down-syndrome infants, speech-sound development differs little from that in nondisabled infants, regardless of differences in cognitive and motor maturity and despite the fact that their language (including phonological) development from the one-word stage onward is delayed to a greater extent than it is in MA-matched, non-Down-syndrome retarded children. Possibly, then, prelinguistic vocal development is largely under the control of factors specific to the task of phonological development.

The delay in phonological development that occurs in Down-syndrome and other mentally retarded individuals beyond the prelinguistic stage does not appear to be accompanied by linguistic or developmental deviance. At the same time, as is the case with nondisabled children, there are wide individual differences among retarded persons, post- and prelinguistically, in phonological performance.

It is interesting that the phonological performance of children with mild mental retardation vis-à-vis phonological processes is indistinguishable from that of MLU-matched, nonretarded, language-disordered children, although both groups use the processes more frequently than do MLU-matched, normally developing children and both appear to be at greater risk for phonological delay than for grammatical delay. Thus, the phonological delay children with mild mental retardation experience is not unique to mental retardation because it also occurs in language-disordered children whose IQ test scores fall within the normal range. This finding, combined with the observation that MA-matched, severely retarded, Down-syndrome and non-Down-syndrome retarded children differ in the frequency and variety of the phonological errors they produce, and the finding of exceptional phonological development in some seriously retarded children tend to weaken claims that the language problems of persons with mental retardation are the result of (or largely the result of) deficits in the nonlinguistic cognitive sphere.

However, one still has to account for the fact that there is a correlation between IQ and the severity of the language delay in persons with mental retardation. Specifically, there is ample evidence of severe and persistent language problems in profoundly retarded persons. One possibility is that some minimal level of functional, nonlinguistic cognitive ability is needed for language (including phonological) development, and such a possibility would be consistent with the version of the innateness hypothesis we presented in chapter 2. Another hypothesis that can be put forward, however, is that because profoundly retarded persons tend to suffer from multiple handicaps (Cartwright et al., 1984, p. 169), their extreme linguistic deficiencies may be the result of problems that are independent of their nonlinguistic cognitive retardation. Evaluation of these and other hypotheses awaits further research.

The research that we reviewed on speech-sound development in persons with Down syndrome and other investigations (Miller, 1987) indicated that phonological development from the one-word stage onward (and language development generally) in this population lags behind (primarily nonverbal) MA, to an increasing extent as time passes. Research by Miller and his associates (Miller, 1988), however, suggested that this is an oversimplification. Miller reported the results of a large-scale study of language production and comprehension in 10-month to 5-year-old Down-syndrome persons, employing a combination of laboratory, naturalistic, and standardized measures. Normative data from nondisabled children made it possible to estimate patterns of language delay relative to MA. Three patterns emerged from the data:

1. Only 5 percent of the subjects evidenced delay in both comprehension and production relative to MA; that is, language comprehension and production progressed at a slower rate than would be expected given the MAs of subjects in this subgroup.

2. Fifty-two percent evidenced a delay in production relative to MA and language comprehension. The delay in this instance did not begin to appear until the second year of life (possibly due to Down-syndrome person's age-appropriate prelinguistic phonological development during infancy) and it tended to increase with increasing CA.

3. The final pattern, in which production and comprehension were consistent with MA, accounted for 43% of the sample.

Miller's findings were unrelated to the hearing or health status of his subjects or to the nature of maternal linguistic input. Forty-six of his 56 subjects displayed structural and functional problems in the vocal apparatus (see also Rosin, Swift, Bless, & Vetter, 1985, for some evidence of speech motor-control problems in persons with Down syndrome). This would predict a larger percentage of production delays relative to MA and comprehension than was observed and, moreover, would lead us to expect retardation relative to CA in prelinguistic speech-sound production among subjects with Down syndrome which, of course, the literature does not support.

Another possibility presents itself, however, that emanates from research on the neurological organization of language functions in the brain. Research on right-handed individuals with Down syndrome, reviewed by Elliott, Weeks, and Elliott (1987; see also Weeks & Elliott, 1992), suggested "that although these individuals perceive speech with their right hemisphere they [like nonretarded and other retarded individuals] depend on left-hemisphere mechanisms for the production of speech as well as other complex movements" (Elliott,

Weeks, & Elliott, 1987, p. 268). Thus, according to Elliott, Weeks, and Elliott, in Down-syndrome persons, speech perception is carried out "with a right hemisphere that is poorly designed for serial, sequential tasks" (p. 268). Given the results for non-Down-syndrome retarded persons, it is not likely that this finding is due to the mental retardation that accompanies Down syndrome.

Unfortunately, as intriguing as these findings are, it does not appear that they can account for:

1. The individual differences that Miller (1988) reports.
2. Exceptional (relative to MA) linguistic achievements in mentally retarded Down-syndrome children (Seagoe, 1965).
3. The fact that language production was the major problem among Miller's Down-syndrome persons.
4. The results of the research on prelinguistic speech-sound production in infants with Down syndrome.
5. The increasing deficit in productive language relative to MA with increasing CA in Down-syndrome children (see also the discussion of language acquisition in Down-syndrome persons in Rondal, 1987, 1988).

Moreover, there were differences in the tasks used in the literature to assess speech production and speech comprehension that might have contributed to the findings, and it is also questionable to what extent the studies that purport to show a left-hemisphere preference for speech production (e.g., Elliott, Edwards, Weeks, Lindley, & Carnahan, 1987) or a right-hemisphere preference for speech perception (e.g., Hartley, 1985) engage Down-syndrome subjects' grammatical competence. In addition, the literature has reported seriously conflicting results vis-à-vis the issue of whether persons with Down syndrome are right-hemisphere dominant for speech perception (e.g., Bowler, Cuffin, & Kiernan, 1985; Hartley, 1985; Obrzut, Boliet, & Obrzut, 1986; Pipe, 1983, 1985; Sommers & Starkey, 1977; Tannock, Kershner, & Oliver, 1984; Zekulin-Hartley, 1981, 1983; and the review in Pipe, 1988). This situation is not surprising, however, given the many differences in methodology among these studies as well as the presence of various methodological problems (e.g., statistics, stimulus materials, task demands, attentional biases). As Tannock et al. (1984) suggested:

> the [left-ear advantage and thus the right-hemisphere advantage] for language stimuli that has been found in [Down-syndrome] persons may have been produced by factors less exotic than reversed cerebral dominance; factors such as contextual arrangements, previous experience, processing strategy, attending and response biases, or concurrent verbal memory load. (p. 222)

We must now strike some cautionary notes regarding the research we have reviewed:

1. Miller's (1988) findings regarding the relationship between production and comprehension, although valuable, are not based upon a systematic comparison of the same linguistic structures assessed in production and comprehension.

2. The various production and comprehension measures he employed may not have been equated on their cognitive information-processing demands (this, of course, is a problem that must be addressed in any comparison of production and comprehension).

3. As Miller (1987) pointed out in an earlier article, "Speech intelligibility remains . . . a consistent problem among individuals with Down syndrome" (p. 243), due to associated anomalies of the face and oral area and problems of speech motor control. He cited, for example, a personal communication of Berry regarding the findings of a large-sample, longitudinal study of children with Down syndrome to the effect that "the majority of his 5- and 6-year-olds were unintelligible" (Miller, 1987, p. 243). Thus, the tendency in much of the literature, which we have not mentioned heretofore, to select only children with Down syndrome whose speech is intelligible may have produced at least some findings that are not representative of most Down-syndrome children.

4. A number of the studies we reviewed reported data based on observations of a relatively small number of subjects, which raises questions of the generalizability of findings as well as the problem of interpreting trends when no statistical tests of differences can be carried out.

5. The intervention programs in which some subjects were engaged may have had effects on their performance.

6. When authors reported information on the reliability of their measures, they tended not to test for the statistical significance of the reliabilities.

7. MA and MLU matching do not necessarily ensure that subjects so matched are equivalent on all relevant nonlinguistic abilities and their mastery of specific linguistic structures, respectively. Thus, many of the findings we reviewed in this chapter (and the studies we will review) must be treated as hypotheses for future research rather than as established empirical generalizations.

4

Semantic Development

The semantic aspects of language development in persons with mental retardation constitute the subject matter of this chapter. The domain of semantics encompasses the cognitive representations (concepts) and relations of perception, thought, action, and affective states that are coded linguistically. According to Rosenberg (1982, p. 351), some of these cognitive phenomena "have their origin in the achievements of nonlinguistic cognitive development; others, apparently, in the impact of adult language on nonlinguistic cognitive development" (Blank, 1975; Bowerman, 1978). Semantics, moreover, includes at least the following phenomena (Rosenberg, 1982):

1. The content and organization of lexical (word) meaning.

2. The basic types of propositional contents (semantic role relations) of simple sentences (e.g., agent–action, object–location).

3. The modalities of simple sentences (e.g., questions, negation).

4. The meanings expressed by such grammatical morphemes as tense and number markers and modal auxiliaries (e.g., *could, would*).

5. The topic-comment (given-new) relation, which in English is signaled by, for example, contractive stress.

6. The semantic dependency relations between the propositions of simple sentences that are expressed through embedding (e.g., *John liked the meal his aunt prepared*) and the use of subordinating conjunctions (e.g., *John was late for school because he forgot to set his alarm*).

7. The semantic dependency relations of connected discourse as signaled by, for example, pronouns and adverbs (e.g., *John went downtown yesterday to*

buy some shirts. When HE got THERE, he found that the store was closed.), and the meanings of the sentences of the discourse as they relate to its topic (although this last item is also of interest to students of pragmatics [see chapter 6]).

8. Metaphor and other types of figurative language (e.g., *This writing assignment is a stone around my neck*).

9. Implication—that is, the meanings derived from utterances through inference (e.g., *It says here that John closed the window; therefore, the window must have been open*).

10. Semantic ambiguity (multiple meanings of words, phrases, and sentences).

Additional considerations pertaining to semantic competence will be addressed later (see also Eco, Santambrogio, & Violi, 1988). We turn first to the topic of lexical-semantic development in nonretarded persons, because the majority of studies of semantic development in retarded persons were concerned with this topic.

LEXICAL-SEMANTIC DEVELOPMENT IN NONDISABLED PERSONS

Reviews of research and theory regarding lexical-semantic development in nondisabled children can be found in Carey (1982), Griffiths (1986), Ingram (1989), Menyuk (1988), and Pease, Gleason, and Pan (1989). Of course, lexical items have not only semantic properties but pragmatic, phonological, morphological, and syntactic properties as well; as a result, their representations develop over a period of time. Young children's first words appear to denote objects, events, and object attributes (Menyuk, 1988). Moreover, the rate at which new words are comprehended and produced increases with age. Approximate times at which nondisabled children have been reported to comprehend their first 10, 50, and 100 words are 12, 14, and 17 months, respectively. The figures that are available for production are 10 words at 15 months and 50 words at 19 months (Menyuk, 1988, pp. 142–143).

A number of phases of early lexical development for a given word are proposed by Menyuk:

1. Comprehension in limited contexts of some words prior to 12 months of age.

2. A phase of *overspecification* or limited use of a word (e.g., *cup* is used to refer to the particular cup a child drinks from).

3. A *slippery* period, during which a child might use a word "to label different aspects of a situation" (p. 144).

4. A period of *overgeneralization*, in which a word is used to refer to a variety of objects that display similar perceptual and/or functional properties (e.g., when *ball* is used to refer to any object that can be rolled—a ball or a tube, for example).

5. A period when words refer to categorically appropriate instances (e.g., *dog* for different dogs).

According to another reviewer (Aitchison, 1987), early lexical-semantic development involves three tasks: (a) *labeling*, (b) *packaging*, and (c) *network building*. "In the labeling task, youngsters must discover that sequences of sound can be used as names for things. In the packaging task, they must find out which things can be packaged together under one label. In the network-building task, they must work out how words relate to one another" (p. 87).

Much of the work on the network-building task in lexical-semantic development was influenced by the research of Rosch and colleagues (e.g., Rosch, 1975; Rosch & Mervis, 1975, and the discussion of the limitations of this work in Carey, 1982, and Gleitman, 1990). According to Rosch, semantic concepts consist of a core of best exemplars (instances) or *prototypes* and a periphery of nonprototypical instances. Prototypical exemplars of a category such as *bird* (e.g., *cardinal, eagle*) differ from peripheral members (e.g., *penguin, ostrich*) in the number of characteristic attributes of the category that they share. Thus, members of a category are said to differ in how representative they are of the category. As a result, a language user is more likely to say that an *eagle* is a bird than that a *penguin* is a *bird*. Rosch has also proposed that in concept hierarchies (e.g., *fruit-apple-Macintosh*), there is a superordinate level (*fruit*), a subordinate level (*Macintosh*), and a basic level (*apple*). The basic level is the one at which exemplars of one category are most distinguishable from exemplars of other categories; as a result, the basic level is likely to be the one most salient for an adult (e.g., Mervis & Rosch, 1981) and the one labeled first by children (e.g., Mervis, 1983).

Children begin lexical-semantic development by referring to present objects and events but soon refer to objects and events that are absent. Labeling, moreover, appears to increase suddenly sometime between a child's first and second birthdays (Nelson, 1973), although individual differences have been reported in this regard (Goldfield & Reznick, 1990). Important aspects of lexical-semantic development that take place beyond the early phases include:

1. Network building, that is, organizing the lexicon into fields of related items (e.g., items of clothing or furniture, means of transportation).

2. Identifying the semantic roles words serve and are combined with in sentences (e.g., agent, instrument).

3. Mastering the meanings of function words (e.g., prepositions, articles).

4. The acquisition of abstract terms (e.g., *honesty, think*).

5. The figurative use of words (e.g., *cold* to refer to someone's personality).

6. Formulating and comprehending word definitions.

Clearly, lexical-semantic development is a huge undertaking for the child and is made even more so by the myriad other tasks confronting him or her, both linguistic and nonlinguistic. How do children manage this task? For some answers, albeit tentative, we turn to a brief discussion of mechanisms of lexical-semantic development.

Mechanisms of Lexical-Semantic Development

In lexical-semantic development, or word learning, conceptual representations are paired with phonological representations. How is this accomplished, given that an unfamiliar word uttered by an adult could refer to any one of a very large number of features of communicative context? Clearly, for word learning to take place, the child's hypotheses concerning such pairings must be constrained. Moreover, word learning presupposes prior independent differentiation of appropriate conceptual and linguistic units. Recall, however, the research reviewed in chapter 2, which indicates that the relationship between cognitive and lexical-semantic development is an imperfect one and that certain conceptual understandings follow lexical-semantic acquisition (Gopnik & Meltzoff, 1986), some of which may actually be shaped by linguistic factors (Bowerman, 1978):

1. Evidence of constraints in word learning comes from studies of the phenomenon of *fast mapping*. Investigators (e.g., Heibeck & Markman, 1987) found that, in a number of domains, young children are able "to rapidly narrow down a word's meaning" (p. 1021).

2. Markman and Wachtel (1988; see also Huttenlocher & Smiley, 1987, and Mervis, 1989) observed a tendency for children to assume that a label refers to an object category as a whole rather than to its parts or other attributes.

3. There is evidence (Locke, 1988) that the child's initial lexical items are constrained by prior phonological competence (i.e., phonemes that appear in the child's first words are those that were evident in the vocal repertoire prior to the appearance of meaningful lexical items).

4. There is increasing evidence (Gleitman, Gleitman, Landau, & Wanner, 1988) of the existence in young children of a predisposition (presumably innate) to segment the incoming speech stream into lexical and other linguistically significant units, as well as an ability to use linguistic context to aid in the identification of the meanings of many unfamiliar words, especially verbs (Gleitman, 1990). Further evidence of biases in word learning can be found in Au and Glusman (1990) and Waxman and Kosowsky (1990).

5. In addition to the factors that facilitate the identification of lexical items in the speech stream and linguistically relevant cognitive representations, and constrain conceptual-phonological pairings, there is the child's learning ability, which is likely to be relevant to word learning, given the fact that such pairings are arbitrary across the languages of the world rather than determined by rule. Consistent with this claim, of course, is the contribution of vocabulary test performance to individual differences in crystallized intelligence.

The Mental Lexicon

What does lexical development achieve for the literate nondisabled language user? Evidence (see Emmorey & Fromkin, 1988, for a review) from studies of speech perception, speech production, and brain-damaged patients supports the view that the mental representation of words (the mental lexicon) consists of independent subcomponents or modules for phonological, orthographic (spelling), semantic, and syntactic information whose outputs can interact during language performance. Phonological and orthographic information, moreover, appears to include morphological structure.

Such findings, it is important to note, articulate well with the modularity claims of Chomsky's (e.g., 1986) most recent theory of grammar, aspects of which include the differentiation of the various subcomponents of grammar and the differentiation of linguistic from nonlinguistic cognitive development. In regard to the latter, the reader will recall our earlier discussion (chapter 2) of the independence of language and cognitive development as it pertained to the cognition-first hypothesis of Piaget and others.

Modularity is thought to characterize language structure and processing and perception in the various senses (Fodor, 1983, 1989; Grodzinsky, 1990). For example, "the language processor is modular, in that the flow of information between it and the other parts of the cognitive system is severely restricted" (Grodzinsky, 1990, p. 19). The modular components of our cognitive system contrast with a central, higher cognitive component that can, for example, attend differentially to the output of the modules, draw inferences, and solve problems in science, math, and philosophy. Central processes cannot interfere with the operation of a module, which runs its course automatically without conscious access to its knowledge systems. Lexical recognition (e.g., Swinney, 1979) and syntactic structuring (Fodor, 1983) appear to be modular, even in brain-damaged, language-impaired adults (Grodzinsky, 1990, pp. 137–141). Thus, lexical processing appears to involve a passive, automatic-recognition stage (the modular component) and an active, strategic-utilization stage (the higher cognitive component).

LEXICAL-SEMANTIC DEVELOPMENT
IN PERSONS WITH MENTAL RETARDATION

An extensive study of early lexical-semantic acquisition in children with Down syndrome was reported by Mervis and associates (Mervis, 1988; see also Cardoso-Martins, Mervis, & Mervis, 1985, and Cardoso-Martins & Mervis, 1985). The study began when the children (3 males and 3 females) were between 17 and 19 months of age and continued until they were approximately 3 years of age. A control group of nondisabled infants was 9 months of age. Interest was in the early acquisition of the names of concrete-object categories. Samples of spontaneous speech in mother–child interactions were collected, followed by production and comprehension testing. Cognitive development was also assessed using Piagetian and standard intelligence scales. Stimuli presented to the children were various possible members of the categories *ball*, *car*, and *kitty*, names that Mervis pointed out "are among the earliest words of children with Down syndrome and normally developing children" (1988, p. 104). (See also Gillham, 1979; Nelson, 1973.)

In the study in question (and in Gillham, 1979), there was evidence that both nondisabled and Down-syndrome children's early categories of objects, which tend to be very general (basic-level) categories, are based on correlated form and function attributes (e.g., if it is spherical and it rolls, it is a ball). However, one child may differ from another and children may differ from adults in the specific form–function attributes they use in the process of sorting objects into different categories. However, the sorting principle is always that of form–function correlations. There is also evidence that a Down-syndrome child as well as a nondisabled child is likely to treat a new object label as referring "to the object as a whole rather than to a part or attribute of that object or an action performed by the object" (Mervis, 1988, p. 116), which suggests that, in this regard, word learning in a child with Down syndrome is similar to that in the typical normally developing child.

Additionally, as Mervis pointed out, there is evidence that nondisabled and Down-syndrome children's very first names for objects refer to a similar, limited set of categories (e.g., people, animals, food, clothing) and exemplars. According to Mervis, Gillham (1979), in a longitudinal study, found considerable overlap in the first 50 words produced by nondisabled and Down-syndrome children. In addition, the basis for these early word choices by nondisabled and Down-syndrome children appeared to be the same, namely, the "children's interest in objects that either move independently or can be manipulated by the child" (Mervis, 1988, p. 119). See also Nelson (1973), which suggests that a cognitive bias contributes to early lexical-semantic pairing in both nondisabled and Down-syndrome retarded children.

An interesting finding of Mervis's investigation was that the level of cognitive development (as assessed by standardized intelligence tests and measures of Piagetian stage of sensorimotor functioning) was similar for her children with Down syndrome and her nondisabled children at the onset of both referential comprehension and referential production. For example, the average MAs for the two groups at the onset of referential comprehension were 14.5 and 13.8 months for the Down-syndrome and nondisabled children, respectively. At the onset of referential production, the average MAs for these groups were 18.9 and 19.5 months, respectively. (Note that in both groups, the onset of referential production lagged behind the onset of referential comprehension.) Nevertheless, the size of the Down-syndrome subjects' vocabularies lagged behind sensorimotor performance, but not MA, up to 20 months. Once again, we find evidence of the risk involved in using MA by itself to assess cognitive status, as is the case in many studies.

According to Mervis' report, a large difference in vocabulary size in favor of nondisabled children exists at a MA of 21 months, which is when nondisabled children begin a spurt in vocabulary acquisition. Thus, it appears "that normally developing children begin their vocabulary spurt at a younger mental age and cognitive level than children with Down syndrome" (p. 122).

In summary, no evidence of linguistic or developmental deviance was forthcoming in the research described by Mervis. Moreover, biases that operate in the word learning of typically developing children also appear to operate in the word learning of children with Down syndrome. However, lexical-semantic development was evidently delayed from the start in the children with Down syndrome, relative to what would be expected from CA-matched, nondisabled children, regardless of whether such development was assessed through comprehension or production. In addition, beyond a MA of approximately 20 months and a certain level of sensorimotor maturity, lexical-semantic development in the domain of concrete-object labels lagged behind cognitive maturity in the children with Down syndrome.

Findings consistent with those reported by Mervis and her associates can be found in, for example, Cunningham and Sloper (1984), Dooley (1976), Glenn and Cunningham (1983), Gopnik (1987, cited in Barrett & Diniz, 1989), Miller (1988), and Thompson (1963).

Studies that included etiological classifications other than Down syndrome tended to investigate older persons with mental retardation. A case in point is a study by Mein and O'Connor (1960) of the oral vocabularies of a large sample of institutionalized retarded persons (CAs 10 to 30; Stanford-Binet MAs 3 to 7) of varying etiologies. The sexes were evenly divided in the sample. The data were collected in interview sessions. Mein and O'Connor found that the vocabularies of their subjects were less diverse than those of a sample of typically developing children of similar MAs. Thus, the exceptional delay in vocabulary acquisition relative to MA that we previously reported may not be limited to individuals with Down syndrome. These investigators also found that MA was a better predictor of vocabulary size than CA or length of institutionalization in their retarded sample. However, it would be of interest to determine whether the delay in question is reduced when the groups that Mein and O'Connor observed are matched solely on verbal MA.

Lexical Definitions

Mentally retarded children's conscious awareness of the meanings of words—a form of what is referred to as *metalinguistic awareness* (i.e., awareness of the nature of linguistic knowledge)—has been examined in a number of studies using tasks that assess the level of abstraction of the definitions of concrete nouns, with *descriptive* or *concrete* being the lowest level, *functional* next, and *abstract* the highest level. For example, "a banana is yellow" is said to be a descriptive or concrete definition, "a banana is something you eat" is a functional definition, and "a banana is a fruit" is an abstract definition.

Unfortunately, such tasks are likely to underestimate a child's lexical-semantic knowledge when compared to a task in which, for example, subjects are given an abstract category label and asked to point to the picture in an array that depicts that category. Moreover, as Mervis' research suggests, form (descriptive) and function attributes of meaning tend to be correlated; thus, it is questionable whether one should precede the other conceptually.

A good example of the research in this area is a study by Papania (1954), in which institutionalized retarded (MAs 6 to 10; mean IQ approximately 70) and CA-matched, nondisabled children were asked to define vocabulary items from the Stanford-Binet Intelligence Test. The typically developing children produced more abstract definitions than the children with mental retardation, whereas the retarded children produced more descriptive-concrete definitions than the nondisabled children. Moreover, as MA (and CA also, apparently) increased, the children with mental retardation produced a larger proportion of abstract definitions. Just the opposite was the case for the concrete definitions (see also Cornwell, 1974). Evidence of a developmental lag in lexical categorical behavior in noninstitutionalized, special-class retarded children was provided by Winters and Brzoska (1976).

Word Relatedness

Word relatedness, or the lexical-semantic network-building task, has been of considerable interest to students of mental retardation, much of it centered on Rosch's (e.g., 1975) work on the typicality of object-category instances. In brief, we see that persons with mental retardation are not differentiated from nondisabled persons in any qualitative way in the domain of concrete-noun relatedness.

In an experiment by Sperber, Ragain, and McCauley (1976), special-class retarded subjects were asked to name as quickly as possible pairs of pictures of objects whose names they already knew. The second item in each of a pair of objects was either in the same conceptual semantic category as the first item (e.g., *cat-horse*) or in a different category. At issue was whether category relatedness would reduce the time to name the second item in a pair, as is the case with children and adults who are not mentally retarded, that is, whether performance would evidence *semantic priming*. Mean IQ, MA, and CA in the group were 60, 7;3, and 16;4, respectively. The results of this study and a second one were consistent with the findings of research with nondisabled persons. Thus, not only was semantic relatedness similar in the two groups but the persons with mental retardation, like nondisabled children, evidenced a facilitating effect of such relatedness in word recognition.

This is not to say, however, that persons with mental retardation are equally efficient in word recognition and production. Elliott (1978), for example, studied object-naming latencies (response speeds) in mildly (M CA = 9.79) and moderately (M CA = 11.75) mentally retarded children, all of whom knew the names of the objects, and reported that the former responded faster than the latter.

Differences in semantic-processing (picture-naming) speed between CA-matched, mildly retarded and nondisabled adolescents (Davies, Sperber, & McCauley, 1981) and CA-matched, mildly retarded and nondisabled adults (Merrill, 1985) have also been reported. Davies et al. found that although the subjects with mental retardation were slower overall than the nondisabled persons on a semantic-priming task, the magnitude of the effect of semantic relatedness was the same for the two groups. Nevertheless, when subjects were given a more active semantic retrieval (from long-term memory) and evaluation task, one in which they were asked to verify the truth of verbal descriptions of pictures with a response of "yes" or "no," the effect of semantic relatedness was greater in the nondisabled group. Merrill speculated that the slower semantic-processing speed in persons with mental retardation is the result of an inefficient central information-processing mechanism. However, given the slow speed of naming pictures in persons with mental retardation, it may be too early to eliminate the possible contribution of an inefficient automatic lexical-semantic processing module in persons with mental retardation.

What happens to the efficiency of semantic processing when retarded and nondisabled persons are matched on MA? According to the results of a study by Sperber, Davies, Merrill, and McCauley (1982), differences in such processing between mildly mentally retarded and nondisabled persons tend to disappear on lexical-semantic tasks when such persons are matched on MA (Wechsler Scale or Stanford-Binet). However, there is also evidence (Merrill & Mar, 1987) that suggests that when more complex linguistic input is involved (i.e., discourse), semantic encoding tends to be less efficient in adolescents with mental retardation than in MA-matched (Stanford-Binet or Wechsler Scales), nondisabled persons. Discourse processing, however, involves factors that transcend lexical and sentential boundaries (e.g., text coherence relative to a topic) and is, therefore, likely to be cognitively more demanding than lexical and sentential processing.

Finally, performance factors in lexical-semantic memory are also implicated in the results of two studies by Glidden and Mar (1978). In the first, a group of students with mental retardation (*M* IQ = 60) and a CA-matched group of nondisabled students (*M* CA = 15;4 and 14;8, respectively) differed less in their underlying knowledge of lexical category instances (*sports* and *animals*) than in their ability to retrieve such instances from lexical-semantic memory. In the second experiment, similar persons with mental retardation were provided cues that facilitated retrieval of category instances, but when these cues were no longer available, the subjects' performance deteriorated.

Prototypes.   Several studies have examined the extent to which the lexical object categories of persons with mental retardation are similar in organization to those of nondisabled persons (Davies, Sperber, & McCauley, 1981; McCauley, Sperber, & Roaden, 1978; Sperber, Davies, Merrill, & McCauley, 1982; Tager-Flusberg, 1985a, 1985b; Weil, McCauley, & Sperber, 1978; Winters & Hoats, 1985, 1986; Winters, Hoats, & Kahn, 1985). This research, which has involved the use of a variety of tasks, indicates that, although delayed in their development (relative to CA), such categories are organized in a manner similar if not identical to those of nondisabled persons.

For example, in a study of referential word meaning in autistic children, Tager-Flusberg (1985b) included a group of retarded children (various etiologies; *M* CA = 11;6; *M* verbal MA = 4;11; *M* IQ = 44) and a group of typically developing children, matched on verbal and nonverbal MA. Tager-Flusberg based her research on the work of Rosch and her associates (e.g., Rosch, 1988; Rosch & Mervis, 1975) and, in a series of two experiments, addressed the question of "the extent to which the children generalized the meanings of words on the basis of prototype representations of the underlying concepts for both basic level and subordinate level categories" (p. 1169). The subjects in the first experiment were shown pictures of objects and asked whether a picture "was an instance of a particular word" (p. 1169). Different items and a nonverbal response task were employed in the second experiment. Selection of stimuli and labels was based upon prototypicality ratings of college undergraduates.

No group or sex differences were found in performance in this study. Moreover, category-membership identification was best for prototypical exemplars and the pattern of errors (overextension and underextension) was the same for each group and consistent with prototype theory. The findings of Experiment 2 were similar to those of Experiment 1. Thus, for the items in question, the lexicons of all three groups appear to be organized similarly. These findings for such widely differing groups of children (as regards organic status, developmental history, and the like) led Tager-Flusberg to propose that there are innately determined constraints on the semantic representations of concrete objects.

These findings were confirmed and extended in a second series of experiments by Tager-Flusberg (1985a). Specifically, prototypicality effects were found in all groups and basic-level concepts were found to be more salient than the more abstract subordinate categories.

Although we must be alert to the possibility of performance differences between nondisabled persons and persons with mental retardation, particularly when matched on CA or when the task is a complex one, none of the findings we have reviewed in this section on lexical-semantic relatedness (nor other findings in the literature on lexical-semantic development in persons with mental retardation) suggest that the semantic competence of persons with mental retardation, although slower to develop, is qualitatively different from that in typically developing persons.

SEMANTIC RELATIONS

Earlier, we discussed Brown's (1973) work on the appearance of semantic relations (e.g., agent–action, possessor–possession, entity–location) in the early multiword utterances of nondisabled children and the observation of similar semantic relations in the early multiword utterances of two children with Down syndrome (Dooley, 1976). However, on the basis of data in the literature on normal language acquisition, it is likely that growth in the mastery of such relations in nondisabled children matched on MA with persons with mental retardation will exceed that of Dooley's subjects. A subsequent study by Coggins (1979; see also Duchan & Erickson, 1976, and Layton & Sharifi, 1979) of the spontaneous utterances of 4 children with Down syndrome (MLUs from 1.22 to 2.06; CAs from 3;10 to 6;3) indicated that, although appreciably delayed in the development of semantic relations, "Down's-syndrome children at Stage 1 of linguistic development . . . [use] the same rather small set of relational meanings as in normal children's early two-word combinations. . . ." (p. 176).

Ideational complexity—the average number of idea units in an utterance—in nonverbal-MA-matched, mildly retarded, nondisabled, and language-impaired (IQs in the normal range) children was investigated by Kamhi and Johnston (1982). The measure in question had to do with the semantic relations or propositions depicted by a verb and the phrase structures with which it can occur. Utterance (sentence) length, however, was not directly related to underlying ideational complexity. However, given the projection principle (e.g., Chomsky, 1986), the authors' claim that "there are few one-to-one relationships between parts of propositions and specific syntactic units" (p. 439) is an oversimplification.

Mean MA and CA in the sample of children with mental retardation were approximately 5;2 and approximately 8;3 respectively; mean IQ was 63.1.

Records indicated that none of the retarded children was suffering from a genetically based disorder. Among other things, it was reported that the retarded and nondisabled children did not differ in the ideational complexity of their spontaneous utterances. Possibly, then, these groups were also matched on verbal MA. Moreover, for both the retarded and nondisabled children, as grammatical errors decreased, the ideational complexity of sentences increased. However, the correlation between these variables for the language-impaired children was positive.

Comprehension (picture choice and acting out) of the semantic relations encoded by *before* and *after* in sentence contexts was studied by Natsopoulos and Xeromeritou (1988). The subjects were verbal-MA-matched, mildly mentally retarded (M CA = 9;7, M MA = 5;3, M verbal IQ = 62.77) and nondisabled children (M CA = 4;3, M MA = 4;5, M verbal IQ = 100.28).

Although the groups were matched on verbal MA, overall performance was found to be significantly higher in the nondisabled group than in the sample of children with mental retardation. However, the pattern of findings suggested that the retarded children in this study may have been hampered by a failure to employ efficient comprehension strategies.

As a final item in this review, we remind the reader that there is evidence of a dissociation of phonological, morphological, and syntactic competence from aspects of semantic and pragmatic competence in some seriously mentally retarded children (Curtiss, 1988b; Yamada, 1990). The formal aspects of language acquisition have been spared relative to aspects dealing with meaning in these individuals. Consistent with these findings is an informal observation we made in our study of grammatical competence in a group of mildly retarded adults (Rosenberg & Abbeduto, 1987), as revealed in naturally occurring conversations among themselves. Although these individuals had evidently achieved a relatively high level of mastery of grammatical morphemes and complex sentence structures, the range of topics they discussed was quite limited. We came away from our experience with the distinct impression that there were significant limitations on their semantic competence. This observation, although informal, is consistent with repeated findings in the literature that the vocabularies of persons with mental retardation are smaller than those of nondisabled persons.

A possible exception to the observation that mental retardation is associated with lower semantic (and pragmatic) achievements is the case of persons with Williams syndrome, a metabolic disorder. Sabo, Bellugi, and Vaid (1986) studied 3 teenage Williams-syndrome persons with mental retardation whose language skills, including their long-term retention of verbally presented information, were far in excess of their MAs (especially their performance MAs), their Piagetian stage of cognitive development, and, quite dramatically, their visuospatial abilities (see also Stiles-Davis, Kritchevsky, & Bellugi, in press). On a number of measures, however, their semantic competence, as well as their related pragmatic competence, was also exceptional. However, on the measure of vocabulary age (vocabulary size), performance was below CA expectation in all of the subjects, and their conversational competence was described as being "somewhat impaired."

Thus, it is likely that the semantic and pragmatic skills of the subjects studied by Sabo et al. were superior to those of the subjects in Curtiss' (1988b) and Yamada's (1990) studies, although it does not appear that Sabo et al.'s subjects were entirely free of problems in the domains in question. However, when we add their exceptional semantic and pragmatic skills to the superiority of their verbal MAs relative to their performance MAs and to their exceptional long-term retention of verbally presented information, we see that their mental retardation is limited primarily to the domain of nonverbal cognitive functions, in particular, visuospatial skills. Therefore, it is possible that Williams syndrome is a disorder in which not only language but also *crystallized intelligence* (Horn, 1976) is spared. Given this possibility, it is questionable whether Williams syndrome constitutes a true case of semantic sparing in the presence of general (both crystallized and fluid-intelligence-impaired) mental retardation.

SUMMARY AND DISCUSSION

Although children with Down syndrome are delayed in their acquisition of the names of concrete-object categories on both spontaneous speech and comprehension measures, the basis for such categories is the same as that found in typically developing children. There is also evidence that children with Down syndrome and nondisabled children share an expectation concerning lexical-semantic pairing, namely, that a new object label refers to the object as a whole.

We noted that the concrete-object categories and the exemplars of such categories are similar in Down-syndrome and nondisabled children. Moreover, we saw that the level of cognitive maturity in these two groups at the onset of referential comprehension and production are similar. Then, up to 20 months of age, vocabulary size in children with Down syndrome lags behind sensorimotor performance but not MA. At an MA of 21 months, however, a large difference in vocabulary size in favor of the typically developed child is apparent. The period during which this occurs corresponds to the onset of the vocabulary spurt in nondisabled children. It is interesting to note that the period in question also coincides with an important period in early syntactic development, namely the period during which children begin to identify the options for combining words and the structures for expressing the underlying grammatical relations in their native language.

It remains to be determined, however, whether these syntactic demands reduce the resources available for lexical-semantic development in children with Down syndrome. The fact that there are some persons with mental retardation who display essentially normal syntax but deficiencies in the semantic domain (Curtiss, 1988b) suggests that such demands, if they do exist, are not the major factors responsible for the exceptional difference in vocabulary size noted between Down-syndrome and nondisabled children at an MA of 21 months. Of course, another possibility is that the exceptional difference in question (and the subsequent exceptional lag in lexical-semantic development) in persons with Down syndrome is due to a cognitive deficit or deficits that is or are not assessed by Piagetian tasks or by the variety of tests used to assess MA. Or these findings may be due to a specifically linguistic deficit affecting lexical-semantic pairing that is still to be identified.

Finally, the reader should be reminded that asynchronies in cognitive and lexical-semantic development are not unique to persons with mental retardation; they are also found in nondisabled children (Gopnik & Meltzoff, 1986; see also Kamhi & Masterson, 1989). Thus, an exceptional slowdown per se in aspects of lexical-semantic development, relative to cognitive status in children who display a variety of cognitive deficits, is not necessarily indicative of qualitatively different development.

To return to our summary and discussion of the literature on semantic development in retarded persons, the picture of exceptional (quantitative) delay in vocabulary acquisition relative to MA in persons with Down syndrome continues in older Down-syndrome persons. Moreover, older institutionalized retarded children and retarded children of varying etiology also appear to be exceptionally delayed in vocabulary acquisition relative to MA. As one would expect, there is a positive correlation between MA and vocabulary size in retarded persons. Thus, persons with mental retardation, regardless of etiology, appear to evidence an exceptional delay relative to MA in lexical-semantic development.

A number of years ago, there was considerable interest in assessing retarded persons' conscious awareness of the meanings of concrete lexical category exemplars via the verbal-definition task. A common but not surprising finding in these investigations was that subjects with mental retardation produce fewer abstract (category-label) definitions than CA-matched, nondisabled subjects.

Our review revealed no qualitative differences between retarded and nondisabled children, adolescents, and adults in the domain of concrete-noun relatedness. A number of studies revealed that persons with mental retardation are able to utilize their knowledge of word relatedness in word-recognition tasks, although more slowly than nondisabled persons (IQ appears to be inversely related to response speed). Moreover, there is some evidence that as task complexity increases, the ability to utilize semantic relatedness decreases in persons with mental retardation. What might be operating here, it has been speculated, is a combination of an inefficient automatic lexical-semantic processing module (which results in slower lexical-semantic coding) and an inefficient central information-processing mechanism that interferes with performance on cognitively demanding tasks (even when retarded and nondisabled subjects are matched on MA). Neither of these possibilities, however, would necessarily result in qualitatively different performance in persons with mental retardation in lexical-semantic processing tasks in which word relatedness is a factor.

Most of this research has been carried out with higher functioning persons with mental retardation, so it remains to be determined whether similar findings will emerge when other subgroups are observed. However, performance and subgroup factors aside, the available research, including the many studies of category prototypes, strongly suggests that the mental lexicons of retarded and nondisabled persons are similarly organized.

There appears to be adequate evidence that children with Down syndrome express the same sorts of semantic relations as do typically developing children in their early word combinations. However, there is also some indication that growth in the mastery of such relations is slower than would be predicated from the Down-syndrome children's MAs. Nevertheless, it has also been reported that older, MA-matched, mildly mentally retarded children and nondisabled children display similar ideational complexity in their spontaneous speech and that there is an inverse relationship between ideational complexity and the incidence of grammatical errors in sentences.

Thus, within the range of phenomena and subjects studied in the research on semantic development in persons with mental retardation, there was no evidence of developmental or linguistic deviance. However, we did find evidence of a significant relationship between cognitive and semantic development, as well as further evidence of a dissociation of linguistic and cognitive development. Moreover, semantic development in both nondisabled and retarded children appears to recruit factors that are not assessed by traditional measures of cognitive development. One question for future research that is raised by this last finding is: How much does the mapping process between meaning and linguistic form–structure contribute to the pace of semantic development in children with mental retardation? Finally, some of the studies reviewed here revealed the presence of task-related performance factors in the semantic behavior of retarded persons, which must be taken into account when attempting to assess their semantic competence.

Although the number of methodological problems we encountered was limited, much is missing from the literature that we reviewed. This fact is difficult to understand, given the relationship between semantic and cognitive development. With few exceptions, the field appears to have concentrated on a limited range of easily researched (relatively speaking) phenomena, having to do primarily with the acquisition of concrete nouns and their interrelationships. Thus, we can only hope that future investigators will address such problems as the development of the modal system (e.g., *would, could, should*), abstract words such as *know, think, believe, justice,* and *honor* (e.g., Abbeduto & Rosenberg, 1985), metaphor (e.g., Winner, 1988), and discourse coherence (e.g., Wright

& Rosenberg, 1993) in persons with mental retardation. It is in the study of such complex phenomena that we are likely to identify the limits of semantic development and performance in individuals whose cognitive capabilities are limited.

5

Morphosyntactic Development

Morphosyntax (i.e., syntax and morphology) is at the center of language competence. It is the vehicle for the expression of semantic relations and dependencies between semantic relations (in complex sentences), the major source of the infinite combinatorial capability of language users, and the strongest candidate for an innate specifically linguistic component in language acquisition (e.g., Chomsky, 1986). In chapter 2, we discussed various aspects of linguistic competence and their acquisition in nonretarded individuals and introduced the reader to the three major theories of language acquisition. On the basis of the material in question, a number of claims can be made concerning language acquisition in typically developing persons that are relevant to the study of morphosyntactic development:

1. Children are able to acquire any human language. Thus, any account of language acquisition must take into account the ease with which children can zero in on characteristics of the local language.

2. Language acquisition takes place on the basis of limited input in a relatively short period of time, with no special training and what appears to be limited or no negative feedback concerning errors.

3. To a large extent, language acquisition is independent of cognitive, social, communicative, and some aspects of semantic development. For example, children master the basics of their native language at a time when their general cognitive capabilities are limited.

4. Related to Claim 3 is the more general observation that knowledge of language and language processing appear to be modular in nature.

5. There is no evidence that language acquisition is constrained by the fact that the linguistic input to which the child is exposed is consistent with a large number of different grammars. Thus, the language-acquisition process and the resulting grammar must be constrained by factors the child brings to the situation.
6. In language acquisition, children acquire a very rich, abstract, and highly complex system of knowledge with an infinite output.
7. Human beings evidence a reduced capacity for language acquisition after childhood.
8. From early in life, for the majority of human beings, grammar is primarily a left-cerebral-hemisphere function. Its neurological organization, moreover, does not appear to be influenced by environmental and sociological factors.

Such considerations led to the claim that there is a strong, specifically linguistic, biological component in language acquisition. Chomsky's principles and parameters theory is an attempt to characterize the nature of the constraints the child brings to the task of language acquisition.

We shall see that the literature on morphosyntactic development in persons with mental retardation is relevant to some of the previous claims regarding language acquisition in nonhandicapped persons. Before we turn to that literature, however, we discuss morphosyntactic development in nondisabled persons.

In an investigation of early language acquisition, Radford (1990a; see also Radford, 1990b) adopted a Chomskyan approach to linguistic competence that allows for the possibility that aspects of Universal Grammar mature at different rates. His data consisted of an extensive body of spontaneous, naturalistic child utterances (including responses to questions) obtained cross-sectionally and longitudinally. According to Radford, at the stage of one-word utterances, children's speech displays phonological, semantic, and pragmatic attributes but no morphosyntactic attributes. The emergence of grammatical structure is seen in the presence of phrases and clauses (single subject-predicate constructions) in the productive multiword utterances that begin to appear between 18 and 24 months of age, whose constituents are lexical-thematic categories (nouns, verbs, adjectives, prepositions, and their semantic roles) and some grammatical morphemes (e.g., plural s attached only to nouns). By thematic, we mean that, although formal, the categories of children's early speech are limited to those that are marked for such basic semantic roles as *agent* and *recipient*. They are thus the first instantiations of the projection principle in syntax acquisition. Moreover, the grammatical structures in which they appear are hierarchically organized and honor the syntactic category-order constraints of English (e.g., that the subject of a clause occurs before its verb and the direct object after its verb). It should be mentioned that some inconsistencies in early word order do occur (Braine, 1976), although they tend to be the exception rather than the rule. Such inconsistencies might be due to, for example, variations in the input available for parameter setting (see Ingram, 1989, p. 327; Pinker, 1984; and the full discussion in Ingram, 1989, of proposals by Braine, Pinker, and others regarding early syntactic development).

Thus, it is possible that the principle of structure dependence is operating in children's early grammar and that the parameter that determines the order of constituents within phrases and clauses tends to be set early. In addition, the child appears to have discovered a significant feature of languages like English with relatively rigid word-order requirements, namely, that they permit hierarchic structure. Soon the child will also discover that languages with such word-order constraints "permit the embedding of sentences and phrases one within the other, resulting in hierarchic structure of potentially infinite depth" (Goodluck, 1986, p. 51). Thus, an important mechanism of language acquisition may be the inferences a child can derive (unconsciously) from one feature of the language concerning another feature of the language.

The reader interested in further examination of evidence for the possible operation of abstract, formal grammatical structures in children's early productive word combinations should read, for example, P. Bloom (1990), Chien and Lust (1985), Chien and Wexler (1990), Hyams (1986), Ingram (1989), Lust and Mazuka (1989), Roeper (1988), and Valian (1986). P. Bloom (1990) presented evidence consistent with the view that from the very beginning children "assign words to syntactic categories like *noun, verb,* and *adjective* and . . . order them by rules and principles that order such abstract categories" (p. 343). Words, moreover, appear to be mapped onto such categories based on certain semantic properties. The term *semantic bootstrapping* is sometimes used to refer to such mapping (e.g., Pinker, 1989; Rondal & Cession, 1990).

The reader will recognize that the appearance of such abstract knowledge at an early stage of cognitive development is clearly inconsistent with the claim that there is a close relationship between nonlinguistic cognitive and linguistic achievements, whether the cognitive achievements necessarily antedate the linguistic achievements or a common prior nonlinguistic cognitive organizing principle necessarily antedates the nonlinguistic cognitive and linguistic achievements.

As Radford (1990a) pointed out, at roughly 24 months of age, we begin to see the emergence of functional nonthematic categories (grammatical morphemes) and the larger structures in which they operate. Examples of these categories are determiners like *the* and *that,* verb tense markers, and modal auxiliaries like *will/would* and *can/could.* Such categories are termed nonthematic because they do not express the semantic roles (e.g., agent, instrument, recipient) that lexical categories express.

Although one-word utterances are agrammatical, there is evidence (e.g., Greenfield & Smith, 1976; Huttenlocher, 1974, cited in Radford, 1990a) that children learn that words like *hit* have an inherent thematic argument structure during the one-word stage of language acquisition. The action depicted by the verb *hit* requires an agent to do the hitting and a recipient of the action (see Ingram's, 1989, discussion of the transition from knowledge of the semantic relations implicit in single words to early syntax). Thus, in order to express semantic relations linguistically, children have to discover how such argument structures are projected onto the syntax of the local language. According to Radford, there is some evidence that the onset of the initial categorical stage of morphosyntactic development, with its thematic concomitants, coincides with the spurt in vocabulary acquisition we discussed in chapter 4. This led him to "conjecture that the ability to develop [the structures in question] facilitates vocabulary growth, since the development of such structures arguably simplifies the task of identifying the argument structure of predicates" (p. 275). However, the reader will recognize that the relationship in question, if it is a causal one, might also operate in the opposite direction; that is, a vocabulary spurt that includes mastery of lexical items' thematic structure might facilitate syntactic development through the operation of the projection principle.

A spurt in syntactic usage in language production, which is correlated with entry into the functional-nonthematic stage of grammatical development, was observed by Anisfeld (1984; cited in Radford, 1990a). As Radford suggested, this spurt may be fostered by entry into the more mature functional-nonthematic stage of morphosyntactic development. If so, some language disorders may reflect problems in reaching this stage. As the reader will recall, Dooley (1976) suggested that children with Down syndrome are exceptionally delayed in the mastery of grammatical morphemes (see chapter 1), but more about this and related research follows.

According to Radford (1990a), the developmental spurts in vocabulary and sentence usage argue for a treatment of grammatical development wherein Universal Grammar "makes different types of principles available to the child at different stages of maturation" (pp. 289–290), but Chien and Wexler (1990) found evidence of the operation of the principles of Universal Grammar right from the beginning, with younger children's linguistic performance hampered by the absence of a pragmatic rule. This again points to the need to consider possible performance factors in our attempts to assess the formal aspects of linguistic knowledge (see also Clahsen, 1990/1991).

MORPHOSYNTACTIC DEVELOPMENT
IN PERSONS WITH MENTAL RETARDATION

A critical review of earlier research on syntactic and morphological development in persons with mental retardation can be found in Rosenberg (1982). Unfortunately, a number of these studies suffer from conceptual, methodological, and reporting (missing-information) problems. Moreover, in this and more recent literature, detailed, systematic cross-sectional and longitudinal studies of the production and comprehension of the same syntactic or morphological structures are virtually nonexistent. The field has shown limited interest in linguistic theory developments that have fueled much of the research on language acquisition in normally developing persons over the last decade. Hence, the literature on morphosyntax in retarded persons that we review here is limited.

Morphosyntactic Development in Persons with Down Syndrome

We saw previously that lexical-semantic development in children with Down syndrome lags behind that in CA-matched, nondisabled children right from the beginning. It also lags behind cognitive development starting at a point relatively early in cognitive development, although the discrepancy between MA and morphosyntactic development in children with Down syndrome may be greater than that between lexical-semantic development and MA (Miller, 1988). According to Miller, children with Down syndrome may display particular "deficiencies in the grammatical marking of their lexicon" (1988, p. 189), a suggestion that fits well into theories such as Chomsky's (e.g., 1986) that assign the lexicon a central role in syntactic development.

However, not all aspects of syntax are projections of underlying lexical-thematic roles; other principles of Universal Grammar (e.g., structure dependence) operate as well. Moreover, the parameters of language variation need to be set in accordance with the particular structure of the local language (Lightfoot, 1991). Thus, it is not surprising that the exceptional delay in language acquisition associated with Down syndrome is greatest for syntax and associated morphology.

Clearly, the lexicon of children with Down syndrome entering multiword speech is less diverse than that of nondisabled children, although we do not know to what extent the words in their lexicon, particularly the verbs, are marked for thematic arguments. However, with no evidence of qualitative differences in the lexical-semantic development of Down syndrome and nondisabled children, it is possible that the former have some appreciation of the thematic argumentation that figures in the operation of the projection principle when they enter the early stage of multiword utterances. More important than this speculation is the fact that the syntactic structure of the early multiword speech of persons with Down syndrome reflects the operation of the projection principle.

Although the development of language in children with Down syndrome is exceptionally delayed (Dooley, 1976; Miller, 1988), their early multiword utterances display a variety of the syntactic structures that express basic semantic relations (Dooley, 1976). In addition, the Down-syndrome children studied by Dooley honored the word-order constraints of English in their early multiword utterances. Was there evidence that the structure of their early multiword speech was similar to that of the earliest multiword utterances of typically developing children (Radford, 1990a)?

Dooley reproduced the multiword utterances generated by his 2 young subjects, Timmy and Sharon, during a number of his early and late observation sessions. Examination of these items suggests that the children were indeed functioning primarily, if not exclusively, at the stage of basic formal lexical-thematic categories:

1. They tended to honor word-order constraints in the vast majority of their multiword utterances, for example:

   I see.
   Goofy sleeping.
   Drop it.
   Man sick.
   They wet.
   Here the hammer.
   I kiss cow.
   Where's daddy?

2. There was some use of inflections attached to appropriate lexical categories, as in:

   It cry*ing*.
   Goofy sleep*ing*.
   He com*ing*.
   Make shoe*s*.

3. They used basic lexical–thematic categories in a variety of contexts in appropriate positions:

   Noun and pronoun subject plus main verb:
   A cow drink.
   They fall.
   It hurts.
   Me bowl.

   Main verb and object:
   Move the book.
   Want a coke.
   Hammering nail.
   Make shoes.
   Need leg.

   Predicate adjective:
   Man sick.
   It heavy.
   They wet.

However, Dooley's subjects had not fully mastered any of the 14 grammatical morphemes made famous by R. Brown (1973). They used determiners such as *the* and *that* very infrequently and they did not use any modal auxiliaries.

In addition, they had not fully mastered the noun phrase in English. According to Lightfoot (1991, pp. 16–17), there are four stages in the acquisition of noun phrases; the first is the single-word stage and the last stage is mature competence. Stage 2 is exemplified by such items as *a coat* and *big foot*, and Stage 3, for example, by *a blue flower* and *your blue cap*. Our examination of the corpus of multiword utterances produced by Timmy and Sharon revealed that Timmy did not produce any noun phrases beyond Stage 2. Examples of items he produced are *more tea, another hat, a cow, the book, the one, three ball, my dad, baby boy,* and *your pockets.* In Sharon's case we noted such Stage 2 noun phrases as *a chair, the paint, another bed, more chalk, baby bed,* and *my comb,* but very limited use of Stage 3 constructions (e.g., *the other side, the kitty shoe*).

We conducted no systematic examination of the verb phrases in Timmy and Sharon's multiword utterances. However, even our brief perusal of the data revealed mastery of a number of intransitive (e.g., *They fell*) and transitive (e.g., *I make cake*) verbs.

Thus, the data that Dooley provided do not suggest anything aberrant in the grammar of his subjects' early multiword speech. However, their progress vis-à-vis grammatical morphemes appears to have been exceptionally slow and may therefore represent a particular stumbling block in their morphosyntactic development.

A common index of early morphosyntactic growth is mean length of utterance (MLU). Rondal, Ghiotto, Brédart, and Bachelet (1988) found that MLU correlates positively and highly with CA (range from 2 to 12 years) in Down-syndrome children ($r = .87$). It also correlates positively with a number of specific measures of grammatical development. Nevertheless, when the sample of Down-syndrome children in Rondal et al.'s study was broken down into three subgroups based on their MLUs (1.00–2.00, 1.50–2.50, 2.00–3.50), significant positive correlations were found only for the first two subgroups. The correlation between MLU and CA in a sample of nondisabled individuals in the CA range from 17 to 59 months was reported to be .88 by Miller (1981).

Based on a variety of morphosyntactic structures, the correlation between MLU and an alternative measure of grammatical maturity in typically developing children (Scarborough, Rescorla, Tager-Flusberg, Fowler, & Sudhalter, 1991) in the MLU range below 3.0 is .93, whereas above 3.0 it is .55 (a repeat of this study produced similar correlations). The correlations in a sample of subjects with Down syndrome showed a similar trend (.93 below 3.0 and .60 above 3.0). In addition, there was a tendency for MLU to overestimate the grammatical maturity of a person with Down syndrome, especially when it was greater than 3.0. The alternative measure of grammatical maturity assessed noun and verb phrase structures, question and negation structures, and sentence structures of varying complexity (from a developmental standpoint).

Research by Fowler, Gelman, and Gleitman (1980), reviewed in Fowler (1988), compared the speech of 12-year-old, MLU-matched ($M = 3.0$), Down-syndrome adolescents (MAs 5 to 6 years) and nondisabled children (CAs 30 to 36 months). The two groups evidenced comparable levels of language development. Overall, the Down-syndrome children's performance on grammatical morphemes, questions, negatives, content words, function words, thematic roles, and sentence structures was similar to that of a 2.6-year-old nondisabled child. This would place them in a stage of normal language acquisition prior to the mastery of the functional-nonthematic grammatical system (e.g., verbal auxiliaries) described by Radford (1990a, 1990b) and the acquisition of complex sentence structures involving subordination.

An examination of the available literature and further observations that the speech of 7- to 9-year-old children with Down syndrome was not distinguishable from that of their Down-syndrome adolescents (Fowler, 1988, p. 220) led to the suggestion that persons with Down syndrome may not progress beyond early morphosyntactic development. This suggestion, it should be noted, is consistent with Dooley's (1976) observation that his subjects with Down syndrome had not yet mastered any of Brown's (1973) 14 grammatical morphemes and Radford's (1990a) prediction that some language-disordered children encounter problems in mastering functional-nonthematic grammatical categories. The end result of this trend is that differences in grammatical competence between persons with Down syndrome and nondisabled persons tend to increase with increasing CA.

Fowler (1988) studied a female child with Down syndrome (IQ = 57) who showed limited, erratic, and very slow progress beyond early grammatical development. Her MLU leveled off for 10 months, followed by sharp fluctuations. Progress on new grammatical morphemes was extremely limited and the use of already mastered items was inconsistent. She also plateaued in the mastery of questions, negation, and aspects of the auxiliary system. Thus, it is possible that mastery of linguistic phenomena beyond the early stage of morphosyntax results in a deterioration of the subsequent acquisition process in persons with Down syndrome. Alternatively, this pattern of language acquisition may result from a change in the innate language-acquisition system as children with Down syndrome approach the end of their critical period for language acquisition.

With respect to the former possibility, because much, if not all, of grammatical morphology is language specific and therefore parametric in nature, one might speculate that there is a significant general (i.e., nonlinguistic) learning component involved in its mastery. Therefore, any condition (such as Down syndrome) that affects learning ability might impact on this aspect of language acquisition as well. However, this explanation is unlikely given the cases of exceptional language acquisition relative to cognitive development in seriously mentally retarded persons, including the case reported by Yamada (1990), in which cognitive development meant MA, Piagetian stage, and information-processing capabilities (e.g., short-term memory). Moreover, although the data were not reported in a form that would satisfy present-day requirements, Seagoe (1965) discovered a case of a Down-syndrome male who may have caught up with his peers in language competence. Also, whatever learning is involved in parameter setting may not involve the operation of general-purpose cognitive abilities (Lightfoot, 1991). A view of morphological development that emphasizes learning would have difficulty accounting for the cases of specific, morphological deficits in nonmentally retarded persons that Gopnik (1990, 1992) reported. Her findings and the results of genetic investigations suggest that we are born with a propensity for the mastery of grammatical morphology. Finally, if research continues to confirm that the subcomponents of language and the processing of linguistic input are modular, it would not be surprising that deficiencies in higher mental processes do not impact on many aspects of language acquisition.

Fowler's (1988) results with 1 Down syndrome child were confirmed in another longitudinal study of morphosyntactic development in which a larger number of children with Down syndrome were observed. In addition, growth rate for grammatical competence was slower and the leveling off referred to previously was more pronounced in lower IQ children. However, according to Fowler, "at least some [persons with Down syndrome] make substantial progress in syntactic development during their teen-age years" (pp. 240–241). Finally, Fowler noted that there is also evidence (Gibson, 1966) of a slowdown in intellectual growth (MA) in Down-syndrome children during middle childhood.

Given this last observation and the likelihood that grammatical development is sometimes spared in persons with Down syndrome, it is possible that Down syndrome can affect both language and cognitive development or language development independently of cognitive status.

The picture that emerges from the studies we have reviewed thus far is not contradicted by the findings of other investigators (Rondal, 1978a; Rosin, Swift, Bless, & Vetter, 1985; Wiegel-Crump, 1981; see also Andrews & Andrews, 1977; Burr & Rohr, 1978; Cunningham, Glenn, Williamson, & Sloper, 1985; Kernan, 1990; Mahoney, Glover, & Finger, 1981; Rohr & Burr, 1978). Rosin et al. compared a group of male adolescents with Down syndrome (M MA = 6.2) to MA-matched, non-Down syndrome mentally retarded adolescents, MA-matched, typically developing children (M CA = 6.1), and CA-matched, typically developing adolescents on a variety of measures.

The performance of the subjects with Down syndrome fell significantly below that of the other groups on MLU, the Miller-Yoder test of language comprehension, and a number of speech measures (intelligibility, consonant articulation, voice quality), despite the fact that, on the Peabody Picture Vocabulary Test, the subjects with Down syndrome did not differ from the groups with which they were matched on MA. Thus, the exceptional delay in grammatical development in persons with Down syndrome may be unique to that population of persons with mental retardation. However, it is important to note that none of the studies reviewed in this section showed evidence of deviance in the grammatical structures the Down-syndrome subjects acquired.

Rosin et al. (1985) suggested that the greatest problems their subjects with Down syndrome encountered were on sequencing tasks. However, a number of studies (e.g., Ashman, 1982; Marcell & Armstrong, 1982; Marcell & Weeks, 1988; Snart, O'Grady, & Das, 1982) have been interpreted to indicate that "the greatest deficit in children with Down syndrome [is] in the area of auditory sequential memory" (Pueschel, 1988, p. 211). However, Lincoln, Courchesne, Kilman, and Galambos (1985) observed that Down-syndrome children "have significant impairments in: (a) the speed of orienting to and categorizing of auditory information, (b) the organization of a motor response, and (c) the processes necessary for effectively utilizing immediate memory" (p. 413) that are not predictable from their MA.

Can such information-processing deficits account for the features of morphosyntactic development in persons with Down syndrome? We think not. First of all, no proponent of an information-processing view of language acquisition has specified a mechanism that could account for the exceptional slowdown in the acquisition of the first sentence structures or the system of grammatical morphemes in English-speaking children with Down syndrome. Second, if the Down-syndrome child's sequential (articulatory and/or auditory) processing deficit affected morphosyntactic development, we would expect its effect to be most pronounced during the stage of mastery of the basic lexical-thematic syntactic structures of the language, when word order is a major factor in sentence structure. Just the opposite is the case, however; the major slowdown occurs in the next stage of morphosyntactic development—the stage of mastery of grammatical morphemes. Indeed, as Rosenberg (1982) pointed out based on his examination of the corpus of multiword utterances produced by Dooley's (1976) Down-syndrome children, there is ample evidence that the children honored the sequential word-order constraints of the adult language in their early combinatorial speech. A sequencing problem would tend to produce word-order errors. Then, of course, the abstract syntax of sentence structure involves more than word order; it also involves, for example, hierarchic phrase structure.

For reasons such as these, we are led to reject the possibility that the morphosyntactic development seen in persons with Down syndrome can be accounted for by their particular information-processing deficits. Given the limited success of attempts to account for language acquisition in terms of the operation of general cognitive deficits, we are left with the hypothesis that the vast majority of persons with Down syndrome suffer from a specific linguistic deficit that interferes more with the acquisition of grammatical morphemes than with the mastery of basic sentence structures. However, we also want to evaluate the possibility that the mastery of basic sentence structures is influenced by the slowdown in lexical-semantic development that is occasioned by their limited learning ability.

Unfortunately, given the limited data available and the limited range of syntactic and morphological phenomena whose acquisition has been studied, we are unable to identify the specific nature of the linguistic deficit (or deficits) in question. However, current linguistic and psycholinguistic theory (e.g., Chomsky, 1986; Grodzinsky, 1990) suggests that future research should examine at least the following possibilities:

1. One or more of the principles of Universal Grammar do not operate, operate partially, or are delayed in the onset of their operation. However, the available evidence indicates that at least the projection principle and the principle of structure dependence are operating in the early grammar of children with Down syndrome, although their operation is exceptionally slowed down.

2. One or more of the parameters of Universal Grammar are lost, not set, or set improperly. Thus far, there has been no evidence of improper parameter setting in persons with Down syndrome, but their persistent deficits in the domain of grammatical morphology suggest that they suffer from other problems of a parameter-setting nature.

3. The linguistic environment does not provide adequate information to set the value of one or more parameters.

4. Down-syndrome children encounter difficulties acquiring certain aspects of morphosyntax solely on the basis of positive evidence.

5. Maturationally, the critical period for language acquisition begins later and/or ends earlier in children with Down syndrome than in other children.

Fragile X Syndrome

Students interested in the role of etiological factors in language acquisition and performance of persons with mental retardation will want to examine the available literature on another common chromosomal abnormality associated with mental retardation—Fragile X syndrome (e.g., Madison, George, & Moeschler, 1986; Paul et al., 1987; Sudhalter, Cohen, Silverman, & Wolf-Schein, 1990). Thus far, however, the research in this area has not produced any findings that are interesting vis-à-vis the question of grammatical development and mature grammatical competence in subgroups of persons with mental retardation. A combination of speech performance and communicative deficits appears to differentiate persons with Fragile X syndrome from other etiologies of mental retardation.

Studies of Other Persons with Mental Retardation

Studies of syntactic and/or morphological behavior in non-Down-syndrome persons with mental retardation present a picture of developmental delay rather than deviance. One of the best known studies of persons with mental retardation is an investigation by Lackner (1968) of special-school, brain-damaged children with mental retardation (CAs 6;5 to 16;2 and MAs 2;3 to 8;10). Samples of speech (spontaneous and controlled) were used to write phrase-structure transformational grammars for the subjects based on earlier versions of Chomsky's theory.

Average sentence length in words increased with increased MA in Lackner's sample, as did the variety of sentence types produced. Moreover, the frequency of use of different sentence types decreased with increased syntactic complexity for each subject. The phrase-structure rules operating in the subjects' spontaneous speech and their performance on a sentence-comprehension and sentence-imitation task became "more differentiated and specific" (p. 190) as MA increased, as well as more sensitive to the linguistic context within which they were used. In addition, the subjects' phrase-structure grammars did not differ qualitatively from the phrase-structure grammar of normal adults. Furthermore, transformational competence also increased as MA increased in Lackner's sample of persons with mental retardation. Grammatical morpheme and complex-sentence usage were also in evidence in these subjects. However, results based on production showed a lower level of syntactic competence than results based on performance on a sentence-comprehension task. Also, the subjects "were unable to repeat correctly sentences which they had been unable to understand" (p. 191). Thus, sentence-imitation performance, like production and comprehension, was grammatically progressive.

Finally, the performance of a group of nondisabled children on the comprehension and imitation tasks did not reveal any qualitative differences between them and the subjects with mental retardation. Clearly, the picture that emerged from Lackner's observations was one of delay rather than developmental or linguistic deviance, although his retarded subjects showed evidence of central-nervous-system involvement. However, from the design of this study, it was not possible to tell how much the retarded subjects' morphosyntactic development was delayed relative to MA.

Individual differences in the syntactic and lexical performance of a group of children with mental retardation in relation to cognitive status (Piagetian stage) were examined by Miller, Chapman, and MacKenzie (1981; see also Chapman & Nation, 1981) in a large-scale study that included comprehension and production assessments. The majority of the children were described as being "multiply handicapped" and "functioning in the moderate to severe range of disability" (p. 131). The authors arbitrarily identified three categories of language performance relative to cognitive status: "within the same range, advanced relative to cognitive grouping, and delayed relative to cognitive grouping'' (p. 132).

Three types of patterns occurred with some frequency:

1. Twenty-four percent of the children fell into the first pattern, which was termed production-only delay. In this instance, only production of syntactic structures was delayed relative to cognitive status; syntactic competence and vocabulary, as estimated from comprehension testing, were consistent with cognitive status.

2. Type 2—delayed comprehension and production (17% of the sample)—included cases "in which all the language measures were delayed relative to cognitive level" (p. 137).

3. Type 3 subjects' (36%) performance was consistent with cognitive status on all of the language measures.

It is interesting to note that in both Miller's (1988) later study that involved children with Down syndrome (see chapter 3) and the study under discussion (Miller et al., 1981), the case in which both production and comprehension were delayed relative to cognitive status contained the smallest percentage of subjects of the three most frequent types of relationship between language-performance measures and cognitive status. The remainder of the subjects were cases in which production-only was delayed relative to cognitive status or both production and comprehension were consistent with cognitive status. Production-only delays, however, were more characteristic of the children with Down syndrome than of those in Miller et al. (1981). The occurrence of such patterns is clearly not consistent with the cognition-first view of language acquisition. The reader will also recall the issues we raised in chapter 3 regarding the study reported by Miller (1988).

A number of investigators examined language-comprehension performance (or performance on a task with a substantial comprehension component) in persons with mental retardation of unspecified, unknown, or variable etiology. The overall scores of verbal-MA-matched, retarded and nondisabled children on a task that assessed a variety of syntactic structures did not differ in a study by Wheldall (1976). This is not surprising, however, given the likelihood of overlap between measures of verbal MA and measures of linguistic knowledge. At the same time, however, the finding is not consistent with Rosin et al.'s (1985) finding of differences in language production and comprehension performance between subjects with Down syndrome and other subjects with mental retardation and nondisabled subjects, even though the three groups did not differ in verbal MA. Such findings may mean that measures of verbal MA assess basic linguistic knowledge to only a limited extent.

Verbal MA in Wheldall's study correlated highly with overall performance in both groups. The order of difficulty of the various structures in the two groups also correlated highly ($r = .87$). Moreover, the order of difficulty of the structures appeared to be consistent with order of acquisition in typically developing children.

Bartel, Bryen, and Keehn (1973) carried out a broad assessment of language comprehension, including syntactic and morphological structures, in special-class children with moderate mental retardation. The MAs (test not specified) of their subjects varied from approximately 2;8 to 6;0. The literature contained data on the same test (Carrow, 1968) from a group of nonhandicapped subjects of similar MAs. However, the test Bartel et al. employed did not constitute a comprehensive assessment of morphosyntax. Nevertheless, their subjects' performance was inferior to that of the MA-matched controls on a number of the syntactic and morphological structures, with their poorest performance on certain grammatical morphemes and more complex sentence structures. Furthermore, on a number of items, the performance of the children with mental retardation showed little or no improvement over the range of MA sampled. Indeed, on some items, performance appeared to decrease as MA increased. Of course, in the absence of production data and longitudinal comparisons, such findings need to be interpreted with care. Nevertheless, it is clearly the case that, overall, the performance of nondisabled children in the literature exceeded that of the retarded persons in Bartel et al.'s study. Further evidence of morphosyntactic processing relative to intellectual functioning can be found in research by Bliss, Allen, and Walker (1978) and Dewart (1979).

The reader will note that there is a discrepancy in the results of these studies of language comprehension vis-à-vis morphosyntactic relative to cognitive status. According to Abbeduto, Furman, and Davies (1989b), the discrepancy may be the result of the particular grammatical structures under investigation, the range of MAs in the studies, and individual differences in rate of language development relative to rate of cognitive development. To these we would add the possibility of differences in the measures of MA.

Abbeduto et al.'s (1989b) subjects were students with mental retardation (IQs 40 to 79) and nonmentally retarded children, all native English speakers, who were similar in socioeconomic status. Each group was racially mixed and contained males and females. The retarded group included cases of organic and psychosocial origin and cases of unknown etiology. None, however, displayed complicating visual, speech, hearing, or motor impairments. Cognitive status was assessed with the nonverbal Leiter International Performance scale, which assesses mainly problem-solving, recognition, and organization skills. Each group contained three levels of MA—5, 7, and 9 years. A developmentally ordered standardized test of language comprehension—the Test for Reception of Grammar (TROG)—was administered to each subject. It contained single lexical items, phrases, simple sentences, and complex sentences.

The TROG had been shown to correlate .77 with the English Picture Vocabulary Test, a popular measure of lexical knowledge and verbal intelligence. This finding confirms our earlier expectation of overlap between measures of verbal MA and linguistic knowledge. The materials in the test were designed to make minimal vocabulary and information-processing demands upon the subjects. However, it is likely that such a test assesses a combination of semantic and morphosyntactic knowledge, mechanisms of linguistic comprehension, and some information-processing demands peculiar to the particular task and items employed in the test. Moreover, it is difficult to tell, from a grammatical standpoint, how the items for testing were selected. For example, the TROG affords a very limited assessment of grammatical morphemes.

Each linguistic item on the TROG is associated with four sets of colored drawings; only one drawing in each set depicts the linguistic input. To be scored "correct," a subject must choose the appropriate drawing in all of the four items in a given set. The test provides a percentile score and a developmental age.

As for the results, for both the nondisabled subjects and the subjects with mental retardation, the higher the average MA in a group, the higher the average TROG developmental age. However, a marginally significant interaction between MA and group suggested that there was no difference at the MA 5-year level between the nondisabled subjects and those with mental retardation. The mean difference in question at MA 5 was approximately 6 months, whereas at MAs 7 and 9, it was approximately 2 years. Thus, it appears that, on average, comprehension performance began to lag behind MA in the children with mental retardation by MA 7 (or possibly between MA 5 and MA 7).

Abbeduto et al. (1989b) next compared their groups on linguistic forms on which the nondisabled subjects at MAs 5, 7, and 9 had shown a significant improvement with MA. Of the 11 forms that were identified, 5 evidenced a significant difference in favor of the nondisabled subjects on number of correct responses, although the 5 forms in question do not lend themselves to a systematic representation in morphosyntactic terms. However, in analyses that were not reported in the published article, for each group at each MA level, there was clearly a substantial negative correlation between mean number correct and the developmental age of an item for the original 11 items. In addition, the rank order of difficulty of the full 20 items on the TROG for the retarded and nondisabled subjects at each MA level were highly similar. Moreover, there were highly significant negative rank-order correlations between the standard developmental age of an item on the test and its difficulty in the various groups of retarded and nondisabled subjects. Thus, both the nondisabled subjects and those with mental retardation in Abbeduto et al.'s study performed at a level consistent with the individual item's developmental age in the original standardization of the TROG.

Using two different criteria of discrepancies between the comprehension age score and Leiter MA (12 months or more and 18 months or more), these investigators identified: (a) subjects whose comprehension age was greater than their MA, (b) subjects whose comprehension age was equal to their MA, and

(c) subjects whose comprehension age was lower than their MA. However, regardless of the criterion, the majority of the retarded and nondisabled subjects at MA 5 had a TROG age equivalent to their MA. Thus, although "approximately half of the subjects with mental retardation at the two highest levels of MA performed more poorly on the test than would be predicted from their performance on the Leiter" (Abbeduto et al., 1989b, p. 541), as a group, the subjects with mental retardation evidenced considerable variability in the relationship between TROG age and MA.

Regardless of criterion, only a small number of subjects with mental retardation had a TROG age greater than their MA. In addition, after MA 5 there was an increase in the number of subjects with mental retardation whose TROG age was less than their MA. Neither of these trends was characteristic of the nondisabled subjects.

Overall, then, the trends in individual differences observed by Abbeduto et al. (1989b) are consistent with the view that, to a significant extent, linguistic-comprehension performance and nonlinguistic cognition follow independent lines of development.

Cromer (1975) used an acting-out sentence-comprehension task to study the acquisition of a complex sentence structure mastered relatively late by nondisabled children. The structure is one in which the subject of an embedded sentence does not appear in its surface structure (e.g., *The wolf is hard to bite*; *The duck is fun to bite*), unlike the structure in which it does (e.g., *The wolf is willing to bite*; *The duck is glad to bite*). Note that in the first pair of sentences, the entity that does the biting is not specified. The participants with mental retardation ranged in CA from 7;1 to 16;6 and in IQ from 36 to 88. On the task in question, they gave evidence of having mastered the construction whose subject was covert at a MA (picture-vocabulary test) similar to that of nondisabled children who had shown mastery of the construction in an earlier investigation (but see the critical comments of Johnson-Laird, 1975, on these studies and some related research by Cromer). The research on the problem Cromer studied originally was extended in a recent longitudinal investigation (Cromer, 1987).

Grammatical Morphology

The morphological competence of persons with mental retardation was the concern of research by Lovell and Bradbury (1967), Newfield and Schlanger (1968), Dever and Gardner (1970), Dever (1972), and Rosenberg and Abbeduto (1987). Lovell and Bradbury studied a large sample of special-school children with mental retardation in the CA range of 8 to 15 years whose mean IQ was 70.1 (test not specified). A somewhat modified version of a well-known test by Berko (1958) was used to assess their knowledge of grammatical morphology that included real and nonsense words accompanied by pictures. In one item, for example, a subject is told:

This is a wug.
Now there is another one.
There are two of them.
There are two _____.

The subject is expected to supply *wugs* as the appropriate plural form of *wug* when this variant of the plural morpheme in English is in his or her repertoire.

Berko had found age-related improvements in performance on such items among nondisabled children. Lovell and Bradbury, however, found exceptional delay relative to MA on a number of items and little improvement with CA.

Newfield and Schlanger (1968) used a somewhat modified version of Berko's test in a study that included children with mental retardation who were residents of a state school (mean CA, MA, and IQ = 10;4, 6;2, and 60, respectively) and nondisabled elementary-school children (mean CA = 6;10). The test used to assess cognitive status was not specified, but it was very likely a nonverbal scale or included nonverbal items, because the authors also administered the Peabody Picture Vocabulary Test to assess verbal MA. The nondisabled children's performance on this test was superior to that of the children with mental retardation. Consistent with their scores on the Peabody test, the performance of the nondisabled children on the Berko items was, in general, substantially superior to that of the children with mental retardation. However, a similar order of difficulty for the nonsense items was found for the two groups (r = .91)—an order of difficulty similar to that reported by Berko for typically developing children.

In order to check on the reliability of these findings regarding order of difficulty against Brown's (1973) results from the spontaneous-speech performance of nondisabled children, Rosenberg (1982) carried out an additional analysis of the available data. He reported,

> I determined . . . the order of difficulty of the five morphemes that had been studied by both Brown and Berko from data on percentage correct in Table 1 of Newfield and Schlanger's article and compared this data with Brown's results. The morphemes in question in order of difficulty from easiest to most difficult in spontaneous speech were the following:
>
> Progressive [*ing*]
> Plural [*s*]
> Possessive ['*s*]
> Past, regular [*ed*]
> Third person, regular [e.g., He walk*s*].
>
> In the case of Newfield and Schlanger's mentally retarded subjects, order of difficulty on Berko's procedure matched order of mastery in spontaneous speech *perfectly* for both the nonsense and the real words. The nondisabled subjects in Newfield and Schlanger's study showed a similar trend, with one reversal on the nonsense items and one on the real words. (p. 347)

Dever and Gardner (1970) used most of the items in Berko's test to compare the grammatical morpheme competence of nondisabled and mildly mentally retarded boys matched on CA in one case and MA (test not specified) in another case. They reported that the overall performance of the MA-matched, nondisabled group was superior to that of the subjects with mental retardation. However, as one would anticipate, the differences were greatest when the children from the two populations were matched on CA.

In partial replication of his earlier investigation, Dever (1972) added free-speech samples from his subjects with mental retardation (IQs 60 to 84; MAs 6 to 10; test not specified) and found that Berko's test clearly underestimated their knowledge of grammatical morphemes. However, Dever did not report his findings relevant to MA. It is interesting to note that Brown (1973) found that free-speech samples from nondisabled children also date the mastery of grammatical morphemes earlier than controlled observation procedures do. Given these findings and Rosenberg and Abbeduto's (1987) discovery of a relatively high level of mastery in free speech of Brown's 14 grammatical morphemes in mildly mentally retarded adults (see chapter 1), it is clear that Berko's test underestimated the mastery of grammatical morphemes in non-Down-syndrome persons with mental retardation. Moreover, it is important to note that in the research we reviewed here, there was no evidence of deviance in the order of mastery of the grammatical morphemes that have been the subject of investigation thus far or in the structure of the morphemes that have been mastered by non-Down-syndrome persons with mental retardation.

The reader will recall that Rosenberg and Abbeduto's non-Down-syndrome subjects with mild mental retardation also evidenced a relatively high level of mastery in spontaneous speech of the system of complex sentence structures in English, an achievement which investigators previously thought was out of their reach (Rosenberg, 1982). Thus, although the requisite longitudinal data are not available, no evidence has appeared thus far that would lead us to conclude that, relative to cognitive status, non-Down-syndrome persons with mental retardation (brain-damaged and nonbrain-damaged alike, evidently) are especially at risk in the domain of grammatical morphology or are exceptionally delayed in the subsequent mastery of complex sentence structures, although there are undoubtedly mentally retarded persons who fail to achieve (to varying degrees) complete mastery of grammar.

Performance Factors

Given the complexity of morphosyntax, it is important to inquire whether there is any evidence that the sentence-performance (production and comprehension) processes of language-delayed persons with mental retardation are responsible for their morphosyntactic delay. There is little research that bears directly upon these questions, but let us see what we have:

1. In the available studies (Bridges & Smith, 1984; Dewart, 1979; Paris, Mahoney, & Buckholt, 1974), there was no evidence of qualitative differences in the manner in which persons with mental retardation performed sentence comprehension tasks.

2. In studies by Abbeduto et al. (1989b) and Wheldall (1976), it was reported that the order of difficulty of linguistic structures in comprehension tasks in persons with mental retardation tended to match their order of mastery in the speech development of nondisabled persons.

3. Regardless of performance mode, no evidence of qualitative differences in the morphosyntactic structures achieved by retarded and nondisabled persons have been reported in the literature (e.g., Rosenberg & Abbeduto, 1987).

4. No evidence has appeared in the literature to suggest that the morphosyntactic errors in the spontaneous speech of persons with mental retardation during the course of language acquisition differ from those that have been noted in the spontaneous speech of nondisabled children (Dooley, 1976; Ryan, 1975, 1977). If there were significant differences between the two populations in morphosyntactic performance processes, one would expect to find some differences in the structures achieved and/or in the types of errors produced in the comprehension or production modes.

Thus, we are led to conclude (albeit tentatively) that, across a wide range of etiologies of mental retardation, delay in the mastery of morphosyntactic structures is not the result of deficits in the mechanisms of morphosyntactic performance.

Exceptional Morphosyntactic Development

Earlier, we reported (Curtiss, 1988b; see also the reviews in Cromer, 1988, 1991) exceptional achievements in morphosyntax relative to cognitive status in some non-Down-syndrome persons with mental retardation. However, the most dramatic and thoroughly documented case is that of Laura, as reported recently by Yamada (1990; see also the brief report in Curtiss, 1988b, under the name of Marta). As we shall see, Laura is a case of relatively intact linguistic competence in the face of serious semantic, nonlinguistic cognitive, pragmatic, and social deficiencies. She was home-reared until 15 and was 16 years old when first encountered by the author. At that time, with the exception of language, her functioning was at a preschool level. According to a diary her mother kept, Laura could comprehend some words at 20 months and produce approximately 15 words at CA 2;11. However, semantic and communicative problems in her speech were apparent early.

Standardized tests over the years have revealed a large discrepancy between her verbal and performance IQs, although her verbal IQ has remained in the range of persons with mental retardation. At CA 14;9, her full-scale, verbal, and performance IQs were 41, 52, and 32, respectively. Laura is mainly right-handed and relatively recent EEGs and CT scans have been normal; however, she has had periods of serious emotional disturbance. From CA 16 to CA 18.5, she was tested extensively on a battery of language, nonlinguistic cognitive, and neuropsychological measures.

On production measures (spontaneous and elicited speech, imitation tasks), Laura displayed a complex and rich morphosyntax including mature use of a variety of complex sentence structures. However, she was unable to deal with many of these structures on comprehension tests, although she could produce them correctly. For example, she was able to produce a variety of grammatical morphemes that she failed to process on comprehension measures. According to Yamada, factors such as attentional and motivational deficits may have been responsible for her comprehension problems.

Yamada (1990) also indicated that "a significant feature of her speech was her propensity to use forms whose meanings she did not seem to grasp fully" (p. 44). Although she produced sentences that were grammatically correct, which appeared to be consistent with the projection principle, in certain domains "she often didn't know the full meanings of the terms she used and the phrases she constructed" (p. 45). A similar picture of semantic deficit appeared in her performance on comprehension tests. For example, her MA on the Peabody Picture Vocabulary Test—a comprehension measure—was only 3;11. Presumably, such performances in the semantic domain were a reflection of her limited conceptual development. However, further testing of spontaneous speech indicated that both her semantic and her pragmatic knowledge were inferior to her morphosyntactic competence. Moreover, she produced more errors in the area of conversational conventions than in the morphosyntactic or semantic areas. On the basis of such observations, Yamada concluded that "Laura's case argues against a linguistic theory that considers communicative functions [and related social-interactive factors] to be the basis for structural and semantic aspects of language" (p. 72).

In the nonlinguistic cognitive domain, Laura demonstrated a relatively high level of sensorimotor competence, but her linguistic capabilities were clearly in excess of her nonlinguistic cognitive maturity on a wide variety of tasks, thus contradicting claims of the cognition-first hypothesis. Indeed, no cognitive ability turned out to be exceptional in Laura, including short-term memory. Yamada (1990) indicated that, consistent with her MA, Laura "could not repeat sequences of more than three items" (p. 99) but could repeat sentences up to nine morphemes in length and produce sentences as long as 20 words in length. Yamada (1990) pointed out that research with nondisabled 3-year-olds show a similar discrepancy between immediate memory span for unrelated words and the length of sentences the children can produce and comprehend (L. Bloom & Lahey, 1978). Thus it is possible that the information-processing factor of short-term memory capacity is not a major factor in morphosyntactic development.

Consistent with her semantic and comprehension problems, Laura showed a pattern of performance on the Boston Diagnostic Aphasia Test similar to that of patients with Wernicke's aphasia. The speech of such patients tends to be morphosyntactically fluent but deficient in meaning, and they also display sentence-comprehension difficulties (Carroll, 1986).

On a test of hemispheric localization of language that involved phonological processing, Laura tended to favor the left hemisphere slightly. The average right-handed, nondisabled person tends to show a similar trend, though stronger. However, her nonlinguistic sequencing ability—also a left-hemisphere function—is poor. Indeed, her performance was generally poor on abilities which are thought to be controlled by the left hemisphere. Only her left-hemisphere language functions appear to have been spared. For example, in spite of her cognitive sequencing problems, she could produce sentences as long as 20 words in length. Thus, we have here further evidence for a dissociation of aspects of language from general information-processing abilities.

Jackendoff (1987) proposed that the innate language-acquisition system consists of a combination of specifically linguistic and general-purpose cognitive abilities, and Chomsky himself (1990) allowed for a possible contribution of memory and attention capacities to language acquisition. Yamada's (1990) findings, however, suggested that the contribution of general-purpose cognitive abilities to first-language acquisition (and to language performance) is quite limited (see chapter 1 for a discussion of research on the information-processing abilities of persons with mental retardation). What this leaves us with, among other ideas, is the intriguing hypothesis that there are information-processing abilities that are unique to language.

A number of conclusions follow from Yamada's observations:

1. In that Laura's linguistic achievements clearly outdistanced her cognitive achievements in the Piagetian domain, it appears "that many nonlinguistic abilities are neither sufficient nor necessary for the emergence and development of grammar" (pp. 109–110).

2. Mental age, nonverbal or verbal, is not necessarily predictive of linguistic maturity. Hence, it is likely that many of the abilities assessed by standardized intelligence tests are also "neither sufficient nor necessary for" language acquisition.

3. It appears that information-processing factors such as short-term memory and the ability to process sequences of stimuli are of questionable significance in the acquisition and utilization of grammatical knowledge.

4. Cognitive and linguistic abilities that are similarly organized are not necessarily governed by a third common cognitive mechanism. For example, "whereas [Laura] was very deficient at building hierarchical structures in the nonlinguistic

domain, she could construct complex hierarchical structures linguistically'' (p. 110).

5. Laura's striking deficits in the domains of semantics (other than that having to do with lexical argument structure), pragmatics, and social competence generally raise serious questions for claims that achievements in one or more of these areas are the basis for the acquisition of morphosyntax.

6. Linguistic and nonlinguistic cognitive capabilities are differentially governed by the brain. Laura, whose exceptional linguistic capabilities were apparent from the earliest stage of language acquisition, is a strong case for the modularity of the formal aspects of linguistic knowledge, which, according to modularity theory (e.g., Garfield, 1987), are inaccessible to the higher mental processes that are assessed by Piagetian, intellectual, and information-processing tasks.

It is necessary to point out that there has been some tendency for persons with mental retardation whose language achievements are exceptional to get off to a slow start to varying degrees and at some point to begin to catch up rapidly (e.g., Laura; Curtiss, 1988b). How might we account for these observations?

1. We may be dealing with unknown nonlinguistic constraints on the utilization of already acquired linguistic knowledge (i.e., performance not competence constraints).
2. There may be factors that can slow down the maturation of the language capacity so that there is a delay in its activation by linguistic input. Once activated, however, it operates in a more or less normal fashion (at least regarding the formal aspects of language).
3. The intellectual limitations of persons with mental retardation may impact on their early syntactic development by slowing down the acquisition of words whose meanings project onto syntactic structures.

There may be other possibilities, of course. Clearly, we need more research in the area of exceptional language competence in persons with mental retardation.

DISCUSSION AND CONCLUSIONS

Despite the fact that only a limited range of syntactic and morphological phenomena in the language of persons with mental retardation has been studied successfully, and although there is still the question of individual differences to be resolved, some tentative conclusions and directions for research are possible.

We hope we have demonstrated the value, indeed the necessity, of approaching the task of understanding the language development of persons with mental retardation from the standpoint of a well-motivated and comprehensive theory of the linguistic competence of mature, nondisabled persons. However, by now the reader will have recognized that there is much more to be learned about mature, linguistic knowledge than we were able to present given the objectives of the present book. For students and others interested in going beyond the linguistic material we have presented, we recommend a general introductory text by Fromkin and Rodman (1988) and a recent text by Haegeman (1991), *Introduction to Government and Binding Theory*.

Grammatical morphemes play an essential role in sentence and phrase structure (e.g., Haegeman, 1991). The great delay in the mastery of the system of grammatical morphemes in English in Down-syndrome persons with mental retardation is, therefore, a likely contributor to their subsequent syntactic problems. Precisely how this occurs, however, will not be known without more extended longitudinal analyses of morphosyntactic development in Down-syndrome persons than have appeared thus far. However, answers to such questions also depend on progress in linguistic theory, in that there are a number of issues in syntactic and morphological theory still to be resolved (e.g., Haegeman, 1991, Lightfoot, 1991, and the references contained therein).

In spite of the particular syntactic and morphological deficits Down-syndrome persons display, they have been observed to express basic semantic relations in a variety of utterance types, they honor the word-order constraints of English right from the beginning, their earliest syntactic structures appear to be as abstract as those of nonretarded children, and we found no evidence of linguistic or developmental deviance in their early morphosyntactic development, even though they evidence an exceptional delay in grammatical development. Moreover, it is possible that even in some Down-syndrome persons, morphosyntax might be spared relative to cognitive status.

Thus far, neither cognitive nor environmental factors nor problems of linguistic performance appear to be implicated in these findings. In particular, nothing we have seen thus far would lead us to suspect that the morphosyntactic problems that most Down-syndrome persons display are caused by their non-linguistic cognitive problems. Rather, it is likely that they are due to a specifically linguistic effect of the chromosomal disorder that constitutes Down syndrome, one that affects, among other things, the parameter settings that determine the system of grammatical morphemes in a language. Of course, this account may have to be adjusted based on the findings of future studies of exceptional language acquisition in persons with Down syndrome.

We saw in chapter 3 that prelinguistic phonological development in Down-syndrome children is similar to that in typically developing infants. However, on the average, phonological development beyond the prelinguistic stage in this population is clearly delayed, although not linguistically or developmentally deviant. Moreover, the lag in question tends to be greater than would be predicted from their MAs, with the difference between phonological and cognitive status tending to increase with CA. Of course, whether this pattern is true of all Down-syndrome persons with mental retardation is still to be determined. Seagoe's (1965) observation of exceptional language achievements in a mentally retarded person with Down syndrome suggested that it is not. However, it appears that, relative to cognitive status, both phonological (beyond the prelinguistic stage) and morphosyntactic development are exceptionally delayed in most persons with Down syndrome, although evidently to a greater extent in the case of morphosyntactic development. In addition, in the case of both components of linguistic competence, the difference between cognitive and linguistic status tends to increase with age.

The picture that emerges from a comparison of morphosyntactic and semantic development in persons with Down syndrome is not unlike that for morphosyntactic and phonological development. It is one of developmental delay rather than deviance. Initially, lexical-semantic competence is consistent with cognitive maturity but, by a MA of 21 months, lexical-semantic acquisition lags behind cognitive status. However, the basis for the lexical categories that have been studied is the same as that for nondisabled persons, and the exemplars of such categories are similar in both populations. Moreover, in identifying the meanings of words, persons with Down syndrome tend to use the same strategies as nondisabled persons do, although not necessarily to the same extent. Furthermore, there was evidence that the mental lexicon of persons with Down syndrome is organized in a manner similar to that in nondisabled persons. Finally, in their early combinatorial speech, persons with Down syndrome express semantic relations similar to those that nondisabled persons express in their early word combinations, although development appears to be exceptionally slow in Down-syndrome persons. Thus, to a large extent, semantic development in persons with Down syndrome also appears to be exceptionally delayed relative to cognitive status, but evidently not to the same extent as in the case of morphosyntactic development.

Why should semantic development be exceptionally delayed relative to cognitive status, given that, to a significant extent, it has its basis in nonlinguistic conceptual development? One possibility is that semantic competence is poorly assessed or assessed to only a limited extent by the instruments used to determine cognitive status. Another is that because meaning is typically not assessed independently of linguistic form, its rate of development will reflect the rate of development of the other components of grammar. Moreover, it is possible that the exceptional delay in question is due to deficit in a specifically linguistic semantic component of the innate language-acquisition system. Of course, another possibility is that semantic development relative to cognitive status is exceptionally slow because of some combination of these factors. Unfortunately, the available research on language acquisition in persons with mental retardation does not allow us to choose among these explanations.

Studies of syntactic and/or morphological competence in persons with mental retardation of unknown or indeterminate etiology or associated with conditions other than Down syndrome (e.g., acquired brain damage, sociocultural deprivation), suggest that, on the average, development in these areas is delayed—although possibly not to the same extent as in persons with Down syndrome—but not deviant. MA is predictive of morphosyntactic maturity in this population and, although direct comparisons were not carried out, there was no suggestion from study to study that overtly brain-damaged persons with mental retardation are at greater risk for morphosyntactic deficits than are other etiologies. However, Miller et al. (1981) reported individual differences in whether linguistic—including syntactic—performance was delayed relative to cognitive status and performance mode (production vs. comprehension). Other studies (e.g., Bartel et al., 1973; Abbeduto et al., 1989b) found differences between persons with mental retardation and MA-matched, nondisabled controls on comprehension measures of syntactic and/or morphological functioning. Abbeduto et al. (1989b) reported evidence of individual differences in the relationship between comprehension and nonverbal MA in nondisabled persons and persons with mental retardation. Overall, comprehension performance tended to lag behind nonverbal MA after MA 5 in the latter subjects.

There is evidence that the order of mastery of grammatical morphemes in non-Down-syndrome children with mental retardation is similar, if not identical, to that in nonretarded children on both controlled observation procedures and measures derived from samples of spontaneous speech. However, controlled observation procedures tend to underestimate the level of mastery of grammatical morphemes in such children.

Cases of exceptional achievements relative to cognitive status in morphosyntax (and phonology) have been found most often among non-Down-syndrome persons with mental retardation, the most dramatic case being that of Laura. As we indicated earlier, Laura is a case of a relatively high level of morphosyntactic competence in the face of serious semantic, cognitive, pragmatic, and social deficiencies. As we suggested previously, any claim that morphosyntax is semantically (in areas other than those that are involved in the operation of the projection principle), cognitively, pragmatically, or socially based is seriously questioned by such findings. Finally, in neurolinguistic testing, Laura did not evidence a serious deficit in the lateralization of language functions.

We reported earlier that phonological and semantic development in non-Down-syndrome persons with mental retardation, although delayed, is not deviant. However, although the phonological maturity of such persons appeared to be consistent with their MA, we found some evidence that both vocabulary acquisition and morphosyntactic development are exceptionally delayed relative to MA in this population. Clearly, the exceptional delays in language acquisition relative to cognitive status and the individual differences that have been reported in the relationship between language competence and cognitive status in persons with mental retardation over a wide range of etiologies also argue against an account of language acquisition that stresses prior nonlinguistic cognitive achievements.

6

Linguistic Communication and Its Development

To this point, we have been concerned primarily with the acquisition of knowledge about the form and content of language. We now turn to the topic of linguistic communication, or how language is used to communicate with others in social interactions (Levinson, 1983). Participation in linguistic communication requires more than knowing the forms and contents of language. We have all known people who were not very good communicators despite having sophisticated knowledge of the contents and forms of language: a friend who always seemed to bring up sensitive subjects at the wrong time; an acquaintance who made you uncomfortable by talking to you as though you were an old friend; or that professor who assumed that the class knew things they did not and whose lectures were, therefore, incomprehensible. The fact is that communication involves not only knowledge of language but also a variety of cognitive and social skills as well as knowledge about the communicative process itself, which is referred to as pragmatic knowledge. The poor communicators you have known may have had problems in one or more of these domains.

In this chapter, we outline important knowledge and skills involved in using language for communication. We also describe the development of linguistic communication in typically developing children. This sets the stage for our review of research on the linguistic communication problems of persons with mental retardation in chapter 7. More detailed discussions of the nature of linguistic communication are found in Cohen, Morgan, and Pollack (1990), Green (1989), and Levinson (1983). Abbeduto and Benson (1992), McTear and Conti-Ramsden (1992), Schiefelbusch and Pickar (1984), Shatz (1983), and Whitehurst and Sonnenschein (1985) provide detailed reviews of research on typical development in this area.

LINGUISTIC COMMUNICATION
AND PRAGMATIC RULES

Linguistic communication requires making choices about language (Rice, 1984). For example, a speaker has to decide on the content and form of a forthcoming utterance. Competent language users make these choices by following *pragmatic rules*. These rules specify the ways in which linguistic utterances relate to their contexts, that is, to the verbal and nonverbal behaviors of the other participants, the nature of the interaction, the previous discourse, the knowledge and experiences of the other participants, and the physical setting of the talk (Bach & Harnish, 1979).

To illustrate, consider the choices we make when directing another person to perform an action. Natural language provides many different means for expressing most any directive. For example, *Help me with this* and *Would you be able to help me with this?* could both be used to seek assistance. The former is a rather impolite form, whereas the latter is fairly polite. Although we might choose *Help me with this* in the context of scolding a disobedient child, we would probably opt for *Would you be able to help me with this?*, or something similar, in the context of seeking a favor from our employer. In this case, the pragmatic rule guiding our choice could be stated as follows: The degree of politeness warranted depends on the degree to which the directive represents an imposition (rather than an obligation) for the addressee (e.g., see Brown & Levinson, 1987; Gordon & Ervin-Tripp, 1984; Levinson, 1983).

Not only our behavior as speakers but also our behavior as listeners is governed by pragmatic rules. One pragmatic rule, for example, dictates that a definite noun phrase such as *that car* is to be used only if the referent can be identified uniquely from the linguistic or nonlinguistic context (Clark, Schreuder, & Buttrick, 1983). Listeners assume that speakers adhere to this rule and search the context accordingly. If the potential referents of *Look at that car* consisted of a pink-and-blue-striped automobile and a more traditionally colored automobile, therefore, a listener most likely would interpret the utterance as referring to the potential referent with the nontraditional paint job.

In summary, successful linguistic communication requires following pragmatic rules to make choices about language use in a contextually appropriate manner. In the next section, we turn to a more detailed description of some choices facing the participants in a social interaction involving spoken language and the pragmatic rules involved in making those choices. Before doing so, however, we must point out that there has been controversy as to whether various rules involved in communicative performance are actually pragmatic in nature or whether they are better thought of as reflecting semantic principles, more general principles of social interaction, or even general patterns of cognitive behavior (e.g., see Brown & Levinson, 1987; Green, 1989; Kempson, 1975; Levinson, 1983). In this chapter and in chapter 7, we focus on rules that have traditionally been considered pragmatic by researchers in the field of child language and language disorders (e.g., Whitehurst & Sonnenschein, 1985).

THE MANY FACETS OF LINGUISTIC COMMUNICATION

Linguistic communication is a multifaceted process. In this section, we analyze important aspects of the process in terms of the choices and pragmatic rules involved. The reader should be aware that our discussion is selective; we focus on those facets of communication for which the performance of persons with mental retardation has been investigated in some detail (see chapter 7).

Establishing referents. A fundamental requirement in any communicative exchange is to establish the persons, places, objects, and events that are being talked about, or referred to, by the speaker (Whitehurst & Sonnenschein, 1985). Unless the participants are clear about what the speaker is referring to, the conversation will not progress very far. Speakers, then, must choose their words so that their referents can be identified. For example, they must know to use *collie* rather than *dog* if a collie and a poodle are visible to the listener and are thus potential referents. For their part, listeners must choose the one object, person, place, or event in the linguistic or nonlinguistic context that best fits the speaker's choice of words and they must notify the speaker when a unique referent cannot be chosen.

Making the choices involved in establishing referents requires knowing a variety of pragmatic rules. These rules include a *difference* rule and a *participant* rule (Whitehurst & Sonnenschein, 1985). The difference rule specifies that an utterance must allow the referent to be discriminated from the other things to which it might refer. If, for example, there are three hats before the listener, only one of which is blue, *Give me the hat* would violate the difference rule, whereas *Give me the blue hat* would conform. The participant rule dictates that speakers should attend to listener cues (e.g., child and adult listeners may require different information in order to identify the speaker's referent) and that listeners should attend to speaker cues (e.g., a child speaker is more likely than an adult speaker to give an ambiguous message).

The reader should be aware that referents need not always be established entirely by linguistic means (Milosky, 1992). For instance, when a speaker's intended referent is an object that is more visually salient than the other potential referents, he or she will often produce an utterance that does not, by itself, uniquely identify the referent (e.g., as we indicated previously, *that car* could be used to refer successfully to a unusually colored automobile rather than a traditionally colored one). In such cases, the speaker will expect the listener to infer that the salient object is the intended referent, and nondisabled adults (Clark et al., 1983) and even children (Ackerman, Szymanski, & Silver, 1990) will make such an inference.

Expressing and understanding speech acts. Speakers intend their utterances to perform particular social functions, or *speech acts* (Austin, 1962; Bach & Harnish, 1979; Levinson, 1983; Searle, 1969). Speech acts include such functions as asserting, promising, requesting information, and directing someone to perform an action. Because speech acts are conveyed only in part by the words that speakers utter, the same utterance can convey different speech acts on different occasions. For example, the sentence *Can you open the windows?* could be used to direct the addressee to perform an action or it could be used to request information in the form of a *yes* or *no* (Abbeduto, Furman, & Davies, 1989a). In addition, it is usually the case that there are many different linguistic forms for expressing a particular speech act. In the right circumstances, for example, *Open the windows, Can you open the windows?*, and *It's hot in here* could all be used to make the same point. The various linguistic options may be appropriate for different contexts, however (Brown & Levinson, 1987). For example, the impolite *Open the windows* probably should be avoided if addressing one's boss. Speakers, then, must be sure that the words they utter accomplish the speech acts they intend and that they do so in a contextually appropriate manner, whereas listeners must determine which of the several speech acts that an utterance could convey is actually intended by the speaker (Milosky, 1992).

Making these choices requires knowledge of various pragmatic rules (Bach & Harnish, 1979; Green, 1989; Levinson, 1983; Searle, 1975). An example is the answer obviousness rule (Abbeduto et al., 1989a; Clark, 1979), which dictates that speakers not ask a question if they already know its answer. Listeners assume that speakers adhere to this rule and thus, they see sentences such as *Can you open the windows?* as being seriously intended as *yes–no* questions only when the context suggests that the answer to the question posed is nonobvious to the speaker. Another pragmatic rule is the *presumption of relevance* (Bach & Harnish, 1979), which dictates that a speaker's utterance provide the listener with some new information. This rule is involved in a listener's recognition that a speaker intends *That's mine* not as a statement of fact but as a directive to act when the listener is holding one of the speaker's prized possessions. That is, the listener already knows the object in question belongs to the speaker, so the speaker would have no reason to inform the listener of this fact. The listener, therefore, reasons that *That's mine* must have some other function, namely, to direct his or her behavior.

Requests for clarification. Communication does not always proceed in an error-free manner. Listeners may fail to attend to a speaker's utterance or err in the application of a pragmatic rule (e.g., they may judge the answer to a question to be obvious when it is not). Speakers may, among other things, misarticulate all or some portion of an utterance, select the wrong word, or fail to follow the dictates of a pragmatic rule (e.g., they may judge the referent of an utterance to be uniquely identifiable from the context when it is not). When problems occur, participants make use of various repair devices, each of which is designed for a specific type of problem (Bedrosian, Wanska, Sykes, Smith, & Dalton, 1988; Fujiki, Brinton, & Sonnenberg, 1990; Gallagher, 1981; Garvey, 1977; Garvey & BenDebba, 1978). For example, a listener can use *Huh?* to elicit a repetition of the queried utterance by the speaker. As another example, if there is a problem in identifying the referent of an utterance, a listener can say something like *Which one?* Thus, repairing conversational problems requires knowledge of the pragmatic rules governing the use of the various repair devices; that is, listeners must know which repair devices are appropriate to which types of communicative problems, whereas speakers must recognize the type of response each repair device warrants.

Conversational organization. A conversation is more than just a string of utterances or even pairs of utterances (i.e., initiations and responses). Conversation has a structure or organization; that is, the utterances fit together in systematic ways. There is organization to allow participants to take turns at talking. This accounts for the fact that instances of more than one participant speaking at a time are rare in the conversations of nondisabled adults (Duncan & Fiske, 1977; Levinson, 1983; Sacks et al., 1974). Achieving this nearly flawless level of turn-taking requires knowledge of a variety of pragmatic rules. For example, speakers cannot simply claim a turn whenever they like; thus, participants must recognize the points at which a change of speaker can occur. These points are defined linguistically (e.g., at sentence boundaries) as well as through the use of gestures, eye gaze, body posture, and intonation (Beattie, 1980; Duncan & Fiske, 1977; Sacks, Schegloff, & Jefferson, 1974). As another example, participants need to know about devices for assigning the next speaking turn to a specific participant (e.g., the current speaker can include the next speaker's name in his or her utterance; Sacks et al., 1974). As is the case with other communicative tasks, effective turn-taking requires knowing rules that dictate how to use context (i.e., the linguistic and nonlinguistic behavior of the other participants) to make choices.

Conversation is also organized into topics. That is, the participants in a communicative exchange produce a series of turns, each of which relates to the same theme or issue (e.g., an upcoming event, a mutual friend, the state of a favorite sports team). Contributing to a topic, however, requires more than the production of turns that overlap in content. Each turn must contribute to the topic in such a way as to ensure that the topic progresses. For example, initial turns are generally devoted to ensuring that all participants have the background information needed to understand the topic; later turns add information to move the discussion toward closure of the current topic (Dorval & Eckerman, 1984). Contributing to a topic in this manner requires knowledge of pragmatic rules, which specify when a new topic can be introduced into the conversation (e.g., after a long silence in the discussion of the current topic), how a new topic is introduced (e.g., by the use of linguistic markers such as *by the way* and *that reminds me*), and how a turn is to relate to previous turns (e.g., it must overlap the content of the previous turn and add new information). Again, the rules involved concern how to make choices about language behavior on the basis of context (i.e., prior turns in the exchange).

In summary, every facet of the communicative process presents the language user with choices, and competent language users make these choices by following pragmatic rules concerning the relation between language and its contexts. It is appropriate at this point to consider an additional complexity facing the participants in a communicative exchange; namely, different sets of pragmatic rules can be applicable to different types of communicative interaction (Abbeduto & Nuccio, 1989). For example, the rules of turn-taking that guide our behavior when we converse with friends are not the same ones we follow when we attend a lecture (Sacks et al., 1974). In the former situation, we have a great deal of latitude regarding our choice of whether or not to speak. When attending a lecture, in contrast, we can indicate our desire to speak by raising our hands, but it is the lecturer who decides whether or not and when we can speak. As another example, participants in a conversation do not usually ask questions for which they already know the answers. But students are constantly faced with questions from their teachers that violate this constraint (Gilmore & Glatthorn, 1982; Wilkinson, 1982). Thus, participating in a full range of communicative exchanges requires learning what pragmatic rules to apply and how to apply them in different contexts.

THE COMPETENCIES SUPPORTING
LINGUISTIC COMMUNICATION

As mentioned earlier, linguistic communication draws on skills and knowledge in four domains: (a) linguistic, (b) cognitive, (c) social, and (d) pragmatic. In this section, we examine in more detail the ways in which the choices involved in linguistic communication require the coordination of skills and knowledge across these domains.

To illustrate the different domains of expertise involved in communication, consider the choice facing a speaker who wishes to obtain assistance. This speaker must choose among a variety of potential forms, including *Help me with this* and *Would you be able to help me with this?* The relative status or power of the speaker and listener and the politeness of the forms in question are important factors in this decision (Brown & Levinson, 1987). If the speaker was an employee of a large company, for example, he or she probably would opt for *Would you be able to help me with this?*, *Could you help me please?*, or something similar, rather than *Help me with this*, when speaking to the president of the company.

This same employee, however, might prefer *Help me with this* when talking to one of his or her co-workers.

To select a directive form in this manner, our employee would obviously need some facility with the linguistic system (Levinson, 1983). For instance, many of the linguistic forms used to issue directives politely are interrogatives (Brown & Levinson, 1987). If the employee in our example had not mastered interrogative syntax he or she might have no choice but to rely on impolite forms such as *Help me with this*, regardless of the social position of the addressee.

Our employee would also require a variety of cognitive skills (Rice, 1984). Memory would be involved, for instance, in the sense that as the employee elected a linguistic form he or she would need to remember to whom the directive was addressed and the status of the addressee. In addition, the employee would need to have stored—and be able to retrieve efficiently—information about the relative politeness of the various linguistic forms in his or her repertoire.

Selecting a directive form would also require a certain level of social knowledge and skill (Bach & Harnish, 1979). Without knowing about or being able to determine differences in social status, for instance, the employee in our example would not recognize the need to choose *Would you be able to help me with this?* over *Help me with this* when speaking to the president of the company. Perspective taking, another aspect of social competence (Shantz, 1983) would also be involved. For example, the avoidance of *Help me with this* when speaking to the president of the company might require anticipating the potentially negative reaction he or she might have to this impolite and imposing form.

Lastly, the employee in our example needs to know a pragmatic rule or two in order to select the right directive form for an addressee (Levinson, 1983). In particular, he or she would have to know that directives impose and that forms that acknowledge the imposition or the fact that compliance is not presupposed (e.g., *Would you mind helping me with this?*, *Could you help me with this?*) are more polite than those that do not (e.g., *Help me with this*). He or she also would need to recognize that relative status and power determine how much of an imposition a directive is and, thus, how polite one needs to be (Clark & Schunk, 1980).

In summary, linguistic communication draws heavily on (a) knowledge of language (i.e., phonology, semantics, and morphosyntax), (b) conceptual knowledge and cognitive skills, (c) social knowledge and skills, and (d) knowledge of pragmatic rules. An important implication is that developmental changes that typically occur in communicative performance may be the result of changes in any or all of these domains of psychological functioning. It is important to recognize, however, that different aspects of communication are certain to require different levels of expertise in these domains (Shatz, 1983). For example, success in some areas of linguistic communication may require the use of highly sophisticated memory skills but little in the way of social knowledge and skills. Other areas of linguistic communication, in contrast, may require only minimal, basic memory skills but draw heavily on knowledge of various aspects of the social system. With these comments in mind, we now describe the development of linguistic communication in nondisabled children.

DEVELOPMENT OF LINGUISTIC COMMUNICATION IN CHILDREN WITHOUT DISABILITIES

Although our focus is on the use of language for communication, it is important to recognize that communication begins prior to the onset of language (Sugarman, 1984). Between 8 and 10 months of age, children begin to include objects and other people within the same behavioral sequences. For example, the 10-month-old may look at a desired object, make eye contact with a parent, gaze again at the object, glance back at the parent, and so on (Bates, Camaioni, & Volterra, 1975). Similarly, the child may tug on a parent's sleeve and, having secured the parent's attention, point excitedly to a plane flying over head (Bates et al., 1975). Behavioral sequences such as these are generally taken as signaling the onset of genuine, intentional, communication (Sugarman, 1984). This is not to say that the infant's behaviors do not carry meaning for an adult observer prior to the age of 8 months, for the difference in infant state signaled by a cry or by a laugh is quite clear. But what is lacking in the behavior of infants prior to this age is evidence of the intention to communicate. *Cries*, for example, are reactions to internal states and will occur whether or not there is someone available to respond (Whitehurst & Sonnenschein, 1985). The inclusion of both objects and people within the types of behavioral sequences we have described leads to the conclusion that the child intends to affect the listener, that is, to communicate (Whitehurst & Sonnenschein, 1985).

Thus, many of the communicative behaviors observed in children who have begun to master language have their roots in the prelinguistic period (Sugarman, 1984). Nevertheless, communicative development during the linguistic period is not simply a matter of learning to do with language what one has previously done with nonverbal signals. There is much knowledge about communication per se (i.e., pragmatic rules) that is yet to be acquired (Whitehurst & Sonnenschein, 1985). We turn now to these developments.

Establishing Referents

Children younger than 6 or 7 years of age often perform poorly in the task of establishing referents (for reviews, see Dickson, 1981, Glucksberg, Krauss, & Higgins, 1975, Robinson & Whittaker, 1986, and Whitehurst & Sonnenschein, 1985). In the role of speaker, they often produce ambiguous messages (Glucksberg & Krauss, 1967; Robinson & Robinson, 1983; Sonnenschein & Whitehurst, 1983) and fail to give redundant messages under task conditions in which the listener would benefit from redundancy (Sonnenschein, 1984a). In the role of listener, they are inappropriately tolerant of ambiguity in the messages they hear. This tolerance for ambiguity is seen in (a) their tendency to respond to ambiguous messages by making a referent selection rather than by requesting clarification (Lempers & Elrod, 1983; Patterson, Massad, & Cosgrove, 1978; Revelle, Wellman, & Karabenick, 1985), (b) their tendency to blame the listener rather than the speaker for the problems caused by the latter's ambiguous message (Robinson & Robinson, 1976, 1977), and (c) their inability to judge as inadequate another person's ambiguous messages when asked to do so (Beal, 1987; Beal & Flavell, 1984; Sonnenschein, 1986a).

These flaws in young children's referential performance are due in part to their limited linguistic, cognitive, and social competencies (Shatz, 1983). Recent research (Roberts & Patterson, 1983; Sodian, 1988), for example, suggests that perspective-taking deficiencies are involved (but see Shantz, 1981). In particular, preschoolers are poor at evaluating the information that listeners must have to make a referent selection; thus, the messages they produce are sometimes not informative. Preschool children are also poor at making the perceptual comparisons among potential referents that are necessary for adequate speaking and listening performance, at least when the comparison demands are relatively high (Glucksberg et al., 1975; Roberts & Patterson, 1983).

The poor referential performance of young children, however, also reflects a lack of knowledge of, or failure to consistently follow, pragmatic rules. Young children do not recognize, for instance, that messages must conform to the difference rule (Whitehurst & Sonnenschein, 1985). This accounts, in part, for their frequent production of ambiguous messages. They also fail to apply the *editing* rule, which requires an appreciation of the fact that the speaker's utterance is crucial to the success of any effort at establishing referents (Whitehurst & Sonnenschein, 1985). As a result, they judge an ambiguous message to be adequate if it is consistent with what they know to be the speaker's intent (Beal, 1987; Beal & Flavell, 1984) or if it fortuitously leads the listener to select the intended referent (Beal & Flavell, 1983). Finally, preschoolers and young elementary school children fail to follow the *comprehension monitoring* rule (Whitehurst & Sonnenschein, 1985), which requires evaluation of one's own understanding of the message, and as a result, they fail to see an ambiguous message as inadequate even when they are not certain that they have understood it (Beal & Flavell, 1984; Sodian, 1988).

Children younger than 6 or 7 are not completely ignorant of the pragmatic rules involved in establishing referents, however. They understand that a referential expression must describe something and thus they will judge a message which fails to describe any of the potential referents before them as inadequate (Beal, 1987; Lempers & Elrod, 1983; Robinson & Robinson, 1977). They have also mastered at least a rudimentary form of the participant rule; that is, the choices these children make in the task of establishing referents are influenced by their partner's age (Sonnenschein, 1986a) and familiarity with the events or objects being discussed (Menig-Peterson, 1975; Perner & Leekam, 1986; Sonnenschein, 1988).

By the age of 7 or 8, children have acquired the major rules involved in establishing referents. This includes rules dealing with situations in which a speaker's intended referents are established not only by the speaker's utterance but also by the context in which the utterance occurs (Ackerman et al., 1990; Bredart, 1984; Jackson & Jacobs, 1982; Surian, 1991). For example, Bredart (1984) found that when confronted with two stimuli (one consisting of the letter Z and the other of the letters Z and X), 7- to 11-year-olds did not judge *It's the one with the Z* as ambiguous; rather, they saw it as referring to the former stimulus. Apparently, children of this age assume that speakers adhere to the quantity maxim, which requires that a speaker should not be more informative than necessary (Grice, 1975); that is, Bredart's subjects reasoned that a speaker intending to refer to the stimulus with the Z and X would have said *It's the one with the Z and X*.

Even during the elementary school years, however, children do not always successfully manage the task of establishing referents. Known rules are frequently not applied in tasks that are especially cognitively or linguistically demanding (Glucksberg et al., 1975; Whitehurst & Sonnenschein, 1985). Moreover, the scope of many rules still needs to be fine-tuned (Whitehurst & Sonnenschein, 1985). In addition, children become effective at using a variety of different forms of context to infer another person's intended referents only gradually during the school years (e.g., Ackerman et al., 1990).

What experiences are necessary for, or facilitate, children's mastery of the pragmatic rules involved in establishing referents? Adult caregiver behavior seems to play some role. Experimental studies (see Whitehurst & Sonnenschein, 1985, for a review) have shown that observation of an adult modeling correct referential performance leads to improvements in children's referential performance. Experimental studies (Robinson & Robinson, 1981, 1982) have also shown that whereas nonspecific signals of noncomprehension (e.g., *Huh?*) do not promote change in children's speaking or listening behavior, specific feedback does (e.g., *I don't understand which little star you mean because there are two. Tell me more*). In fact, the rate at which parents provide such explicit feedback has been associated with their children's level of referential skill (Robinson & Robinson, 1981). Interestingly, however, most parents provide such feedback infrequently (Robinson & Robinson, 1981). Thus, although explicit feedback may facilitate development, it may not be a necessary condition for such development.

Schooling may also play a role in promoting the development of referential pragmatic rules. For instance, it has been suggested (Beal & Flavell, 1984; Olson & Nickerson, 1978) that reading, which requires a careful analysis of written expressions, prompts children to attend more closely to spoken linguistic expressions as well (i.e., to follow the editing rule). Others (e.g., Robinson &

Whittaker, 1986) have suggested that teacher behavior also fosters the development of children's referential skills. For example, because teachers are constantly testing their young charges' comprehension, a student's comprehension failures will be more apparent to both the teacher and the student.

Expressing and Understanding Speech Acts

By the time they are producing multiword utterances (around 18 months of age), if not before, children use language to perform a variety of speech acts (Abbeduto & Benson, 1992). Dore (1976), for example, categorized the utterances produced by 3-year-old children engaged in a variety of activities at preschool. Dore identified the following types of speech acts in the children's language: (a) requests, (b) responses to a prior speech act of another participant, (c) descriptions of observable events or properties of the environment, (d) statements about mental states or normative constraints on behavior, (e) conversational devices, which were utterances that served to initiate, maintain, regulate, or end communicative exchanges (e.g., *mm-hmm* as an acknowledgment), and (f) performatives, which were utterances that accomplished social ends simply by virtue of being said (e.g., *I'm going to be the teacher*). Other researchers, using somewhat different taxonomies to describe the utterances of 2- to 3-year-olds, have also provided evidence that these children use language to achieve a variety of social ends (e.g., Chapman, 1981b; Coggins & Carpenter, 1981; Dale, 1980; Dore, 1975, 1977; Pelligrini, 1984; Reeder, 1983; Roth & Davidge, 1985; Van Kleeck, Maxwell, & Gunter, 1985). It is important to note that although preschoolers recognize that language can be used to perform many different speech acts, they may construe these acts in more narrow and less sophisticated ways than do older children and adults (Abbeduto & Benson, 1992; Astington, 1988, 1990).

Much research on children's expression of speech acts has focused on the linguistic forms used to issue directives to act. This research has demonstrated that children as young as 2 years of age do not rely exclusively on the imperative (e.g., *Gimme another toy*), which is the prototypical directive form; instead, they select from a fairly large pool of potential directive forms (Gordon & Ervin-Tripp, 1984; Read & Cherry, 1978). Preschoolers, for example, use the imperative, elliptical imperative (e.g., *Another toy*), and various embedded imperatives (e.g., *Can you give me another?*) to convey their directives. On occasion, they also mitigate their directives by adding *please* or by varying the harshness of their intonation (Bock & Hornsby, 1981). The pool of linguistic forms used does increase with age, however, and some of the forms used in the preschool period come to be produced more frequently by school-age children. For instance, the use of permission requests (e.g., *Can I have another toy?*), conventionalized hints (e.g., *Is there any juice left?*), and embedded imperatives (e.g., *Could you give me some more?*) increases during the early school years, whereas imperatives and *want* statements (e.g., *I want another book*) become less frequent (Ervin-Tripp, Guo, & Lampert, 1990; Garvey, 1975; Gordon & Ervin-Tripp, 1984; Nippold, Leonard, & Anastopolous, 1982). School-age children also use a greater variety of modal verbs in their embedded imperatives and permission requests than preschoolers (Axia & Baroni, 1985; Nippold et al., 1982). Young school children also use *please* more often than preschoolers (Nippold et al., 1982), although not in all types of communicative interactions (Ervin-Tripp et al., 1990). The use of hints (e.g., *It's freezing in here*, when intended to mean something like *Raise the heat*) increases throughout the early school years (Ervin-Tripp, 1977; Gordon & Ervin-Tripp, 1984). Finally, school-age children are more likely than preschoolers to include as adjuncts a clause containing an explicit rationale for their directives (e.g., *Do you have any markers. . . . Mine's broken*; Ervin-Tripp et al., 1990; Gordon & Ervin-Tripp, 1984).

No doubt these developmental changes are reflections of the advances in children's linguistic, cognitive, and social sophistication that occur during the preschool and school years. For example, improvements in certain areas of perspective taking and in knowledge of social roles are correlated with children's increasing use of *please* and various polite directive forms (Nippold et al., 1982). As another example, the embedded imperatives and permission directives commonly used in English contain a variety of auxiliary verbs, the complete set of which is mastered only gradually over the course of the preschool and school years (Coates, 1988).

Age-related changes in the directive forms children use, however, are also due to changes in children's pragmatic knowledge. For example, knowledge of the relative politeness of many commonly used directive forms (e.g., the permission directive) and of various softeners (e.g., *please*) and intensifiers (e.g., *you have to*) continues to develop well into the school years (Becker, 1986; Nippold et al., 1982). This new pragmatic knowledge, together with parental encouragements to be polite (Becker, 1988, 1990; Greif & Gleason, 1980; Snow, Perlmann, Gleason, & Hooshyar, 1990), probably leads young school-age children to abandon impolite forms such as the imperative in favor of more polite forms like the permission request.

Another important advance in children's pragmatic knowledge occurs at age 8 or 9. At this age, children recognize that a directive represents an imposition on the listener and that a listener may not comply (Axia & Baroni, 1985; Gordon, Budwig, Strage, & Carrell, 1980). This, in turn, motivates them to use forms which minimize the imposition or indicate that compliance is not assumed (Gordon et al., 1980). For example, through the use of adjuncts, 9-year-olds indicate that they would not be imposing were it not for circumstances beyond their control (e.g., *Do you have another marker? Mine's broken*).

Although children have a number of directive forms available to them, they do not choose among them at random when they wish to issue a directive; instead, they follow pragmatic rules and select a form appropriate to the context.

Preschoolers, for example, are more likely to use a polite form for their directives if the listener is older or of higher social status than they are (Camras, Pristo, & Brown, 1985; Gordon & Ervin-Tripp, 1984; James, 1978; Olson & Hildyard, 1981). They are also more apt to select a polite form if they do not know the listener well than if he or she is familiar to them (Ervin-Tripp et al., 1990; Gordon & Ervin-Tripp, 1984). In addition, preschool-age children are more polite when seeking a favor than when seeking to end some infringement on their rights, and when they are angry than when they are happy (Camras et al., 1985; Ervin-Tripp et al., 1990; Gordon & Ervin-Tripp, 1984; James, 1978; Olson & Hildyard, 1981). Although preschoolers adjust their directive production to the context, there is evidence (Axia & Baroni, 1985; Baroni & Axia, 1989; Gordon et al., 1980; Gordon & Ervin-Tripp, 1984) suggesting that not until 7 to 9 years of age do children recognize the rationale behind the adjustments (e.g., that listeners varying in social status warrant varying degrees of politeness because they differ in how likely they are to see a directive as an imposition).

The reader should note that although politeness is an important consideration in selecting contextually appropriate directive forms, speakers must consider other factors as well (Ervin-Tripp et al., 1990). In highly task-oriented activities such as math work groups in school, for example, speakers often opt for imperatives or other forms, which are unambiguous as to their intent yet impolite, rather than opting for hints or other forms, which are polite but leave room for multiple interpretations. Children gradually become better at balancing considerations of politeness and clarity in such activities during the school years (Wilkinson & Calculator, 1982; Wilkinson & Spinelli, 1983; Wilkinson, Wilkinson, Spinelli, & Chiang, 1984).

Children's comprehension of speech acts conveyed by the utterances of other people shows significant development over the preschool and early school years (Abbeduto & Benson, 1992). Initially, children are best characterized as "responders" to, rather than "interpreters" of, spoken language. That is, they search for cues that will tell them how to respond to the utterances they hear but show little understanding of what those cues indicate about the speaker's intent (i.e., about the speech act being performed). One-year-olds, for instance, adopt a variety of sometimes idiosyncratic strategies for responding (Shatz & McCloskey, 1984). Their choice of strategy is sensitive to intonation and the presence of "special" sentence-initial words (e.g., wh- words), and thus they respond differently to questions and nonquestions, and to wh- questions and yes–no questions. However, they largely ignore the context and the literal meaning of the utterance when deciding on a response; as a result, their responses are not consistently appropriate to either the literal meaning of the utterances they hear or to the speech acts those utterances express (Shatz, 1978; Shatz & McCloskey, 1984). Between 2 and 2½ years of age, children begin to respond differentially to a variety of wh- questions and show evidence of attending to some aspects of the context (Shatz & McCloskey, 1984). Nevertheless, children under 2½ are still guided, for the most part, by response strategies whose application is triggered by a limited number of utterance or contextual features (Shatz & McCloskey, 1984). These children, for example, tend to respond to any adult utterance that refers to an action by carrying out the action, even if the adult is not expressing a directive to act.

By the age of 3, children become capable of recognizing the intent behind a speaker's utterance (e.g., Reeder, 1980; Reeder & Wakefield, 1987). That is, they are now interpreters of language rather than simply responders to language. Even well into the school years, however, children sometimes search for cues about the response the speaker expects rather than try to determine the speaker's intent (Elrod, 1983; Olson & Hildyard, 1981).

As children become more concerned with identifying the intent of a speaker's utterance, they rely more heavily on the context of an utterance. Near the age of 3, for example, children can use a speaker's previous utterances to them (Shatz, 1978) and the spatial arrangements of the participants and referents in a conversation (Reeder, 1980) as context for interpreting a speaker's sentence. However, preschoolers and even young elementary-school children do not always take full advantage of the information conveyed by the context (Abbeduto, Davies, & Furman, 1988; Abbeduto, Nuccio, Al-Mabuk, Rotto, & Maas, 1992; Ackerman, 1978; Elrod, 1983). This finding suggests that these children do not recognize: (a) the relevance of some types of contextual information for understanding speech acts, or (b) all of the interactions in which context is relevant (Abbeduto & Benson, 1992).

Although understanding speech acts requires using context, the speaker's utterance cannot be ignored and there is improvement over the preschool and early school years in the ability to make appropriate use of the information in utterances (Abbeduto & Benson, 1992). For instance, it is not until well into the school years that children consistently recognize that negative directives such as *Won't you color the circle blue?* are not prohibitions but rather requests for performance of the action named (Carrell, 1981; Eson & Shapiro, 1982; Leonard, Wilcox, Fulmer, & Davis, 1978). Moreover, once children start using context as a basis for their decisions about speech acts, they sometimes ignore the speaker's utterance and look only at the context (Bernicot & Legros, 1987; Reeder, 1990; Reeder & Wakefield, 1987).

Age-related changes in children's comprehension of speech acts are due in large measure to concurrent developments in linguistic, cognitive, and social functioning (Shatz, 1983). For example, Reeder (1990; Reeder, Wakefield, & Shapiro, 1988) suggested that progress in the area of metalinguistic awareness (i.e., the ability to reflect on and evaluate linguistic expressions) promotes the shift from an excessive dependence on context at 3 years of age to a more balanced consideration of a speaker's utterance and its context a few years later. As another example, Ledbetter and Dent (1988) provided evidence that advances in the domain of receptive syntax are related to improvements in the comprehension of speech acts over the preschool years. Improvements in pragmatic competence are also involved, however. New pragmatic rules, such as the presumption of relevance (Ackerman, 1981; Conti & Camras, 1985), are acquired; others, such as the answer obviousness rule (Abbeduto et al., 1988), are fine-tuned during the school years.

What experiences are necessary for, or facilitate, young children's development in the area of speech-act expression and comprehension? Parental behavior may play a role. For example, parents devote considerable time to teaching children about politeness markers such as *please* and about the contexts in which polite requests (e.g., *May I be excused?*) should be used (Becker, 1988, 1990; Gleason, Perlman, & Greif, 1984; Snow et al., 1990). This teaching takes a number of forms, including: (a) deliberate modeling, (b) the prompting of politeness (e.g., *Say "thank you"*), (c) comments on politeness errors (e.g., *You didn't say "please"*), and (d) the verbal reinforcement of correct politeness behaviors (Becker, 1988, 1990; Gleason et al., 1984). Parents also behave in a way that may promote the development of speech-act comprehension skills. For instance, Schneiderman (1983) found that mothers made greater use of hints (e.g., *It belongs here*), which require some inferential skill on the listener's part, as their children aged and became more cognitively and linguistically sophisticated. The mothers in Schneiderman's study were also more likely to rephrase their requests in a more direct form after their original requests to their children met with noncompliance (e.g., they shifted from an embedded imperative to an imperative). Other investigators (e.g., Olson-Fulero & Conforti, 1983; Schaffer, Hepburn, & Collis, 1983) have also observed that mothers adjust their requesting behaviors to their children's comprehension skills. Unfortunately, researchers have not yet demonstrated that parental politeness instruction or adjustments to their sons' and daughters' levels of comprehension play a causal role in the development of children's speech-act skills.

Another potential environmental influence on the development of speech-act comprehension may be the types of early literacy experiences made available to children. In particular, Reeder (1990; Reeder et al. 1988) found that variations in the literacy environment of the home (e.g., number of children's books available, parental modeling of reading and writing) was associated with differences in the rate of development of comprehension skills. Reeder et al. argued that early experiences with printed matter foster metalinguistic skills, which then prompt preschoolers to base their decisions about speaker intent on both linguistic and contextual information rather than to rely on the latter exclusively.

Requests for Clarification

Children as young as 2 years of age consistently reply to some but not all types of requests for clarification (Anselmi, Tomasello, & Acunzo, 1986; Brinton, Fujiki, Loeb, & Winkler, 1986; Tomasello, Farrar, & Dines, 1984; Wellman

& Lempers, 1977). If, for example, an adult queries a 2-year-old's utterance (e.g., *I want a cookie*) with a request for confirmation (e.g., *A cookie?*) or a nonspecific request for repetition (e.g., *What?*), the 2-year-old will usually respond in some way (Gallagher, 1981). Children of this age, however, are unlikely to respond (Gallagher, 1981) to specific requests for repetition (e.g., *A what?*) or requests for specification (e.g., *Which cookie?*). Moreover, even when 2-year-olds respond to clarification requests, they do not always supply the information sought; their most frequent response is to repeat verbatim their original message (Gallagher, 1981; Wellman & Lempers, 1977), and this is often not sufficient to resolve the communication failure (Shatz & O'Reilly, 1990). In fact, learning to provide precisely the information sought in another person's request for clarification appears to be a long and gradual process. In referential communication tasks, for instance, 4-year-olds often respond to a listener's *I don't understand* by including an additional, but uninformative, adjective in their descriptions of the referent (Peterson, Danner, & Flavell, 1972); even children as old as 9 years of age typically respond to queries such as *Which ball?* by including one adjective in their descriptions even when two or more adjectives are required to identify the referent (Deutsch & Pechmann, 1982).

Although they are not always successful, even very young children try to reply to clarification requests in a manner appropriate to the situation at hand. For example, Tomasello et al. (1984) found that 2-year-olds responded in a more informative way to the clarification requests of a stranger than to those of their mothers. It seems reasonable to assume that a stranger, who lacks data on the linguistic nuances and other idiosyncracies of the child, would require more information to understand what the child has said. Whether 2-year-olds make such an assumption about the knowledge states of their listeners or whether their adjustment is based on a consideration of other, more concrete factors remains to be determined (Shatz & O'Reilly, 1990).

Two-year-olds also request clarification of messages produced by other people, although they do so fairly infrequently (Revelle, Karabenick, & Wellman, 1981; Shatz & O'Reilly, 1990). In fact, as we saw in our review of research on referential communication, even children as old as 6 years of age produce requests for clarification at a low rate, at least in experimental settings (Cosgrove & Patterson, 1977; Flavell, Speer, Green, & August, 1981). Moreover, young children fail to request clarification even when there are indications (e.g., a puzzled facial expression) that they have had difficulty understanding a message they have heard (Ironsmith & Whitehurst, 1978). Young children also produce such queries in only some of the many situations in which they are required (Lempers & Elrod, 1983). For instance, Revelle et al. (1985) found that although 3-year-olds produced clarification requests when confronted with an unintelligible message, an impossible request (e.g., *Bring me the refrigerator*), or an utterance for which no referent could be identified, only children who were 4 or older requested clarification of messages that were referentially ambiguous or that were especially long and thus taxing of their memories. In addition to failing to use clarification requests in many of the circumstances calling for them, preschoolers also produce them when there is, in fact, no communication problem to be solved (Revelle et al., 1981).

What factors account for the limited effectiveness with which young children produce and respond to clarification requests? Cognitive and linguistic limitations are certainly involved. Nonspecific requests for repetition, for example, require only that the child repeat the original utterance, whereas specific requests for repetition necessitate a comparison of the query to the child's original utterance to determine the particular constituent to be repeated (Shatz, 1983). This difference in processing difficulty may explain why 2-year-olds are more likely to respond to nonspecific than to specific requests for repetition.

A recent study by Shatz and O'Reilly (1990) suggests that social-cognitive development also plays an important role. These researchers pointed out that adults recognize that communication is a process whereby people with different perspectives come to have a shared understanding of the world, and that clarification requests are essentially linguistic devices for ensuring that this "meeting of the minds" occurs. Shatz and O'Reilly argued that 2-year-olds, and perhaps even older children, lack the sophisticated theory of the human mind that is the basis for this view of communication and clarification requests. Support for this claim came from Shatz and O'Reilly's finding that toddlers are more likely to respond appropriately to queries about their requests for desired objects than to queries about their assertions, and that they have relatively little interest in responses to their own clarification requests. This suggests that they view the clarification request as a tool for obtaining concrete goals and for participating in conversation, not as a means for achieving a shared understanding with another person. This may, in turn, account in part for their limited ability to produce and respond to such requests. (For an opposing view about the social-cognitive sophistication of 2-year-olds, see Golinkoff, 1983, 1986.)

Limited pragmatic knowledge, however, may also be a factor in the failure of under-7-year-olds to produce and understand clarification requests (Whitehurst & Sonnenschein, 1985). In particular, as indicated in our review of referential skills development, young children are simply not as adept as older children or adults at recognizing when a message has led to a misunderstanding. Even children as old as 9 do not recognize the functions and power of all the linguistic devices available for requesting clarification (Patterson, Massad, & Cosgrove, 1978).

We understand little about the particular types of experiences required to master the full range of clarification requests. Recent data (Shatz & O'Reilly, 1990) suggest that the ways in which parents use clarification requests is not particularly well suited to teaching their children about these devices. For example, parents use queries such as *A ball?* not only as clarification requests but also as rhetorical (i.e., insincere) questions. Does this contribute to the difficulty children have in learning the clarification function of such forms? At present, we do not know the answer to this question.

Conversational Organization

Turn-taking. Initially, children do not engage in much turn-taking. The vocalizations of 3- to 4-month-olds frequently overlap with those of their adult "conversational" partners (Anderson, Vietze, & Dokecki, 1977). However, this overlap is probably not indicative of a lack of turn-taking skill; nor is it likely that it is a precursor to the development of turn alternation (Shatz, 1983). Instead, these early overlaps probably serve to maintain interpersonal contact and a sense of togetherness (Stern, Jaffe, Beebe, & Bennett, 1975), which explains why they are often intentionally initiated by the adult.

Nondisabled infants do display some turn-taking behaviors at an early age, however. Three-month-olds often vocalize when their mothers pause (Bateson, 1969; Snow, 1977) and this alternation of speaking turns increases dramatically in frequency over the first year of life (Snow, 1984). Moreover, the likelihood of an infant vocalizing is affected by many of the same variables that influence the turn-taking behavior of adult conversationalists, such as the partner's direction of eye gaze, facial expression, and intonation (Trevarthen, 1986). For example, infants are more likely to vocalize when an adult stops speaking if the adult has been using the high-pitched, sing-song intonation of child-directed speech (Snow, 1986) than if the adult's intonation has been that of adult-to-adult talk.

The presence of such systematic turn alternation in the interactions of infants and adults, however, probably does not mean these infants know the types of turn-taking rules attributed to adults (Shatz, 1983). An infant may refrain from vocalizing when the mother talks, for example, only because information-processing limitations prevent vocalizing and attending to the mother's speech simultaneously (Schaffer, Collis, & Parsons, 1977). Moreover, much of the turn alternation may be due to the efforts of the highly skilled and attentive adult who adapts his or her behavior to that of the infant (Schaffer et al., 1977).

Although it is not clear precisely what infants know about the system of rules involved in conversational turn-taking, there is evidence to suggest that by the end of the third year of life, children have grasped at least the basics of that system. In particular, it is near the age of 3 that children display many of the same reactions to turn-taking errors as do nondisabled adults. In dyadic interactions with adults, for instance, these children respond to overlapping turns by ending their utterance abruptly (Bedrosian, Wanska, Sykes, Smith, & Dalton, 1988). Even when interacting with other children, "stopping short" is the predominant reaction for 3-year-olds (Garvey & Berninger, 1981). This is also the predominant response in adult-to-adult talk (Sacks et al., 1974). What remains to be determined, however, is when children master the complete adult system of turn-taking rules.

We know little about the specific causal factors involved in the development of turn-taking. However, parents interact with their infants and toddlers in ways that seem well suited to teaching young conversationalists about turn-taking. For example, parents prompt their children to participate in the conversation and they pause to allow such participation (Snow, 1977). Parents' criterion for what counts as an acceptable turn on their child's part is also based on the child's response capabilities (Snow, 1977). The highly routinized games that parents play with their children (e.g., peek-a-boo) are a particularly rich source of information about turn-taking (Snow, 1984). Although such descriptions of parent-child interaction are suggestive, the causal role of parental behavior in the development of turn-taking remains to be demonstrated.

Topic organization. The talk of even 1½- to 2-year-olds engaged in conversation with adults displays some organization at the level of topic in that these children often tailor their utterances in accordance with their partner's preceding conversational turn. For example, Bloom, Rocissano, and Hood (1976) found that the 4 toddlers they studied were more likely to produce syntactically contingent utterances in response to questions from an adult than to the adult's nonquestions. Similarly, Folger and Chapman (1978) found that imitations of an adult utterance by 1- to 2-year-olds were more likely if the adult utterance was an imitation of the child, a description, or a request for information than if it was a request for action. As another example, Boskey and Nelson (1980) studied young children who were frequent imitators of adult talk, and found that imitations by the children were more likely following questions that they could not answer than following questions for which they knew the answer. Finally, it was found (Chapman, Miller, MacKenzie, & Bedrosian, 1981) that children are more likely to respond to an adult utterance that continues the child's topic than to an adult initiation of a new topic.

Toddlers also demonstrate some skill in organizing sequences of discourse that extend beyond two turns in length. For instance, Scollon (1976) reported on a girl at the one-word stage of development who produced, in a series of one-word utterances, the same content she would later produce within a single multiword utterance. Shatz and Gelman (1977) provided examples of preschoolers who produced numerous consecutive turns on the same topic within the context of explaining the operation of a toy to a younger child.

Although young children have some appreciation for the fact that their contribution to the talk must be contingent on what has already been said and that topics should be maintained, they still have much to learn about the topical organization of conversation. For instance, their contributions are frequently inappropriate on pragmatic grounds (see the earlier section on "Expressing and Understanding Speech Acts") and noncontingent with the topic of the prior adult utterance (e.g., Bloom et al., 1976). Similarly, many of the strategies they use to produce extended discourse do not lead to topical coherence. For instance,

Keenan (1974) studied the naturally occurring interactions of a set of 2-year-old twins and found that they frequently "maintained" the conversational topic beyond two turns by repeating all or part of a prior turn. They also relied heavily on phonological substitution to achieve this effect. For example, one member of the pair would produce a word that rhymed with that produced by his brother. In her review of the literature on discourse coherence, Shatz (1983) concluded that toddlers manage a "fit on formal grounds without achieving a semantic or pragmatic match" (p. 858).

The failure to achieve topical coherency no doubt reflects limits on what young children comprehend of other people's messages. A lack of mastery of the means for contributing to a topic and the organizational principles underlying coherent discourse are probably also involved, however, as demonstrated by Dorval and Eckerman's (1984) extensive study of the discussions of small groups of acquainted peers. We turn now to this study.

Dorval and Eckerman's discussion groups covered the age period between second grade and adulthood. These investigators found that a relatively high proportion of the conversational turns of second graders were *unrelated* or only *tangentially related* to the topic of the turn of the preceding speaker. Progress between the second and fifth grades consisted of a proportional increase in what Dorval and Eckerman called *minimally related* turns. These are turns which are on topic but which do not expand on the point made in the preceding speaker's turn. Minimally related turns are illustrated by the following excerpt from Dorval and Eckerman (p. 21):

Speaker 1: I always do crummy at P.E.
Speaker 2: Um—well, me and Joey don't do good either.

In contrast to minimally related turns, a *factually related* turn expands on the content of the previous speaker's turn. Such a turn is exemplified by the contribution of Speaker 2 in the following excerpt from Dorval and Eckerman (p. 21):

Speaker 1: I always do crummy at P.E.
Speaker 2: It's 'cause ya miss a lot ah school. Don't get no practice.

Factually related turns were found to show a proportional increase throughout childhood and into adolescence.

Dorval and Eckerman also found that not only does the topical coherence of discussion change with age, but so do the ways in which speakers achieve coherence. For example, Dorval and Eckerman found that factually related turns that elaborated on a previous turn increased with age after the ninth grade, whereas factually related turns that expressed an opinion about the content of a previous turn decreased over this same age span. Similarly, they found that directives were used to control who talked at the lower grades, whereas directives were used to solicit particular types of information at the higher grades. Finally, younger children began and ended topics abruptly. The younger discussion groups did not, for example, mark the boundaries of topics by long pauses or by tangentially related turns to the same extent as the discussion groups comprised of older children and adults.

Dorval and Eckerman's analysis also indicated that topic length (i.e., the number of conversational turns devoted to the same topic) increased with age. This was due in large measure to the ways in which speakers responded to the previous turns of their partners. For example, the production of minimally related turns was inversely related to topic length, whereas continuations of a story begun in a previous turn and repetitions of a previous turn were positively correlated with topic length. Thus, the topics of young children may be short-lived not so much because these speakers lose interest in the topic but because they are not particularly skilled at keeping the topic alive.

Dorval and Eckerman interpret their results as indicating that young speakers must learn increasingly more mature means of contributing to the topic. For example, they must acquire devices for signaling topic boundaries. In fact, Dorval and Eckerman argued that all speakers, even adults, generate talk by following various procedures that are sensitive to the topic of a previous turn, being only minimally constrained by the speech act that turn conveys. Although there is good reason for rejecting Dorval and Eckerman's extreme view (e.g., see Ervin-Tripp, 1984), their research nevertheless makes clear that producing topically coherent talk requires more than just the comprehension of speech acts.

The factors that are causally involved in the development of topical coherence have not been identified yet, although suggestions have been offered. Games and other interactions that are highly structured and repetitive may serve as a "scaffold" for learning the participatory procedures identified by Dorval and Eckerman; that is, rules for participating in such routine interactional sequences may eventually be generalized to less stereotypical, conversational interactions (Ervin-Tripp, 1984; Furman & Walden, 1990). Parental behavior may be particularly important in facilitating the early development of topical coherence (e.g., Messer, 1980). Finally, it seems certain that advances in cognitive, linguistic, and social-cognitive functioning are involved (Dorval & Eckerman, 1984), although the details of such cross-domain relationships remain largely unexplored.

CONCLUSION

As a group, persons with mental retardation evidence developmental delays in most if not all aspects of language (see previous chapters), cognition (Brooks, McCauley, & Merrill, 1987; Brooks, Sperber, & McCauley, 1984), and social competence (Simeonsson, Monson, & Blacher, 1984; Zigler & Hodapp, 1986), although a few of these individuals display age-appropriate skills in some facets of psychological functioning. As we have seen in this chapter, linguistic communication depends critically on skills and knowledge in these domains; thus, developmental changes in linguistic communicative performance can be expected to occur more slowly in most persons with mental retardation than in nondisabled individuals. In fact, as we have seen in previous chapters, even those individuals with mental retardation who display exceptional levels of skill in some areas of linguistic competence continue to have problems in the domain of linguistic communication. In chapter 7, we examine research designed to describe more precisely the extent, nature, and causes of the linguistic communication problems of persons with mental retardation.

7

Development of
Linguistic Communication

In this chapter, we review studies designed to describe and understand the performance of persons with mental retardation in the domain of linguistic communication. This has been an especially active area of research over the last decade or so. In part, this activity is a reflection of renewed interest in the social aspects of language evident in developmental psychology since the pioneering work of Elizabeth Bates in the mid-1970s (Bates, 1976). It also reflects three recent trends in the field of mental retardation:

1. There has been an increased emphasis on the importance of deficits in adaptive functioning to the definition and identification of mental retardation (Grossman, 1983). Problems in linguistic communication are central to most empirical and theoretical investigations of adaptive functioning in persons with mental retardation (Abbeduto, 1991).

2. There has been a very active effort to increase the nondisabled community's acceptance of persons with mental retardation (Lipsky & Gartner, 1989). Data suggest that problems in linguistic communication can interfere with the process of social acceptance (Black & Hazen, 1990; Gallagher, 1991a; Hemphill & Siperstein, 1990).

3. As we discuss in chapter 9, researchers and practitioners in the field of mental retardation have become frustrated with the failure of language-intervention efforts during the 1960s and 1970s. Rightly or wrongly, many of these individuals believe that this failure is tied to a focus on the formal aspects of language and the neglect of the communicative aspects of language use.

These trends led to a proliferation of studies on linguistic communication and mental retardation. As the reader shall see, these studies are concerned largely with describing the problems shared by individuals with mental retardation in the area of linguistic communication. The potential causes of those problems have been addressed infrequently.

PRELINGUISTIC COMMUNICATION

Our interest lies in the development and use of natural language by persons with mental retardation. As seen in chapter 6, however, many of the social functions for which we use language (e.g., requesting an object or action, indicating recognition of an object or person) are performed through gestural and other nonverbal means prior to the development of language (Bates, 1976). Even children who have yet to acquire any language at all must conform to at least some of the rule systems that constrain linguistic performance (e.g., those involved in turn-taking; Snow, 1984). It is possible, therefore, that many of the difficulties that persons with mental retardation have in communicating through language will be manifested during, or even have their roots in, the prelinguistic period. For this reason, we begin with a brief consideration of the nonverbal communicative skills of persons with mental retardation who are prelinguistic or who have just begun to crack the linguistic code.

Prelinguistic Communication and Cognition

Most studies of prelinguistic individuals with mental retardation have focused on the relationship between their communicative performance and cognitive functioning. By and large, these studies were based on Piaget's theory of the development of children's thinking (e.g., Piaget, 1952; see chapter 1 for a discussion of the essential features of Piaget's theory). The basic Piagetian claim about the prelinguistic period is that advances in representational skill underlie a wide range of superficially disparate achievements in infancy including, for example, those in communication, play, tool use, and imitation. Therefore, researchers in the field of mental retardation have been interested in whether delays in communication are linked to delays in other areas of cognitive functioning as predicted by Piagetian theory.

In one of the first of these studies, Greenwald and Leonard (1979) compared the communicative performance of 1- to 4-year-olds with Down syndrome to that of typically developing children matched to them on level of cognitive maturity. Cognitive maturity was measured using several subscales of the Uzgiris-Hunt Ordinal Scales of Psychological Development (Uzgiris & Hunt, 1975). These scales are based on Piaget's views about the nature of normal intellectual development during the first 2 years of life (e.g., Piaget, 1952). Subjects were assigned to either sensorimotor Stage 4 or 5 according to their performance on the subscales used. The Stage 4 child is considered capable of extending existing behaviors to cover a wider range of problems than was previously possible (e.g., they can now imitate facial expressions and other actions they cannot see themselves perform), whereas the Stage 5 child is thought to be capable of creating new behavioral sequences when confronted with novel problems (e.g., using a toy as a stick to obtain another, out-of-reach, object).

Greenwald and Leonard (1979) assessed the communicative functioning of their subjects using the imperative and declarative tasks originally developed by Snyder (1978). In the imperative task, several interesting objects are visible to the subject but out of reach. Attaining the objects, therefore, requires that the child somehow request help from the experimenter. In the declarative task, the child repeatedly performs an act on a single class of objects (e.g., putting blocks into a bucket one block at a time). The child is then asked to perform the same act on a new type of object (e.g., a doll) so as to prompt the production of behaviors indicating the change (e.g., pointing to the doll). A numerical developmental score is assigned to each requesting and indicating behavior on the basis of the mode of communication (e.g., verbalization is considered more mature than gesturing) and the extent to which the child has incorporated both the experimenter and the object of interest into the same behavior (e.g., pointing at a desired object is judged to be a less sophisticated communicative behavior than first making eye contact with the experimenter and then pointing at the object).

Greenwald and Leonard (1979) found no difference in the imperative task performance of the children with and without Down syndrome at either sensorimotor Stage 4 or 5. However, children with Down syndrome who were at Stage 5 on the Uzgiris-Hunt subscales exhibited less mature behaviors on the declarative task than did the Stage 5 typically developing children. This difference between the groups, however, seems to have been a reflection of variations in linguistic skill rather than pragmatic skill. In particular, Greenwald and Leonard suggested that their subjects with Down syndrome made less frequent use of words and other vocalizations than did the nondisabled children. Moreover, although this was true on both the declarative and imperative tasks, these researchers point out that verbalization is weighted more heavily in scoring performance on the former task than on the latter.

In a study motivated by these same questions, Smith and von Tetzchner (1986) studied Norwegian-speaking children at sensorimotor Stages 5 and 6. Like Greenwald and Leonard (1979), these researchers found that children with Down syndrome did more poorly on the declarative task than nondisabled children matched to them on Uzgiris-Hunt stage. In contrast to Greenwald and Leonard, however, Smith and von Tetzchner found that the children with Down syndrome were no less verbal in the declarative task than were the nondisabled subjects. There are several possible reasons for this difference between the studies, including the fact that the subjects were learning different languages.

The declarative-task performance of persons whose mental retardation was due to factors other than Down syndrome was also found to be immature relative to performance on the Uzgiris-Hunt scales (Lobato, Barrera, & Feldman, 1981). Moreover, this declarative deficit in children with mental retardation is seen as early as sensorimotor Stage 3 (Lobato et al., 1981). Thus, persons with mental retardation, regardless of etiology or level of sensorimotor functioning, perform poorly on even the most primitive aspects of declaration, although the source of this poor performance is not clear.

At this point, it is important to note two shortcomings of the Uzgiris-Hunt scales. First, like many of Piaget's original tasks, the tasks comprising this instrument underestimate the progress of typically developing children on the path from reflexive, nonrepresentational thought to rudimentary, symbolic reasoning (Smith, Sera, & Gattuso, 1988). This is because the tasks are heavily influenced by children's motoric capabilities, motivation, and memory, as well as by their level of representational functioning. Unfortunately, it is not known whether Piagetian tasks such as those on the Uzgiris-Hunt scales underestimate cognitive ability to the same extent in nondisabled children and persons with mental retardation. As a result, the value of the scales for comparing the prelinguistic communicative performance of children with and without mental retardation is unclear.

The second shortcoming of the Uzgiris-Hunt scales is that the intercorrelations among the subtests are not particularly high for typically developing children (Bretherton, Bates, Benigni, Camaioni, & Volterra, 1979). That is, children often perform at different stages on scales tapping different domains (e.g., causality and imitation). Moreover, there is evidence that for nondisabled children (Bretherton et al., 1979), as well as for children with mental retardation (Mundy, Seibert, & Hogan, 1984), different aspects of prelinguistic communicative performance (e.g., requesting, indicating) are related to performance on different Uzgiris-Hunt subscales. These findings are contrary to Piaget's claim that performance across all sensorimotor tasks is determined by a single, underlying mode of thought. More importantly for our purposes, these findings suggest that matching subjects with and without mental retardation on the basis of their average performance across several Uzgiris-Hunt subscales, as was done in the studies discussed to this point, might obscure the true relationship between cognition and prelinguistic communication (Mundy, Seibert, & Hogan, 1984).

Because of these and other criticisms directed at the Uzgiris-Hunt scales, some researchers have begun to move away from an exclusive reliance on them. For example, Mundy, Sigman, Kasari, and Yirmiya (1988) compared the nonverbal communicative performance of children with Down syndrome to that of nondisabled 16- to 28-month-olds matched to them on mental age (MA), as determined from their performance on standardized, psychometric measures of intelligence. Communicative skills were assessed using several tasks from the Early Social-Communication scales (ESCS; Seibert & Hogan, 1981). In each

ESCS task, the child participates in an interaction with an experimenter who encourages the child to perform a particular communicative behavior. Mundy et al. selected tasks designed to prompt requesting, indicating, and social-interactional behaviors (i.e., attempts at initiating and sustaining interactions such as turn-taking in games and inviting the experimenter to play). Mundy et al. examined only nonverbal communicative behaviors, despite the fact that all of their subjects were producing at least some linguistic utterances.

Mundy et al. (1988) found that the children with Down syndrome produced more social interactional behaviors (especially turn-taking and inviting the experimenter to play) but fewer requesting behaviors than did the nondisabled children. This finding may indicate, as Mundy et al. suggested, that children with Down syndrome have special difficulty acquiring control of the nonverbal means for requesting. Alternatively, it may simply reflect their lack of motivation to make requests in the semistructured situation presented to them.

In a second study, Mundy et al. (1988) found that the pattern of results displayed by their subjects with Down syndrome was not characteristic of a group of children with mental retardation who were heterogeneous as to etiology but included no children with Down syndrome. This was true despite the fact that the groups were matched on MA and chronological age (CA). Further, the non-Down-syndrome children with mental retardation did not differ in communicative performance from mental-age-matched, nondisabled children. Thus, Down syndrome may be associated with a unique profile of strengths and weaknesses in nonverbal communicative performance. Whether this profile reflects something about the pragmatic skills and knowledge of these children, their motivation and interests, or other factors, however, is not clear.

In summary, the most striking finding of the studies we have considered is that although persons with mental retardation display delayed development in all domains of prelinguistic communication, the delay is greater in some domains than in others. How these asynchronies are to be interpreted is not at all clear, however. The asynchrony may reflect the linguistic deficits of these children in combination with the varying linguistic demands of different communicative tasks. Alternatively, the motivations and interests of children with mental retardation may differ from those of their nondisabled peers and these differences may play a role as well. It is also possible that there are cognitive differences between children with and without mental retardation that are simply not captured by Piagetian or psychometric measures of intelligence; these cognitive differences may account for their different profiles of communicative performance. Variations in pragmatic knowledge and skill, perhaps reflecting an unusual pattern of caregiver behavior, may also play a role in producing the asynchronous communicative performance characteristic of children with mental retardation. Research to date, however, does not allow us to decide between these and other possible explanations. Finally, there is some evidence of etiological differences in the studies we have reviewed.

Prelinguistic Communication and Language

In some of the studies described in the preceding section, the relationship between communicative skill and mastery of the linguistic system was also investigated. In particular, the researchers computed correlations between their measures of communicative functioning and one or more measures of linguistic maturity. The basic rationale is that a significant correlation between prelinguistic communication and language is evidence that deficiencies in the former domain are somehow responsible for deficiencies in the latter. Most often, the claim is that the prelinguistic behavior is a prerequisite for the development of the linguistic behavior. That is, if the prelinguistic behavior does not develop or develops slowly, linguistic behavior will be affected negatively. The problem with this approach is that there are usually several equally plausible interpretations of any such correlation. In addition, as seen in chapter 2, prelinguistic developments are thought to play a minimal role in many linguistic achievements according to a number of recent theoretical treatments of language acquisition (e.g., the parameter theory of Chomsky).

In the Smith and von Tetzchner (1986) study, a Norwegian version of the Reynell Developmental Language scales (Hagtvet, 1979) was administered to the subjects in addition to the measures of communicative functioning described earlier. The Reynell scales are designed to tap attainment of developmental milestones in several areas of language (e.g., syntax, the lexicon) and in both the receptive and expressive modes. These researchers found that the declarative and imperative task performance of the subjects with Down syndrome at age 2 years was positively correlated with their Reynell scores at age 3 years.

Although these correlations could arise if, as Smith and von Tetzchner (1986) claimed, prelinguistic indicating and requesting behaviors are prerequisites for mastering certain facets of the linguistic system, other possibilities exist. For instance, recall that some of Smith and von Tetzchner's subjects had some facility with language and that linguistic attempts at indicating or requesting received higher scores than did nonlinguistic attempts. This raises the possibility that the predictive correlations observed by Smith and von Tetzchner mean only that there is some consistency over time in the rate at which children with Down syndrome attain various linguistic milestones.

In the study described earlier, Mundy et al. (1988) also administered the Reynell scales to their subjects. These researchers, however, examined concurrent relations between nonverbal communicative performance and language skill (i.e., relations at one point in time) but not predictive relations (i.e., relations between a measure taken at one time and another measure taken at a later time). They found few significant correlations among measures for the most cognitively advanced half of their subjects (i.e., those with an average MA near 28 months) in each group. For the less cognitively advanced subjects (i.e., those with an average MA near 16 months), the frequency of nonverbal requesting was correlated with Reynell receptive and expressive scores for the Down-syndrome group, whereas nonverbal indicating was correlated with these two language measures for the nondisabled group.

Mundy et al. (1988) took these findings to indicate that nonverbal communicative skills, such as those involved in requesting and indicating, are prerequisites for the acquisition of language for Down-syndrome individuals and intellectually normal children, respectively. However, interpreting these correlations in terms of causal relationships is simply not warranted. At a minimum, the identification of developmental prerequisites would require examining relationships among variables over time (i.e., longitudinal data), not concurrent relationships. A more reasonable interpretation of the Mundy et al. (1988) correlations is that the Reynell scales tap pragmatic skills involved in the nonverbal communicative tasks that were employed.

In short, the correlational nature of the studies reviewed in this section leaves the matter of prelinguistic prerequisites for language very much in doubt. Moreover, it seems unlikely that much will be learned by examining the relation between prelinguistic achievements and measures of language such as the Reynell scales that average across performances in the different components of language (i.e., lexical semantics, syntax, etc.). The work of Curtiss (1988b), Yamada (1990), and others (see chapter 2) showed that development is determined by at least partly different mechanisms across these different components. This suggests that prelinguistic achievements will be involved differentially in the various components of language, with some components not depending on such achievements at all and others, perhaps, building on those achievements (e.g., later pragmatic developments). Uncovering such relationships, however, will require the use of a battery of highly differentiated, theoretically motivated measures of language rather than a simple, global language score. It will also require that those relationships be examined within the context of a longitudinal design.

REFERENTIAL COMMUNICATION

In this section, we discuss research on the performance of persons with mental retardation in the area of referential communication, which, it will be recalled, is concerned with the way speakers indicate the person, place, or thing to which they intend their utterance to refer and with the way listeners determine the entities to which an utterance refers (Whitehurst & Sonnenschein, 1985). Most of the investigations in this area employed a variant of a laboratory procedure developed by Glucksberg and Krauss in their research with nondisabled children (Glucksberg & Krauss, 1967; Glucksberg, Krauss, & Higgins, 1975). In this procedure, one member of a dyad—the speaker—is shown several stimuli (e.g., pictures), one of which is arbitrarily designated as the referent by the experimenter. The same stimuli are presented to the other member of the dyad—the listener. However, the experimenter does not tell the listener which stimulus has been designated as the referent. The speaker and listener are separated by an opaque partition so that the speaker can see neither the listener nor the listener's stimuli and vice versa. Thus, the communicative situation is a non-face-to-face one. The speaker's task is to produce a verbalization that will contain all the information the listener needs to select the referent. The listener's task is to select a stimulus on the basis of what the speaker says.

Typically developing children perform nearly flawlessly as both speaker and listener on many variants of this task by age 9 or 10 years (Dickson, 1982; Glucksberg et al., 1975; Robinson & Whittaker, 1986; Whitehurst & Sonnenschein, 1985). Most of the studies we shall review were designed to determine whether persons with mental retardation reach a similar level of proficiency on this task. The subjects in these studies were adolescents and adults for the most part and, as a result, relatively little is known about the early developmental course of linguistic reference in persons with mental retardation. Moreover, the reader shall see that the subjects in most of these studies have not been described in terms of etiology of retardation. This is not surprising because etiology cannot be determined for the vast majority of individuals who have IQs between 50 and 70 (McLaren & Bryson, 1987). Nevertheless, this makes it difficult to determine to which segment of the population of persons with mental retardation the results of work on referential communication are generalizable.

Longhurst (1974) was the first investigator to use the Glucksberg and Krauss (1967) paradigm to study referential communication in persons with mental retardation. His subjects were adolescents with moderate, mild, or borderline mental retardation (IQs 40 to 55, 56 to 69, and 70 to 90, respectively). Same-sex dyads were formed, with the members of each dyad having the same level of retardation. One member served as speaker and the other as listener. As in the original Glucksberg and Krauss (1967) work, the stimuli were unfamiliar, nonsense designs.

Longhurst (1974) found that the adequacy of the dyads' referential performance decreased with increased severity of retardation. More importantly, it was found that even the subjects with borderline mental retardation, many of whom had mental ages of 10 or above, did not approach the nearly flawless level of performance usually demonstrated by nondisabled 10-year-olds in this task (Glucksberg et al., 1975). In fact, listeners with borderline mental retardation selected the correct referent on only about half of the trials. Moreover, additional studies led Longhurst to conclude that the failures of the dyads were due, in large measure, to the production of inadequate messages by speakers, although several design problems make this conclusion tentative at best (Rosenberg, 1982). In any case, it is clear from the Longhurst study that the task of referential communication, at least in its Glucksberg and Krauss (1967) variant, is an especially difficult one for persons with mental retardation (Abbeduto, 1991; Abbeduto & Rosenberg, 1987, 1992).

What is not clear from the Longhurst (1974) study, however, is why the Glucksberg and Krauss (1967) task is so difficult for persons with mental retardation. One possibility is that these individuals lack the requisite pragmatic skills (see chapter 6 for the skills involved), which, in turn, could result from some inadequacy in the social experiences provided them by their caregivers (Abbeduto, 1991; Abbeduto & Rosenberg, 1992). A second possibility is that the below-MA-level referential performance of individuals with mental retardation is a reflection of their linguistic deficiencies, which, it will be recalled, are often more severe than their cognitive impairments (Chapman, 1981a; Miller, Chapman, & MacKenzie, 1981; Rosenberg, 1982; chapter 5 of this book). This possibility could have been ruled out had Longhurst pretested his subjects to ensure that they had command of the linguistic skills (e.g., vocabulary) needed to formulate and understand descriptions of the stimuli (Rosenberg, 1982). A third possibility is that the cognitive requirements of the Glucksberg and Krauss (1967) task are simply beyond the ken of individuals with mental retardation. That is, the task may require cognitive skills that are especially deficient in these individuals relative to the skills tapped by the standard psychometric measures of intelligence commonly used to determine MA. Fortunately, several researchers have tried to decide among these and other possible explanations.

For example, in a study by Beveridge and Tatham (1976) the subjects were dyads of adolescent males with moderate mental retardation. A pretest indicated that the subjects could produce and comprehend verbal descriptions of the simple scenes (e.g., a picture of a girl cutting a cake) used as stimuli. Nevertheless, it was found that the efforts of the dyads seldom led to the selection of the correct referent by the listener. This suggests that the problems affecting persons with mental retardation in the area of referential communication are not simply a reflection of their linguistic deficits, although those deficits no doubt contribute something to their poor referential performance (Abbeduto, 1991).

Rueda and Chan (1980) tested the hypothesis that persons with mental retardation are poor at making the careful, perceptual comparisons among potential referents on which successful referential communication depends. To do this, they employed a Glucksberg and Krauss (1967) -type task and examined the performance of dyads of adolescents with moderate mental retardation under two conditions: (a) the referent and nonreferent were from different categories (e.g., a bear and a bell), and (b) the referent and nonreferent were from the same category but differed in their physical attributes (e.g., the pair consisted of a clown with a hat and a clown without a hat). Rueda and Chan argued that this latter condition required more careful perceptual comparison of the members of each stimulus pair than did the former condition. The dyads did far worse in achieving a correct referent selection by the listener in the condition thought to require more careful perceptual comparison. A subsequent study led Rueda and Chan to conclude that the poor performance of the dyads in the original study reflected the difficulty that perceptual comparison posed for speakers rather than for listeners.

In interpreting this result, there is a question as to whether these problems in comparison are reflective of pragmatic or cognitive impairment. It is possible, for example, that speakers with mental retardation failed to make appropriate comparisons among the potential referents because they did not recognize the need to do so, as would be the case if they had not acquired knowledge of the difference rule. (It will be recalled from chapter 6 that the difference rule captures the generalization that a referential expression should be designed to be appropriate for one and only one member of the set of potential referents.) Limited knowledge of the difference rule would be a pragmatic problem. Failure to make the requisite perceptual comparison among potential referents could also be reflective of a host of cognitive problems (e.g., unsystematic scanning of visual stimuli, failure to extract relevant perceptual dimensions from visual stimuli). Deciding between these and other alternative explanations is important because each suggests a different type of intervention. Unfortunately, the Rueda and Chan (1980) data do not allow this decision to be made.

Beveridge, Spencer, and Mittler (1979) were also interested in determining what it is about referential communication that individuals with mental retardation find so problematic. They employed an interesting variant of the Glucksberg and Krauss (1967) paradigm. In particular, the dyad consisted of a person with mental retardation and an experimenter, and the two alternately played the role of speaker and listener. In the "failure" phase of the procedure, the experimenter purposely erred on each and every trial; as speaker, the experimenter would produce a referentially ambiguous message, whereas he or she would select the wrong stimulus when in the role of listener (even if the subject's message was unambiguous). On each failure trial, the subject was asked to say who was at fault. The failure phase was preceded and succeeded by a block of baseline trials (i.e., trials on which the experimenter was an accurate and cooperative partner). Beveridge et al. were interested in whom the subjects blamed for the communicative failures and how their referential behavior changed (if at all) after experiencing repeated failure. The subjects were adolescents with mild to moderate mental retardation, with a variety of etiologies represented.

Beveridge et al. (1979) found that although some subjects appeared haphazard in assigning blame, many saw a consistent source for the failure—either the listener or the self (i.e., the subject took responsibility for the failure regardless of whether he or she was speaker or listener). No subject consistently attributed the failure to the speaker. It is interesting to note that nondisabled children younger than about 6 years also fail to blame the speaker for a referential problem (Robinson & Whittaker, 1986). This pattern of assigning blame has typically been thought to reflect a pragmatic problem such as a failure to understand the importance of the "very words" of the message to the success of a communicative exchange (e.g., Beal & Flavell, 1984). A similar limitation in pragmatic knowledge may have been the basis for the blaming behavior of Beveridge et al.'s subjects. It is important to note, however, that at the outset of the study, Beveridge et al. gave their subjects practice in, and feedback about, the identification and description of the various referential failures that would occur in the experiment. It is possible that the subjects' later decisions about who was to blame for the referential failures were determined more by the practice and feedback than by any conception of the communicative process they held prior to participating in the experiment.

It is important at this point to note three features of the Glucksberg and Krauss (1967) task that make unclear the extent to which results obtained from it are generalizable to the real-world communicative situations that confront persons with mental retardation:

1. Listeners in the studies we have described were often not told that they should or could request clarification of problematic messages; speakers were seldom told which objects their listener had chosen. This is very different from everyday conversation, which requires that speakers and listeners work together over a number of conversational turns to make clear the objects, people, or events being talked about (Clark & Wilkes-Gibbs, 1990). That adolescents and adults with mental retardation operate in a similar manner is suggested by the finding (to be discussed in more detail later) that they produce and respond to requests for clarification of problematic messages in at least some situations (Abbeduto & Rosenberg, 1980; Longhurst & Berry, 1975; Paul & Cohen, 1984; Zetlin & Sabsay, 1980). Thus, persons with mental retardation may be more adept at referential communication when allowed an opportunity to collaborate with their partner over the course of a conversation. In fact, young, nondisabled speakers have been found to benefit from such collaboration as well (Deutsch & Pechmann, 1982).

2. The Glucksberg and Krauss (1967) task, as we have mentioned, is a non-face-to-face one. Although adolescents with mental retardation no doubt encounter non-face-to-face communicative situations in their daily lives (e.g., when they have to talk on the telephone), it seems clear that face-to-face encounters predominate. Moreover, the demands of referential communication in face-to-face and non-face-to-face tasks are not identical. In the former but not the latter, for example, a speaker has to coordinate an utterance and nonverbal signals (e.g., direction of eye gaze and gestures). Therefore, there is no guarantee that the results of the foregoing studies tell us anything about how individuals with mental retardation will perform in the majority of the referential tasks they face, that is, the face-to-face ones (Abbeduto & Rosenberg, 1987).

3. The Glucksberg and Krauss task is designed so that the dyad can succeed only if: (a) the speaker's message describes the referent but none of the

other potential referents, and (b) the listener selects a referent solely on the basis of the speaker's message (Abbeduto, 1991; Abbeduto & Rosenberg, 1987, 1992). This is quite unlike the situation in everyday conversation in which speakers often produce messages whose words are consistent with more than one potential referent (Clark, Schreuder, & Buttrick, 1983). Such ambiguities seldom cause problems for nondisabled adult listeners, who rely on the context in which the messages occur to disambiguate them (Clark et al., 1983). As indicated in chapter 6, however, learning to use disambiguating context is a lengthy process that extends well into the school years for typically developing children (Ackerman, Szymanski, & Silver, 1990). Therefore, studies that have employed a Glucksberg and Krauss (1967) -type task may tell us little about the performance of persons with mental retardation in situations like everyday talk, which allow the production of ambiguous referential descriptions.

Limitations of Glucksberg and Krauss (1967) -type tasks no doubt explain why performance in such tasks is not a good predictor of referential performance in more natural, conversational situations for children with and without language problems (Bishop & Adams, 1991). It is encouraging, therefore, that recent studies of the referential performance of individuals with mental retardation have involved the use of tasks designed to avoid many of the limitations of the Glucksberg and Krauss procedure. Several investigations involved face-to-face communicative tasks and there has even been an attempt to examine the ability of persons with mental retardation to deal with referential ambiguity. We describe a few of these recent studies.

In a study by Loveland, Tunali, McEvoy, and Kelly (1989) on face-to-face referential communication, adolescents and adults with Down syndrome learned a novel board game and then explained the game to an experimenter. The experimenter followed a standard protocol and asked questions when the subject did not provide critical information about the game spontaneously. The experimenter's initial questions were general (e.g., *Tell me how to play the game*), with more specific questions (e.g., *Tell me where to start*) following if an adequate answer was still not forthcoming. Loveland et al. found that their subjects with Down syndrome needed to be asked fewer questions, particularly highly specific questions, than did a group of adolescents and adults with autism. Of course, it cannot be determined from this study whether the former subjects performed at a level consistent with their CAs or MAs because the research questions of interest to Loveland et al. did not require inclusion of a nondisabled comparison group.

The ability of children with mild to moderate mental retardation to deal with referential ambiguity was the subject of a recent investigation by Abbeduto, Davies, Solesby, and Furman (1991). These researchers focused on listener, rather than speaker, performance. In their task, the child played the role of storekeeper and responded to the face-to-face requests of a nondisabled adult customer. Each request was nominally ambiguous in that it described each of two objects for sale equally well. Some requests, however, were embedded in a disambiguating context. For example, before saying *Show me that cup* on a trial on which the objects for sale included a child's cup and an adult's cup, the speaker indicated that she was searching for a gift for a small child. Abbeduto et al. found that the children with mental retardation were as likely to use the context to resolve ambiguity as were nondisabled 5- to 10-year-olds matched to them in terms of nonverbal MA. This suggests that although children with mental retardation may be delayed in dealing with referential ambiguity (compared to CA expectations), the delay is no more than that displayed in other domains of psychological functioning (e.g., nonverbal cognition).

Before concluding this section, it is important to recognize that the nature and difficulty of reference making probably vary across different types of communicative tasks (Abbeduto, 1991; Abbeduto & Rosenberg, 1987). One task which would appear to place unique and particularly heavy demands on referential performance is narration, or storytelling (Feagans & Applebaum, 1986; Peterson & McCabe, 1983). Recent investigations (e.g., Hemphill, Picardi, & Tager-Flusberg, 1991; Kernan & Sabsay, 1987; Nwokah, 1982) suggest that individuals with mental retardation do quite poorly at making their referents understandable when retelling or creating stories. In fact, children with mild mental retardation do more poorly in this regard than would be expected on the basis of their MAs (Hemphill et al., 1991). Moreover, reference making appears to be one of the more difficult aspects of narration for these children. For instance, Hemphill et al. found that, when telling the story from a wordless picture book, their MA-matched subjects with and without mental retardation did not differ on measures of narrative length, morphological and lexical diversity (e.g., proportion of nouns, number of clausal connectives, number of tense and aspect shifts), or use of narrative devices (e.g., attention getters, exclamations, qualifiers). However, these same groups differed in terms of measures of referential adequacy (e.g., the use of indefinite articles to introduce new characters), with the subjects with mental retardation doing less well. These findings suggest that the referential inadequacies that persons with mental retardation display in their narratives are not simply a reflection of problems in encoding or recalling the stories to be told, contrary to previous claims (e.g., Abbeduto & Rosenberg, 1992). It should be noted, however, that Hemphill et al.'s subjects were matched on MA as determined by their full-scale scores on the WISC-R, which taps various linguistic performances as well as cognitive ability. As we have indicated previously (chapter 1), this complicates interpretation of the results.

In summary, the results of numerous investigations have demonstrated that persons with mental retardation display developmental delays in every facet of referential communication that has been examined. These individuals perform poorly for their CAs (a) in the roles of speaker and listener, (b) in face-to-face as well as non-face-to-face interactions, and (c) across a variety of tasks associated with a range of information-processing and communicative demands (e.g., narration, description of physically present objects). However, some aspects of referential communication are more problematic than others for persons with mental retardation, with the speaking performance of these individuals often falling below mental-age expectations. The extent to which the various referential problems associated with mental retardation are due to linguistic, cognitive, pragmatic, or other factors is not entirely clear, although we offer some speculations in this regard at the conclusion of this chapter. Finally, we know little about the developmental course of referential development during childhood for persons with mental retardation or about etiological differences in referential performance.

SPEECH ACTS

As mentioned in the previous chapter, the speech act is a core concept in the study of linguistic communication and it has stimulated a good deal of research in the field of mental retardation. Recall that a speech act is the social function a speaker intends an utterance to perform in a communicative interaction (Austin, 1962; Bach & Harnish, 1979; Green, 1989; Levinson, 1983; Searle, 1969). Examples include: (a) commitment to a future course of action (e.g., *I promise to be home early*), (b) the issuance of a threat (e.g., *I'll get you for this*), and (c) the provision of a warning (e.g., *You'll hurt yourself if you try to jump over that*). We now consider research on the expression and comprehension of speech acts by persons with mental retardation.

Expressing Speech Acts

Researchers interested in the expression of speech acts by persons with mental retardation have sought to answer three questions:

1. Do persons with mental retardation express the same types of speech acts, at the same relative rates, as do typically developing individuals?
2. Do individuals with mental retardation express their speech acts through the same linguistic means as do typically developing persons?
3. Are the conditions that elicit or motivate the expression of different speech acts similar for persons with and without mental retardation?

We consider research on each of these questions in turn.

Numerous investigations address the first question, that is, the speech acts that persons with mental retardation express and the relative frequencies with which they express those acts. The typical approach in these studies has been to record the language produced by a subject interacting with a peer or a care provider. Each of the subject's utterances is then classified into one or more categories of speech acts, based on a consideration of the words it contains and its linguistic and nonlinguistic context (e.g., the ways in which the other participants react to it). The category systems employed in the field of mental retardation were based on coding systems used to describe the speech-act use of nondisabled children and adults (Abbeduto & Benson, 1992). The rationale underlying this approach is that an analysis of this type provides data on the subject's conception of the social world and the social ends to which language can be put (Abbeduto & Benson, 1992). Before describing these studies, it is worth noting that this approach has been plagued by a number of methodological problems (Chapman, 1981b; Reeder, 1983; van Kleeck, Maxwell, & Gunter, 1985), not the least of which is the failure to provide evidence that the speech-act categories employed have any psychological reality or meaning for the subjects (Abbeduto & Benson, 1992).

This approach has characterized several studies of speech-act development in children with mental retardation. Owens and MacDonald (1982) developed a taxonomy of speech acts, which they used to analyze the language produced by 4- to 6-year-olds with Down syndrome and nondisabled 2- to 3-year-olds during dyadic play with their mothers. Half of the children in each group were in Brown's Stage I (i.e., MLU between 1.0 and 2.0) and half in Stage III (i.e., MLU between 2.5 and 3.0). The categories of speech act scored included: (a) question, (b) answer (to a question), (c) declaration (i.e., an assertion), (d) practice (i.e., unprompted imitation, babbling, singing, and other instances of "playing with the language"), (e) suggestions/commands (and other requests for action), (f) naming an entity (i.e., the child spontaneously labels an object or event),and (g) continuant (i.e., acknowledging a maternal utterance without adding semantic content to the topic of conversation; e.g., *Oh!*, *mm-hmm*).

Owens and MacDonald (1982) found few differences between the children with and without Down syndrome and between children at different language levels in terms of the relative frequency with which the various speech acts were used. Some speech acts, however, were expressed more often than others by all groups. The most frequently occurring speech act for both the Down syndrome and nondisabled groups was the answer, whereas the question category was among the least frequently used. This, no doubt, reflects the fact that during the early stages of language development, conversation is controlled by the adult, who devotes most of his or her conversational turns to eliciting the participation of a partner who has limited linguistic, conversational, and cognitive skills (Snow, 1984).

The fact that the mothers in the Owens and MacDonald (1982) study were probably controlling the conversation and thus the behavior of the children raises an interesting question about how we should interpret the results of this investigation. In particular, do the results tell us more about the children or about their mothers? That is, the mothers of Down-syndrome children may have worked very hard to structure the interaction so as to avoid some of their children's performance limitations. The mothers of the nondisabled children may not have had to work as hard to get their children to look conversationally skilled. For example, the mothers of the children with Down syndrome may have introduced topics that they knew were especially likely to elicit comments or questions from their children, whereas the mothers of the nondisabled children may have been less selective in their topic choices. If the children were left to their own devices, as they would be with a nondirective adult or with another child, the children with Down syndrome may have appeared even less skilled than in the Owens and MacDonald study. Without analyzing the behavior of the mothers in the Owens and MacDonald study, such an interpretation cannot be ruled out.

Results similar to those of Owens and MacDonald (1982) were obtained in a study by Coggins, Carpenter, and Owings (1983), who used the Communicative Intention Inventory (Coggins & Carpenter, 1981) to categorize the verbal and nonverbal behaviors of Stage I children, including those with Down syndrome and those who were developing typically. The Coggins and Carpenter scoring system includes many of the same categories used by Owens and MacDonald (1982). Here again, however, we must ask whether the results tell us more about the conversational behavior of the children or their mothers.

Researchers have also examined the speech acts spontaneously produced by adolescents and adults with mental retardation. For example, in a study by Abbeduto and Rosenberg (1980), the subjects, who were all males, ranged in CA from 20 to 31 and evidenced borderline to moderate mental retardation. Estimated MAs for the sample ranged from 8 to 13 years. An analysis of medical, educational, and personal records indicated that etiology of retardation had not been determined for any subject, except that none displayed the signs of Down syndrome. Three triads were formed from various combinations of the subjects. The data for the study consisted of three 15- to 45-minute mealtime conversations for each triad.

Abbeduto and Rosenberg (1980) first segmented the conversations into turns. A turn included all the utterances begun by a speaker prior to the initiation of speech by another participant. Each turn that initiated an exchange between two participants was then scored as conveying one of the following broad categories of speech acts: (a) assertion, (b) commissive, (c) expressive, (d) question, or (e) request. In an assertion, the speaker made a statement of fact (e.g., *But you made it*). In a commissive, the speaker committed to some future course of action (e.g., *So we're extra late, I'm gonna buy some beer and . . .*). An expressive was scored if the speaker indicated feelings about, or evaluated, a proposition (e.g., *She's more important than this lousy meeting*). Questions and requests both sought a specific response from the listener—a verbal response in the former case (e.g., *Who's invited them?*) and a nonverbal one in the latter (e.g., *Pass your applesauce*). These categories were derived largely from previous work on nondisabled adults (e.g., Searle, 1969, 1976).

It was found that each triad of subjects produced all five categories of speech acts. Assertions and questions were the most frequently occurring speech acts; these two categories accounted for better than 47% and 43%, respectively, of the initiating turns, which demonstrates that adults with mental retardation were especially interested in giving and receiving information. Although expressives and commissives were relatively infrequent (4% and 3%, respectively), that they occurred at all suggests that adults with mental retardation are able to encode fairly abstract content in their utterances; that is, they can talk about their future plans and their feelings. Similar results have been obtained for adolescents with organically based retardation (Zetlin & Sabsay, 1980) and, in a case study, for an adult with moderate retardation (Owings & McManus, 1980; Owings, McManus, & Scherer, 1981). In fact, there is even some anecdotal evidence (Price-Williams & Sabsay, 1979) that adults with profound retardation (i.e., IQs below 20) competently express a variety of speech acts in their conversational interactions.

At this point, we mention two limitations of the studies of speech-act expression in adolescents and adults with mental retardation:

1. Because no normative comparison was included in the studies cited, we do not know whether the subjects with mental retardation used the various categories of speech acts at rates appropriate for their CAs or levels of functioning in other domains (e.g., cognition, linguistic competence).

2. The speech-act categories scored in these investigations were quite broad and each encompassed a number of different subtypes (Abbeduto & Benson, 1992). For example, within Abbeduto and Rosenberg's (1980) category of requests, a distinction could be made between those seeking an action and those seeking termination of an ongoing action (Abbeduto, 1984). Whether adolescents and adults with mental retardation make use of all subtypes of request (or any other category of speech act), therefore, cannot be determined from the studies we have considered.

The studies of speech-act expression considered to this point, then, are not without their methodological and conceptual problems. Nevertheless, they are consistent in suggesting that although their progress in this area of communicative functioning is slower, persons with mental retardation come to conceive of social interaction and of the social uses of language in ways that are highly similar to that of nondisabled children and adults. That is, individuals with mental retardation perceive various types of beliefs, desires, commitments, and feelings as the substance of social interaction and recognize that language is an appropriate medium for expressing that substance. It is important to appreciate that this similarity emerges despite the fact that nondisabled individuals and persons with mental retardation experience very different environments (e.g., see Zigler & Hodapp, 1986). This raises the possibility that speech acts emerge from social-cognitive concepts that "reflect universal features of cognitive growth and of human social interaction" (Abbeduto & Benson, 1992, p. 262).

We now turn to studies that have focused on the second question, that is, on the linguistic means by which persons with mental retardation express their speech acts. Recall that mature speakers typically have available to them many different linguistic forms for the expression of a given speech act and that they select a form on the basis of various social considerations. For example, the imperative (e.g., *Give me another*) is an impolite form of request. Competent speakers thus avoid the imperative in situations in which they wish not to offend the addressee (Brown & Levinson, 1987), as would be the case if they were seeking a favor or addressing a supervisor at work. They might use the imperative, however, in a situation in which they were less concerned about offending the addressee, as might be the case when chastising a disobedient child. The results of several studies suggest that persons with mental retardation evidence delays in using the linguistic forms appropriate for the expression of particular speech acts.

In one of these studies (Bliss, 1985), persons with mild to moderate retardation (of unspecified etiology) were asked to produce requests in two different hypothetical contexts. In one context, the subject was to pretend to request that his or her mother allow an overnight party. In the other, the subject was to ask an unfamiliar adult to keep a lost puppy. The experimenter played the roles of mother and unfamiliar adult. The reader should note that these contexts varied on two dimensions: (a) the subject's familiarity with the addressee (i.e., mother vs. unfamiliar adult), and (b) the magnitude of the imposition represented by the request (i.e., agreeing to a one-night party vs. agreeing to care for a pet for an indefinite period of time). This complicates interpretation of any effect of context on the subjects' messages; that is, subjects with and without mental retardation might both vary the form of their requests as a function of differences in the context, while basing their decisions on different dimensions of the context.

Bliss (1985) assigned each request a numerical score based on the extent to which the speaker was sensitive to the addressee's perspective. For example, because *I need you to keep this puppy* refers only to the subject's perspective, it would receive a lower score than *You would really enjoy this puppy*, which acknowledges the addressee's perspective by indicating how he or she might benefit through compliance with the request. The former is a less polite request than the latter. As a result, nondisabled adults are more inclined to make requests through linguistic forms that acknowledge their addressee's perspective if: (a) the addressee is unfamiliar rather than familiar, and (b) their request represents a major rather than a minor imposition (Gordon & Ervin-Tripp, 1984).

Bliss (1985) found that the subjects received higher scores for the stranger-puppy context than for the mother–party context. Thus, persons with mental retardation learn to consider addressee familiarity or degree of imposition (or both) when deciding how to express their speech acts, although they are delayed in this regard (i.e., the subjects with mental retardation were chronologically older than the nondisabled comparison group in the Bliss investigation).

Like Bliss (1985), Abbeduto (1984) elicited requests to hypothetical scenarios from subjects with mental retardation. Abbeduto found that children with mild to moderate mental retardation (of unknown etiology) varied the politeness of their requests in accordance with several dimensions of the context. For instance, they used polite forms (e.g., *Could you stop singing?* or *Will you stop singing, please?* rather than *Stop singing*) more often when the cause of the request was the speaker's desires rather than the behavior of the addressee and for an adult addressee rather than a 2-year-old addressee. Moreover, the children with mental retardation behaved in much the same way as a group of younger, nondisabled children who were matched to them on nonverbal MA and measures of linguistic competence. Again, we have evidence that persons with mental retardation learn to select linguistic forms for their speech acts on the basis of the same social considerations (e.g., politeness, the identity of the addressee) as do typically developing children, albeit at a slower rate.

Nuccio and Abbeduto (1993) also conducted a study to investigate the ways in which children and adolescents with mild to moderate mental retardation expressed their speech acts. As in the previous studies, these investigators focused on requests. This study is noteworthy, however, for two reasons:

1. In the studies described previously, the subject produced requests in response to hypothetical scenarios involving people the subject did not know. Moreover, the subject's request had no real effect (i.e., the request led to no real change in the world, nor did the subject really want to effect such a change). As a result, it is not clear whether the subjects' behavior in these studies tells us anything about their behavior in actual communicative interactions. In the Nuccio and Abbeduto investigation, in contrast, requests were elicited from the subjects within the context of an actual interaction with another person and each request served a real purpose for the subject. In particular, each subject worked with various construction materials for a specified time period, at the end of which he or she requested new materials from an adult.

2. The previously described studies focused largely on the subjects' sensitivity to relatively static dimensions of the context (e.g., addressee age and familiarity). In everyday communication, however, it is often the case that speakers consider aspects of the context that are more dynamic. For example, polite requests are more likely if the addressee is sad or angry rather than happy and

if he or she is busy with a task rather than unoccupied. Nuccio and Abbeduto examined the impact of variations in addressee affect (i.e., sad or happy) and activity (i.e., occupied or unoccupied with a task) on the requests of their subjects with mental retardation.

Nuccio and Abbeduto (1993) found that their subjects with mental retardation varied the politeness of their requests in accordance with the addressee's affect and activity level, as did a group of nondisabled children whose CAs were such that they could be expected to be similar in mental age to the group with mental retardation. It was also found that, regardless of the addressee's affect and activity, the subjects with mental retardation tended to use request forms that were less polite than those used by the nondisabled subjects. For example, the former were less likely to use interrogative requests such as *Can I have another?*, which are fairly polite, and more likely to use elliptical forms such as *Another one*, which are relatively impolite. These differences emerged despite evidence that the subjects with mental retardation could produce the more polite forms. The results of this study, then, are important because they suggest that even when persons with mental retardation attempt to adjust their language use to the social situation, they may not always be completely successful and, thus, they may be seen as rude or as socially inept.

We have seen that researchers have been interested in the types of speech acts persons with mental retardation express and the manner in which they express those acts. But what about the factors that motivate a speaker to express a particular speech act in the first place? For example, what leads a person to decide to request an action from another person, criticize another, or make an assertion?

A study by Bray, Biasini, and Thrasher (1983) was designed to address this question. In particular, these investigators sought to identity the situations that prompted adolescents and adults with moderate to severe mental retardation to issue verbal requests for objects. The 4 subjects, whose etiologies are not reported by Bray et al., varied greatly in their linguistic skills, with one subject producing largely one- and two-morpheme utterances and another producing numerous utterances containing six or more morphemes. Bray et al. used a game in which the subject was a customer in a store and an experimenter played the part of the storekeeper. Two objects (e.g., a cup and a battery) were placed on the store counter on each trial. The subject was then asked to obtain the object that went with a third object (e.g., a radio without a battery). In the baseline phase of the study, the objects were within reach of the subject. In this phase, then, the subject could obtain the object by reaching for it or by asking the storekeeper. In contrast, in the experimental phase, the objects were covered by a transparent barrier; the subject could obtain the desired object only by asking the storekeeper for it. Each subject was tested in both phases, with the phases being presented in an alternating sequence.

Bray et al. (1983) found that the subjects were able to obtain the appropriate object in both conditions. In the baseline phase, however, the subjects usually just reached for the desired object. In the experimental phase, in contrast, 3 of the 4 subjects typically made a verbal request for the object. The subjects' verbalizations included single-word utterances, such as object labels (e.g., *battery*) or diectic utterances (e.g., *that*), as well as multiword requests (e.g., *Gimme that*). The subject who failed to vary her behavior across conditions was an adolescent with severe mental retardation.

The Bray et al. (1983) investigation suggests that some persons with mental retardation quite sensibly decide that a verbal request is in order when they cannot achieve the desired goal on their own. What we do not know from these results, of course, is how their performance in this area compares to that of nondisabled persons at the same chronological age or developmental levels.

In summary, persons with mental retardation display delayed development in all areas of speech-act expression that have been investigated. These individuals may have special difficulty (i.e., perform below MA level) in the area of linguistic politeness, that is, in using appropriately polite forms for their requests. The source of these problems in politeness is not clear, although it does not appear to be due to linguistic deficits per se. This latter finding is consistent with the work of Curtiss (1988a) and Yamada (1990) in suggesting that linguistic and pragmatic development involve at least partly independent processes. Despite delays in speech-act development, persons with mental retardation who achieve some level of language proficiency eventually come to use language in ways suggesting that they have fairly detailed knowledge about the social uses to which language can be put and the listener characteristics and other contextual factors that affect speech-act expression. However, the extent to which this knowledge approaches that of the mature, nondisabled speaker has not yet been determined.

Comprehending Speech Acts

As mentioned in chapter 6, most sentences can be used to perform different speech acts in different contexts. For example, *That's mine* would be a directive to act if addressed to a child who was caught with one of the speaker's prized possessions. This same sentence would be an assertion, however, if uttered by an executive who was giving some associates a tour of the properties he or she had amassed. Therefore, understanding speech acts requires following pragmatic rules and using the clues provided by a speaker's sentence and the context in which it is spoken (Levinson, 1983). Research on the comprehension of speech acts by persons with mental retardation has consistently yielded evidence of delays in this area of communicative functioning.

An experiment conducted by Abbeduto, Davies, and Furman (1988) was designed to determine whether children and adolescents with mild to moderate mental retardation (and nonverbal MAs between 5 and 9 years) use a pragmatic rule referred to as the *answer-obviousness rule* (Abbeduto, Furman, & Davies, 1989a; Clark, 1979) to understand speech acts. This rule captures the generalization that speakers usually ask a question only if they do not know its answer. This generalization leads competent listeners to interpret a sentence such as *Could you make this roll?* more often as a directive to act and less often as a yes–no question when the answer to the literal question it poses seems obvious to the speaker.

In the Abbeduto et al. (1988) investigation, the experimenter addressed a series of interrogatives to the subject. Each interrogative could convey a directive and/or a question intent and each asked about the ability of the subject to perform the action named (e.g., *Could you tear the telephone book in half? Do you think you could squeeze the air out of the ball?*). The interrogatives were spoken in either a *compatible* or an *incompatible* context. In the compatible context, the ability of the subject to perform the action named and, thus, the answer to the question posed, was obvious. For example, *Could you turn the flashlight on?* referred to a flashlight that the experimenter had already turned on and off several times before placing it on the table in front of the subject. In the incompatible context, in contrast, the materials were selected so that the subject's ability to perform the action and, thus, the answer to the question posed, was nonobvious. For instance, *Could you roll the shoe box?* referred to a standard size shoe box on the table before the subject. Abbeduto et al. (1988) expected that subjects who used the answer-obviousness rule in comprehension would be more likely to interpret the interrogative as a question and, thus, respond with "yes," "no," or other "answering" behaviors, in the incompatible context than in the compatible context.

It was found that the subjects with mental retardation, even those at the lowest MAs studied, varied their responses to the interrogatives across contexts in a way that was consistent with the use of the answer-obviousness rule. However, their use of the rule was not CA appropriate but instead was similar to that of nondisabled children matched to them in terms of nonverbal MA. Although delayed in this area of speech-act comprehension, mastery of the answer-obviousness rule is nonetheless an impressive accomplishment for persons with mental retardation. In particular, such mastery indicates that they have recognized consistencies in the behavior of other people (i.e., that people do not normally ask questions that have obvious answers) and that they exploit these consistencies when faced with an utterance that allows multiple interpretations.

One final result of the Abbeduto et al. (1988) study should be mentioned. This is the finding that the subjects with mental retardation kept pace with non-disabled children who were matched to them on nonverbal mental age in the area of speech-act comprehension, despite the fact that they performed more poorly than them on a standardized test of receptive language—the Test for

Reception of Grammar (TROG; Bishop, 1982). The TROG mainly indexes mastery of syntax. Thus, mastering at least some aspects of the linguistic system may be more problematic for persons with mental retardation than the task of speech-act comprehension.

Developmental delays in the speech-act comprehension of children with mental retardation have also been documented in several observational studies. It was found, for instance, that in the context of dyadic free play, children with mental retardation responded to parental requests for action at rates equivalent to those seen for MA-matched, nondisabled children (Hanzlik & Stevenson, 1986; Sigman, Mundy, Sherman, & Ungerer, 1986) but below the rates seen for their nondisabled, CA matches (Leifer & Lewis, 1984). At the same time, however, Down-syndrome preschoolers were found to respond in a more mature fashion to a variety of maternal requests than did nondisabled children matched to them in terms of MLU (Leifer & Lewis, 1984). This latter finding is consistent with that of Abbeduto et al. (1988) and, again, suggests that the pragmatic achievements of at least some persons with mental retardation may outdistance their achievements in other aspects of language.

Although development of speech-act comprehension is delayed in persons with mental retardation, studies by Zetlin and Sabsay (1980) and Abbeduto and Rosenberg (1980) suggest that, by adulthood, these individuals have become effective listeners, at least in some situations. Recall that these studies involved an analysis of the naturally occurring conversations of persons with mental retardation. These studies are informative because the manner in which the participants in a conversation respond to the utterances of a partner tells us about the interpretations they have assigned to the utterances. A subject who responds by carrying out the action named in another person's sentence, for example, is providing evidence that he or she has reached a directive interpretation.

In their study, Zetlin and Sabsay (1980) examined the responses of adolescents with moderate mental retardation to the obligating speech acts of peers and staff familiar to them. (Obligating speech acts are those that require a response from the addressee.) A question (e.g., *Who's going?*) is an example of an obligating speech act; not replying to a question is socially unacceptable. Zetlin and Sabsay found that their subjects responded appropriately to the majority of the obligating speech acts addressed to them during unstructured cleanup activities. Similarly, Abbeduto and Rosenberg found that better than 90% of the obligating turns that occurred in the mealtime conversations of triads of adults with borderline to moderate mental retardation were responded to appropriately. In the Abbeduto and Rosenberg (1980) investigation, even the majority of nonobligating turns (e.g., assertions) received appropriate replies (e.g., acknowledgments such as *mm-hmm*) rather than nonreplies.

The reader should note that the situations in which Zetlin and Sabsay (1980) and Abbeduto and Rosenberg (1980) assessed speech-act comprehension were highly familiar to the subject (e.g., the speakers were familiar peers, the topics of conversation were those the subjects selected, the physical setting was familiar). Successful comprehension may not require a detailed analysis of the context or of the speaker's words in such situations (Abbeduto, Furman, & Davies, 1989a). Therefore, there is no guarantee that adolescents and adults with mental retardation will be successful listeners in less familiar situations that require more careful analysis of the linguistic and contextual information available to them (Abbeduto, 1991; Abbeduto & Rosenberg, 1992). Moreover, it is difficult to interpret the level of performance exhibited by the subjects in the Zetlin and Sabsay (1980) and Abbeduto and Rosenberg (1980) studies without an appropriate normative comparison. The lack of a normative comparison group also limits the conclusions that can be drawn from other investigations of the speech-act-comprehension skills of adults with mental retardation (e.g., Paul & Cohen, 1985).

To summarize, developmental delay characterizes the performance of persons with mental retardation in the area of speech-act comprehension. Despite the delays, individuals with borderline to mild mental retardation, whether children or adults, use the speaker's utterance and the context in which it occurs according to various pragmatic rules to make decisions about the speaker's speech act. Moreover, persons with borderline to moderate mental retardation eventually become quite skilled as adults at understanding speech acts in highly familiar interactions associated with minimal cognitive, linguistic, and pragmatic demands. Whether these adults evidence mature comprehension in other, more demanding, types of communicative exchanges has yet to be determined, although this seems unlikely. Finally, the performance of children and adolescents with mild to moderate mental retardation in the task of speech-act comprehension is at a level appropriate for their MAs but exceeds some aspects of their linguistic development, most notably their syntactic development.

REPAIRING COMMUNICATION FAILURES

Communication does not always proceed smoothly, even when the participants are adults of average intelligence. For instance, a speaker may assume background knowledge that his or her listeners do not possess or may fail to articulate the words of the message clearly. A listener, on the other hand, may momentarily fail to attend to a speaker or make an incorrect inference about the speaker's intent. As discussed in chapter 6, when these types of communication failure occur, there are devices available for identifying and correcting the problem (e.g., *Which one?* to signal that another participant's *Hand me that pen* was ambiguous). In this section, we discuss research on the ways in which persons with mental retardation produce and respond to these repair devices.

Requesting Repair

There is ample evidence from observational studies that persons with mental retardation produce repair devices when they have problems understanding another person's message, at least in some situations (Abbeduto, 1991; Abbeduto & Rosenberg, 1992). For example, Zetlin and Sabsay (1980) found that their adolescent subjects with organically based mental retardation produced a variety of repair devices when interacting with a teacher. These investigators reported no data on the frequency with which the repair devices were used, however. In their study of the mealtime conversations of adults with moderate to borderline retardation, Abbeduto and Rosenberg (1980) found that verbal requests for repair accounted for some 5% of all responses to a prior conversational turn.

Although these observational studies suggest that some persons with mental retardation are capable of producing repair devices, they do not indicate whether these individuals use such devices appropriately (Abbeduto, 1991; Abbeduto & Rosenberg, 1992). For example, it is possible that Abbeduto and Rosenberg's (1980) subjects failed to understand a large number of utterances, but that they requested repair in only a small proportion of those cases. Additionally, these subjects may sometimes have used the wrong repair device (i.e., one that would not solicit the specific information needed to resolve a given misunderstanding).

Experimental studies have avoided this problem by directly manipulating the adequacy of the messages addressed to the subjects with mental retardation and thereby the need for a repair device or the type of device that is appropriate. These studies suggest that persons with mental retardation do not request repair in all instances in which they should. In a study described previously, Abbeduto et al. (1991) found that children with mild to moderate mental retardation seldom requested clarification of an adult speaker's ambiguous messages (i.e., utterances that described two physically present objects). Instead, the children appeared to guess at the speaker's intended referent in this face-to-face situation. Similar results were reported by Ezell and Goldstein (1991). In another study mentioned earlier in this chapter, Rueda and Chan (1980) examined the non-face-to-face referential performance of adults with moderate mental retardation and found that they seldom requested clarification from a peer who had produced a referentially ambiguous message. In contrast to the preceding studies, Warne and Bedrosian (cited in Bedrosian, 1988) found that adults with moderate mental retardation did request clarification if the speaker was talking about physically absent referents that were unrelated to the current conversational topic. They were less likely to do so, however, if the speaker stayed on topic. Thus, there is variability across situations in the use of repair devices by persons with mental retardation.

There are several possible explanations for the tendency of persons with mental retardation to use repair devices in only some of the situations in which they are needed (Abbeduto, 1991). The most likely explanation is that various performance factors prevent these individuals from making use of the repair devices in their repertoires. In the Abbeduto et al. (1991) investigation, for example, the speaker who produced the problematic messages was a nondisabled adult. It is possible that the subjects with mental retardation recognized that a request for clarification was in order but refrained from making such a request because they wished to avoid offending the adult by pointing out the error. A performance explanation such as this is plausible because young, nondisabled children attend to factors such as speaker age and ability when evaluating the adequacy of spoken messages (Sonnenschein, 1986a).

In summary, persons with mental retardation, even as adults, do not request repair in all situations in which it is appropriate. The particular situational factors affecting their production of repair devices are not well understood. Additionally, most investigations in this area have focused on adolescents and adults and, as a result, we know little about the early developmental course of this aspect of linguistic communication in persons with mental retardation. The delay in this area of communicative functioning may be especially great, as evidenced by below-MA performance in the study by Abbeduto et al. (1991).

Responding to Requests for Repair

Several published studies focused on the effectiveness with which persons with mental retardation respond to requests for repair of their own inadequate messages. As was true of the production of repair devices, this research has also uncovered developmental delays. For example, Coggins and Stoel-Gammon (1982) studied 4 children with Down syndrome who averaged 5.4 years in CA and were in Brown's Stage I of language development (i.e., they produced multiword utterances but not much in the way of grammatical morphemes). The children's responses to the repair requests of an adult (whose identity is not reported by the investigators) in a variety of everyday encounters (e.g., mealtime, book reading) were analyzed. Coggins and Stoel-Gammon found that the children responded in some way to every adult repair request; more often than not, they responded by revising their original, problematic utterance (as opposed to simply repeating it verbatim). A similar level of expertise was evidenced by three of the four 5- to 6-year-olds with Down syndrome studied by Scherer and Owings (1984). The authors of both of these studies suggested that the pattern of responding displayed by the children with Down syndrome was similar to that seen in younger, preschool-age, typically developing children (Gallagher, 1977, 1981; Garvey, 1977).

Research also suggests that responding to some repair devices poses greater difficulty for persons with mental retardation than does responding to others.

This was demonstrated nicely in a study by Longhurst and Berry (1975). These investigators included persons ranging in age from 10 to 22 years who were divided into three groups according to the severity of their mental retardation: (a) borderline, (b) mild, and (c) moderate. A referential communication task was used in which the subject's task, on each of several trials, was to produce a description of a nonsense drawing that would allow the experimenter to select that drawing from among several alternatives. The experimenter and subject could see each other's faces, but not each other's drawings. The experimenter responded to a predetermined number of the subject's descriptions by requesting a repair. The experimenter produced three types of repair devices: (a) nonverbal (i.e., the experimenter responded to the description with a puzzled facial expression), (b) explicit verbal (i.e., *Tell me something else about the picture*), and (c) implicit verbal (i.e., *I don't understand*). Because the explicit repair request made the response requirements the clearest, one would expect it to elicit the highest proportion of adequate responses. In fact, Longhurst and Berry found that the three groups all made adequate responses to most of the explicit requests for repair. Only the subjects with borderline mental retardation, however, were able to deal effectively with the other types of repair device. Thus, the specificity of the feedback provided in a repair device influences the ability of persons with borderline to moderate mental retardation to repair a conversational failure. Recall that this finding characterizes the performance of very young, typically developing children as well (Shatz, 1983).

Although the development of persons with mental retardation in this area of communicative functioning is delayed, there is evidence to suggest that they become fairly skilled by the time they are adults in responding to a variety of requests for repair. For example, Paul and Cohen (1984) investigated the extent to which adults with mental retardation, whose average age was near 30 and average performance IQ was 68, were able to meet the varying response requirements of different verbally expressed repairs. While conversing with each subject, the experimenter produced three types of repair request: (a) a request for confirmation (e.g., *You watched "Dynasty"?* after a subject's *I watched "Dynasty" last night*), (b) a request for repetition (e.g., *What?*), and (c) a request for repetition of a specific constituent (e.g., *You left what in your dream?* after the subject's *I left the hospital in my dream*). The subjects not only responded to every request for repair, they also tailored their response to the specific type of repair device employed. For example, the most frequent response to a request for confirmation was a *yes* or *no*, whereas the most frequent response to a request for repetition of a specific constituent was to repeat the constituent queried. Although no nondisabled comparison group was included, the high level of performance the subjects exhibited suggests that they had mastered the specific repair devices Paul and Cohen studied. Abbeduto and Rosenberg (1980) also observed that their adult subjects with moderate to borderline

mental retardation nearly always responded appropriately to repair devices directed to them by peers.

Despite the high level of performance exhibited by the adults in the Paul and
Cohen (1984) and Abbeduto and Rosenberg (1980) studies, it is important to
recognize that not all types of repair devices were included in these studies. For
example, these studies did not involve an examination of the implicit verbal requests for repair studied by Longhurst and Berry (1975), which were problematic for many of the children and adolescents who participated. Such requests
may continue to pose problems for individuals with mental retardation even in
adulthood. Moreover, recall our discussion of the possible effect of performance
factors on the production of repair devices by persons with mental retardation.
It is possible that the ability of these individuals to respond appropriately to various repair devices is also affected by setting, topic, and partner variables.

In summary, persons with mental retardation evidence developmental delays not only in requesting repair of conversational failures but also in responding to requests for repair directed at them. Variability is apparent in the responses
of these individuals to repair requests, as it was in their production of such requests; persons with mental retardation respond more effectively to some repair
devices than to others. By adulthood, many individuals with mental retardation
are quite skilled at responding to a variety of requests for repair. This last finding should be interpreted cautiously, however, because the issue of variability
in performance across situations and across types of repair devices has not been
adequately addressed by research directed at adults with mental retardation.

ORGANIZING THE CONVERSATION

To this point in our discussion of linguistic communication, we have focused on
certain characteristics of the utterances produced (e.g., their referential adequacy, the speech acts they express) and on the ways in which individual utterances are understood and responded to. But a conversation is more than simply
a string of utterances or even pairs of utterances (e.g., question and answer).
A conversation has a structure or organization; that is, the utterances fit together
in systematic ways. For example, we take turns at talking rather than all speaking at once. In this section, we consider how persons with mental retardation
manage the task of organizing a conversation.

Taking Turns

A conversation is usually organized so that only one person speaks at a time.
As indicated in chapter 6, instances of overlap between the turns of different
speakers or of one speaker interrupting another are infrequent in the conversa-

tions of nondisabled adults (Duncan & Fiske, 1977; Levinson, 1983; Sacks, Schegloff, & Jefferson, 1974). In fact, it has been estimated that only about 5% of the transitions between speakers involve an overlap or interruption in the conversations of intellectually normal adults (Levinson, 1983).

Studies of the turn-taking behavior of children with mental retardation have focused, for the most part, on loosely structured (e.g., free play) dyadic interactions with parents (Davis & Oliver, 1980; Davis, Stroud, & Green, 1988; Tannock, 1988). The results suggest that the rate of turn-taking errors (e.g., interruption of one speaker by another) for these children is similar to that seen for younger, typically developing children matched to them on measures of linguistic and/or cognitive functioning (e.g., MLU, mental age). Despite this delay, the rate of turn-taking errors is quite low, even for children with mental retardation as young as 2 or 3 years of age, which suggests that this may not be a major problem area for these individuals (Abbeduto, 1991).

However, the results of these studies of children's turn-taking must be viewed cautiously (Abbeduto, 1991; Abbeduto & Rosenberg, 1992). As we pointed out previously, the parents of children with mental retardation may work especially hard (compared to the parents of typically developing children) to structure the interaction to ensure optimal conversational performance from their children. As a result, children with mental retardation may be far less adept at taking turns when engaged in conversation with, for example, their peers. Relevant data from peer interactions are not available, however.

In contrast to studies involving children with mental retardation, research on the conversational turn-taking of adults with mental retardation has, in fact, focused on interactions with peers. In a study we have referred to earlier, Abbeduto and Rosenberg (1980) found that their adult subjects with borderline to moderate mental retardation managed the vast majority of speaker changes appropriately: Overlaps or interruptions occurred in only about 10% of the speaker changes observed, a rate that is not appreciably different from estimates for nondisabled adult conversation. Abbeduto and Rosenberg also found that most of their subjects' overlaps were short (i.e., less than three words) because one or both of the parties who overlapped halted their utterances prematurely. Nondisabled adults handle instances of overlap in the same way (Sacks et al., 1974). Together, these findings suggest that turn-taking is not a major problem area for adults with milder forms of mental retardation.

The nearly flawless nature of the turn-taking of nondisabled adults has been attributed to the fact that speaker change is highly rule-governed (Sacks et al., 1974). The turn-taking of the adults with mental retardation in the Abbeduto and Rosenberg (1980) investigation likewise seems to have been rule-governed. This is suggested by an analysis of the types of turn-taking errors that occurred. Many of the errors involved a speaker adding an optional element after what could have been the end of a turn, just as another participant started to speak.

The following is an example from Abbeduto and Rosenberg's subjects (the arrow indicates the point at which the overlap began):

Speaker 1: . . . Where's that new bowling alley of
     yours . . . by the way?
Speaker 2:   ↑What are you?

Such errors also account for a large proportion of the turn-taking errors of non-disabled adults (Sacks et al., 1974). Sacks et al. suggested that these errors occur because potential speakers are under pressure to claim a turn as soon as it is appropriate to do so and, as a result, they sometimes claim a turn at a point that could be, but is not, the end of the current speaker's turn. Apparently, adults with mental retardation are under a similar pressure and are aware of the rules defining the potential ends of turns.

In short, despite early delays, the turn-taking behavior of children and adults with mental retardation is highly systematic and rule governed and appears to be an area of relative strength. This conclusion should be considered tentative, however, given the limited number of situations in which the turn-taking behavior of these individuals has been examined. Sacks et al. (1974) pointed out that different rules characterize turn-taking in different communicative formats (e.g., conversation, debate, and lecture). We pointed out several times before that situational factors, such as familiarity of the participants, influence the pragmatic performance of persons with mental retardation. It seems probable that the turn-taking performance of persons with mental retardation will be subject to similar situational variation.

Contributing to the Topic

The utterances of a conversation are generally organized into topics. That is, we often take a series of turns at speaking, each of which relates to the same topic (e.g., an upcoming event, a mutual friend, the state of our favorite football team). The ability of individuals with mental retardation to organize their contributions to the conversation at the level of topic has been examined in only a few studies.

In their study, Abbeduto and Rosenberg (1980) found that although some of the topics brought up by their adult subjects with mental retardation were discussed only briefly, many occupied a substantial number of consecutive conversational turns. The mean number of consecutive turns by different speakers ranged from 7 to 21 for the three triads studied. Moreover, the longest uninterrupted discussion of a topic by each triad ranged from 36 to 157 turns. This study, then, demonstrates that some adults with mental retardation are capable of sustaining a topic over an impressive span of conversational time.

We should be cautious in attributing a high degree of topic-related skill to Abbeduto and Rosenberg's (1980) subjects, however (Abbeduto, 1991). One reason, of course, is that these investigators included no normative comparison; thus, it is not clear whether their subjects with mental retardation stayed on topic as long as would be expected on the basis of their CAs or developmental levels. A second reason is that good topic skills involve more than simply staying on topic. As discussed in chapter 6, nondisabled adults formulate their turns to add new information to the topic, they establish background information before introducing a new topic, and they contribute in a way that ensures that the topic moves in a logical manner or at least toward some form of closure (Dorval & Eckerman, 1984). Moreover, one may perseverate on an event and, thus, actually stay on a topic too long. In short, topic length may not be a good measure of topic quality (Abbeduto, 1991).

Therefore, a study by Warne and Bedrosian (cited in Bedrosian, 1988) is noteworthy because it involved an examination of the nature of the contributions to the topic made by adults with mental retardation. These investigators examined the conversations of 4 adults with moderate retardation as they were engaged in a popcorn-making activity. Although 3 of the subjects tended to produce utterances that were on the topic, their contributions did not seem to add much to the progression of the topic. For example, they often continued a topic simply by acknowledging the contribution of the previous speaker (e.g., by saying *mm-hmm*). (Acknowledgments allow the topic to continue but they provide no new information.) This suggests that adults with mental retardation, at least those in the moderately impaired range, have the desire to keep a topic going, but they lack the skills needed to advance the topic. Whether adults with less severe impairments evidence similar difficulties remains to be determined.

We know very little about the topic-continuation skills of children with mental retardation. Tannock (1988) was concerned with several aspects of the conversational behavior of children with Down syndrome as they engaged in dyadic free play with their mothers. Unfortunately, Tannock's only measure of topic-related behavior was topic length. Beveridge, Spencer, and Mittler (1979) also examined topic-related behaviors. These researchers found that those children with mental retardation who were more advanced on several measures of communicative functioning (e.g., frequency of conversational initiations to others) were also more likely than their less advanced peers to produce utterances that were related to the academic task at hand. Because Beveridge et al. did not include a normative comparison group, however, there is little else we can say about this study. Moreover, the ability to stay involved in academic tasks probably reflects more about the subjects' academic abilities and interest in academics than about their topic skills.

Clearly, more work is needed on the development of topic organization in persons with mental retardation. It is hoped that future work will involve the use of a wider variety of measures and reflect the multifaceted nature of topic management.

GENERAL DISCUSSION

Persons with mental retardation display developmental delays in every area of linguistic communication investigated to date. Delays can be seen in the areas of referential communication, speech acts, conversational repair, and conversational organization. Both speaking and listening performance fall below CA expectations. In addition, developmental delays in communicative functioning are seen even during the prelinguistic period, although the relation between problems in the prelinguistic period and later linguistic and pragmatic achievements is a matter of controversy. The delays evident in communicative performance are at least as great as those in the cognitive domain.

Despite such delays, individuals with mental retardation achieve impressive levels of skill in many areas of linguistic communication. For example, they are able to use various dimensions of the context to make decisions about another person's intended referents and speech acts and to decide when to express a particular speech act and how to express it. Individuals with mental retardation also use context to judge the appropriateness of another person's contributions to the talk (Oetting & Rice, 1991). They also acquire pragmatic rules (e.g., the answer-obviousness rule), which requires that they recognize regularities in the communicative behavior of others and use those regularities to guide their own linguistic performances. As adults, persons with mild to moderate mental retardation appear to manage quite well in many areas of linguistic communication, at least when they are participants in familiar situations associated with minimal task demands.

Some aspects of linguistic communication pose greater difficulties than others for persons with mental retardation. For example, turn-taking appears to be an area of relative strength for these individuals, with a low rate of turn-taking errors whether one considers conversations between parents and their preschoolers with Down syndrome or between adult peers with milder forms of mental retardation. Linguistic politeness in speech-act expression and referential communication, in contrast, are especially problematic for persons with mental retardation, with their performance in these areas sometimes below expectations based on their MAs.

Abbeduto (1991) pointed out that the pattern of asynchronous communicative development characterizing persons with mental retardation is consistent with expectations derived from work on typical development. Those areas in which typically developing children acquire the bulk of the requisite pragmatic knowledge and skill early (e.g., turn-taking) are the least problematic for persons with mental retardation. In contrast, the greatest problem areas for individuals with mental retardation are those for which the developmental course for nondisabled children continues into the school years (e.g., linguistic politeness; Abbeduto & Benson, 1992). This suggests that the mechanisms involved in the acquisition and use of pragmatic knowledge and skills may be similar for persons with and without mental retardation (Abbeduto, 1991).

Persons with mental retardation have, on occasion, been found to be more communicatively skilled than would be expected on the basis of global measures of their linguistic competence such as MLU and receptive-language age. This finding is important for two reasons:

1. It suggests that not all achievements in the domain of grammar are necessary for success in the communicative domain and, thus, persons with mental retardation can succeed at many everyday communicative tasks in spite of their linguistic impairments (Abbeduto, 1991; Abbeduto & Rosenberg, 1992).

2. This finding suggests that the mechanisms involved in the acquisition of pragmatic knowledge and skills are not the same as those underlying other aspects of language development, particularly syntactic development (Abbeduto & Rosenberg, 1987). This is consistent with claims about the modularity of the various components of language (e.g., Chomsky, 1986), and is further supported by the work of Curtiss (1988), Yamada (1990), and others (see chapters 1, 2, and 5).

In none of the studies we have considered have persons with mental retardation displayed communicative performance that was more developmentally advanced than expected on the basis of global measures of their cognitive functioning, such as MA (also see Abbeduto, 1991; Abbeduto & Rosenberg, 1992). On a host of tasks involving linguistic communication, persons with mental retardation perform at levels equivalent to, or below, those of their nondisabled MA matches. This has been true across studies differing in terms of the characteristics of the individuals studied and the procedures used to assess communicative and cognitive functioning. We have suggested elsewhere (Abbeduto, 1991; Abbeduto & Benson, 1992; Abbeduto & Rosenberg, 1992) that this pattern of results indicates that there are important cognitive prerequisites for many pragmatic achievements. Precisely which aspects of cognition function as prerequisites for particular pragmatic achievements has yet to be determined, however.

We also lack data concerning other factors that might constrain the pragmatic development and performance of persons with mental retardation. For example, it is clear that various aspects of a person's social knowledge and skill (e.g., knowledge of social-status differences, ability to impute various mental states to others) contribute to his or her communicative performance (Astington, Harris, & Olson, 1988; Bach & Harnish, 1979; Gallagher, 1991a; Rice, 1984; Shantz, 1981). Unfortunately, there have been few attempts to examine the relation between the social and social-cognitive impairments that characterize persons with mental retardation (Simeonsson, Monson, & Blacher, 1984; Siperstein, 1992) and their pragmatic difficulties. In addition, there is evidence that parents may play an important role in at least some aspects of nondisabled children's pragmatic development (see chapter 6). Despite numerous investigations into the nature of the linguistic and communicative interactions that occur between children with mental retardation and their caregivers (see chapter 8), we know little about caregiver contributions to the delays in pragmatic development described in this chapter. Finally, recent studies (Abbeduto, Nuccio, Short, & Benson, 1992; Brownell & Whiteley, 1992) demonstrated that persons with mental retardation often do poorly in linguistic communication not because they lack the requisite skills but because they fail to apply the skills in their pragmatic repertoires. An important task for future research is to determine why these performance failures occur.

8

Adult–Child Interaction and the Development of Language and Communication

Proponents of the social-interactionist perspective (e.g., Bohannon, MacWhinney, & Snow, 1990; Bohannon & Warren-Leubecker, 1989; Bruner, 1981; Furrow & Nelson, 1986; Ninio & Bruner, 1978; Snow, 1984, 1986; see also chapter 2) contend that adults and other competent language users play a crucial role in children's acquisition of a first language. In particular, they argue that the special Child Directed Language (CDL) register we use when talking to young children (i.e., motherese) helps, and may even be necessary for, children to become linguistically and communicatively competent. Thus, the social-interactionists have interpreted the adjustments that define CDL as simplifying the task of acquiring linguistic and communicative competence for the child. These adjustments (compared to adult-to-adult talk) include the following: (a) a more concrete and less diverse vocabulary, (b) the virtual absence of grammatical errors and false starts, (c) a slower rate of articulation, (d) a higher pitch and exaggerated intonation, (e) a preponderance of utterances concerned with the here-and-now, and (f) a focus on the objects and events to which the child is attending (Bohannon & Warren-Leubecker, 1989; Hoff-Ginsberg & Shatz, 1982; Menyuk, 1988; Snow, 1984, 1986). Among other things, the social interactionists believe that these adjustments: (a) capture and hold the child's attention, (b) facilitate segmentation of the speech stream into linguistically relevant units, and (c) allow the child to "bootstrap" his or her way into syntax via meaning and context. The social-interactionists have also claimed that CDL involves interactional sequences that are not characteristic of adult-to-adult talk and that these special sequences assist children in mapping linguistic forms onto meanings. An example of such a sequence is provided by the observation (Bohannon & Stanowicz, 1988; Bohannon et al., 1990; Demetras, Post, & Snow, 1986;

Hirsh-Pasek, Treiman, & Schneiderman, 1984) that adults are more likely to repeat (and thus mark as "special") ill-formed child utterances than well-formed ones. For the social-interactionists, the need to endow the child with the linguistic predispositions and knowledge suggested by Chomsky (1988) and others working within the framework of Universal Grammar and the theory of parameters (see chapter 2) is greatly diminished by these and other observations concerning CDL (Bohannon et al., 1990).

The social-interactionist perspective has been embraced wholeheartedly by many researchers in the field of mental retardation; thus, we find numerous studies that focus on the interactions that occur between persons with mental retardation and their parents. The hypothesis motivating these studies is that at least some of the delay seen in the linguistic and communicative development of persons with mental retardation can be traced to the ways in which their parents talk to and interact with them. The approach has typically been to make comparisons between the language produced by parents interacting with their children with mental retardation and that produced by parents interacting with their typically developing children. If the two groups of parents differ in any way, the interpretation is that the parents of the subjects with mental retardation are behaving in a way that is less than optimal for their children's development. Thus, the assumption guiding this research is that the communicative environment that works best for nondisabled children is the one that works best for persons with mental retardation, too.

The appeal of the social-interactionist perspective to the field of mental retardation may lie in what is perceived, rightly or wrongly, as the optimism of this perspective. That is, the emphasis on the environment as the critical agent of developmental advance has been taken to imply that intervention is not only possible but rather straightforward. Improving the language and communication skills of persons with mental retardation requires only that one determine the ways in which the linguistic and social environments of these individuals are atypical, so that their environments can be changed to more closely resemble those of nondisabled children. Unfortunately, in their rush to embrace the social-interactionist perspective, many in the field of mental retardation have overlooked its methodological and theoretical shortcomings as well as the fact that not all of the claims emanating from this perspective have received empirical support (see chapter 2). As a result, researchers in the field of mental retardation have made many of the same mistakes as those studying typical development from the social-interactionist perspective. In addition, the former researchers have not typically attempted to give a plausible account of how the pattern of parental behavior they have observed could account for the specific pattern of language and communication development that characterizes persons with mental retardation (e.g., delay rather than deviance, especially severe problems in the area of morphosyntax for persons with Down syndrome). No doubt this explains why research to date has not been particularly successful in confirming the hypothesis that adult caregivers contribute significantly to the linguistic and communicative problems of persons with mental retardation.

In this chapter, we review research on the linguistic and communicative behavior of the parents of persons with mental retardation. We begin by considering the extent to which these parents exhibit those features of the CDL register that social-interactionists claim are important simplifications (compared to adult-to-adult talk). In subsequent sections, we consider the interactive and discourse aspects of caregiver behavior.

CHILD-DIRECTED ADJUSTMENTS

Numerous studies have examined the extent to which the parents of persons with mental retardation make the same types of child-directed adjustments in their talk as do the parents of nondisabled children. It should be noted that although some of the parental adjustments directed at nondisabled children involve explicit attempts on the part of parents to teach their children about language and communication, such as the politeness instruction that occurs at the dinner table (Becker, 1988, 1990; Snow et al., 1990), most do not. Instead, the vast majority of these adjustments are thought to reflect parental attempts to communicate with a relatively unskilled conversational partner (Snow, 1986). Nevertheless, the social-interactionists argue that the net effect of these adjustments is to provide a series of "language lessons," with the complexity of the lessons linked to the current linguistic and other competencies of the child. In fact, some aspects of parents' language and communication behavior (e.g., MLU) do change in the direction of increased complexity as their children progress developmentally (e.g., Bohannon & Marquis, 1977; Cross, 1977; Newport, 1977). The correlation between the two, however, is far from perfect. In addition, it is not clear (for reasons outlined in chapter 2) which, if any, of these child-directed adjustments affect the course or rate of children's progress in particular areas of language and communication. Therefore, the reader should keep in mind, as we review the following studies, that merely demonstrating that the parents of children with mental retardation do not display the typical child-directed adjustments in their talk is not in and of itself evidence that these parents cause the language and communication problems of their children. In fact, as we mentioned in chapter 2, children in many other cultures become linguistically and communicatively competent despite the fact that their parents do not display the typical CDL adjustments.

Among the first studies concerned with child-directed adjustments and mental retardation was that of Buckhalt, Rutherford, and Goldberg (1978). These researchers examined the language that mothers directed to their children with Down syndrome in two situations: (a) where the mother attempted to teach the child to perform a task, and (b) where the mother and child were left to wait for the experimenter. The children ranged in CA from 9.5 to 17 months, with an average MA of 8 months (estimated from the Bayley Mental Development scale). Although not reported, it is probable, given the MAs of the children with Down syndrome, that all were prelinguistic. The behavior of the mothers of the children with Down syndrome was compared to that of women who interacted with their nondisabled children in the teaching and waiting situations. The two groups of children were matched in terms of CA; thus, on the average, the nondisabled children could be expected to be more developmentally advanced than the children with Down syndrome in most, if not all, areas of linguistic and communicative competence (see chapters 3, 4, 5, and 6), as well as in other domains of behavioral and psychological functioning (see chapter 1).

Buckhalt et al. (1978) found that there were no differences in the MLUs of the two groups of mothers, a result similar to one obtained in a case study by Gunn, Clark, and Berry (1980). Recall that one of the claims of the social-interactionists is that the CDL adjustments made by the parents of nondisabled children are linked to their children's levels of linguistic and communicative competence (although just what dimensions of these competencies parents attend to have seldom been specified). Therefore, the Buckhalt et al. results suggest that the parents of the children with Down syndrome had not simplified their talk in consideration of their children's developmental status. Instead, the mothers of the children with Down syndrome made simplifications more in line with a consideration of their children's chronological ages. What, if anything, this pattern of maternal behavior contributes to the language and communicative delays of persons with Down syndrome remains to be determined.

Buium, Rynders, and Turnure (1974) also examined parent–child interactions for children with Down syndrome and nondisabled children matched to them on CA, but the children they studied were older than those in the Buckhalt et al. (1978) investigation (i.e., a mean of 24 months compared to a mean of 13.5 months). Moreover, many of the children with Down syndrome in the Buium et al. study were probably producing at least a few single-word utterances. In contrast to the Buckhalt et al. study, Buium et al. observed a number of differences in the language of the two groups of mothers when they were engaged in dyadic free play with their children. For example, the mothers of the children with Down syndrome had lower MLUs and produced more single-word utterances than did the other mothers. The different results of the Buium et al. and Buckhalt et al. studies may be due to the different developmental levels of the children involved.

Surprisingly, Buium et al. (1974) took their results as an indication that the mothers of the children with Down syndrome were contributing to their children's language-learning problems by providing an overly simplified linguistic environment. This conclusion, however, is not warranted. Buium et al.'s design is simply not adequate for demonstrating a causal connection between any aspect of maternal behavior and rate of child progress in language or communication. Moreover, the differences observed between the two groups of mothers in this study may well reflect an attempt on the part of the mothers to adjust to the very different levels of competence displayed by their children, which, from the social-interactionist perspective at least, would be expected to facilitate rather than hinder their children's language and communication development.

It should be noted at this point that in both the Buium et al. (1974) and Buckhalt et al. (1978) studies, the mothers of the children with Down syndrome were significantly older than the mothers of the typically developing children. In fact, this is true in many of the studies involving subjects with Down syndrome reviewed in this chapter. This nonequivalence of the two groups of parents can be traced to the fact that the incidence of Down-syndrome births is positively correlated with maternal age (Robinson & Robinson, 1976). Randomly selecting children with Down syndrome and nondisabled children of the same CA (or younger) will result in a higher mean maternal age for the former group than for the latter. This confounding of maternal age and child diagnostic category makes it difficult to interpret the results of such studies. We simply do not know whether differences in the behavior of the two groups of mothers should be interpreted as differences in the linguistic environments of children with and without Down syndrome or as differences in the linguistic environments of children with younger and older mothers.

In contrast to the studies of Buium et al. and Buckhalt et al., more recent investigations involved comparisons between mothers whose children with and without mental retardation were matched in terms of one or more developmental indices (e.g., MLU, mental age). This shift to developmental-level matching represents an attempt to deal with a major interpretative problem facing studies involving CA-matched subjects; namely, differences in the linguistic behavior of parents of CA-matched children with and without mental retardation may reflect CDL adjustments on the part of the two groups of parents to the very different competencies of their children. The assumption underlying developmental-level matching is that if parents are making child-directed adjustments and these adjustments are somehow linked to the linguistic and other competencies of their children with mental retardation, then these parents should behave similarly to the parents of the developmental-level-matched, nondisabled children.

The most comprehensive investigation involving developmentally matched children and their parents is that of Rondal (1978b). Rondal's subjects were 21 children with Down syndrome and their mothers and 21 nondisabled children and their mothers. The CAs of the former children ranged from 3 to 12 years, whereas those of the latter ranged from 20 to 32 months. The two groups of children were matched on MLU, with subjects in each group falling into three MLU ranges: 1 to 1.5, 1.75 to 2.25, and 2.5 to 3.0. Maternal education was similar across the two groups. The mother–child dyads were recorded as they engaged in free play at home. The measures of maternal language in these sessions tapped, among other things, lexical-semantics (e.g., type-token ratio), propositional semantics (e.g., the relative rates at which state, action, process, and other semantic relations were expressed), and syntax (e.g., MLU, number of modifiers per utterance, proportion of multiclause sentences). Also examined was the occurrence of various interactional sequences, including explicit approval/disapproval of child utterances, expansions and corrections of child utterances, and prodding (e.g., *Can you say. . . ?*), all of which have been claimed by social-interactionists, although not necessarily shown empirically, to have facilitative effects on the rate of linguistic development in nondisabled children.

Two results of the Rondal investigation are of interest here:

1. There were no meaningful, significant differences between the mothers of children with and without Down syndrome.

2. There were numerous significant differences related to the children's MLU for most measures of maternal language; this was equally true for both groups of mothers. Similar results were obtained by several other investigators (e.g., Petersen & Sherrod, 1982). Such findings suggest that mothers of children with Down syndrome make the adjustments typical of CDL and, moreover, that these adjustments are linked to aspects of their children's linguistic competence in the same manner as seen in nondisabled populations. Again, however, the precise effect of the specific adjustments studied by Rondal on the developmental progress of the children, with or without mental retardation, remains to be determined.

It is worth noting at this point that the failure to find a difference between the language behavior of the mothers of developmental-level-matched groups of children with and without mental retardation does not imply that changing the behavior of the former group of mothers would not benefit their sons and daughters. For example, in chapter 5, we raised the possibility that the syntactic problems of persons with mental retardation may result, at least in part, from impairments that are specifically linguistic in nature. Presumably, this would involve problems in identifying and/or analyzing those parental utterances that are necessary for the setting of various parameters. It may be, then, that children with mental retardation would benefit from changes in their linguistic environments that serve to make these crucial, parameter-setting utterances more salient, frequent, or systematically presented than they are typically.

The reader should also be aware that the fact that the parents of children with mental retardation make the typical CDL adjustments at one point in their children's development does not mean that they do so at earlier or later points. In fact, Rondal (in press) recently suggested that after children with mental retardation achieve an MLU of 3.0, their mothers are less likely than mothers of nondisabled children with similar MLUs to make the typical CDL adjustments.

The evidence for this claim is his finding that the former mothers produce language that is more complex (as indexed by MLU) than do mothers of nondisabled, MLU-matched children. What role, if any, this pattern of maternal behavior plays in the delayed language and communicative development of persons with mental retardation remains to be determined.

The lexical usage of mothers of children with Down syndrome was the focus of an investigation by Cardoso-Martins and Mervis (1985). The mothers' language was recorded as they interacted with their children in a dyadic free-play situation involving toys from each of three categories (i.e., cats, cars, balls). The 2- and 3-year-olds with Down syndrome who participated were prelinguistic (although their MAs were in the range at which nondisabled children begin speaking). Three groups of nondisabled children who were matched to the children with Down syndrome on several dimensions were also included (along with their mothers): (a) a group matched on CA, (b) one matched on MA, and (c) one matched on language level (i.e., they were prelinguistic, but near the age at which they could be expected to begin talking).

Cardoso-Martins and Mervis (1985) found that the mothers of the children with Down syndrome differed from the mothers of the language-matched and MA-matched, nondisabled children on a number of measures. These differences included significantly lower proportions of deictic utterances (e.g., *This is a ball*) and nouns (as opposed to pronouns) for the mothers of the children with Down syndrome. The mothers of the children with Down syndrome, in contrast, did not differ from the mothers of the CA-matched, nondisabled children. Cardoso-Martins and Mervis concluded that the former mothers contribute to the delayed lexical development of their children by failing to provide them a sufficient number of referent-label pairings.

Cardoso-Martins and Mervis' (1985) conclusion is simply not warranted. In this study, these researchers have not established any relation between maternal labeling behavior and subsequent child lexical development, let alone a causal relation between the two. Moreover, Cardoso-Martins and Mervis (1990) recently reported that they failed to replicate some of these findings with a new sample of subjects. Although they attribute this failure to differences in the competence of the children in the two investigations, it may also be the case that the differences observed in the 1985 study are simply not reliable. Therefore, further research on this issue is required.

In this section, we considered whether the parents of children with mental retardation make adjustments typical of talk directed to nondisabled children. This research has indicated that, like the parents of nondisabled children, the parents of children with mental retardation adjust many aspects of their language to fit their children's linguistic capabilities rather than their CAs. This research has also shown that the parents of children with mental retardation do not display all the adjustments expected on the basis of their children's levels of linguistic competence. There is no evidence, however, that the language and communication problems of persons with mental retardation can be traced to the CDL adjustments that their parents make or fail to make. In the remaining sections of this chapter, we focus on the interactional features of the talk between parents and their children with mental retardation.

RECOGNIZING AND INTERPRETING
PRELINGUISTIC INTENT

Adults interpret many of the behaviors produced by nondisabled, prelinguistic infants as attempts at communication long before the child is capable of intentional communication (Snow, 1984). Moreover, adults respond verbally to infant behaviors to which they attribute communicative intent and do so in a manner that is consistent with that intent. This is illustrated in the following sequence:

Adult: Try this new food. It's so good.
Child: (vocalizes)
Adult: Oh, you want more, huh?

Some theorists (e.g., Harding, 1983) believe that such adult behavior facilitates the infant's transition into language and linguistic communication. For example, it has been argued that such parental behavior prompts the child to recognize that speech sounds have meaning (Harding, 1983). There is, however, little empirical support for this claim. In fact, the finding (Goldin-Meadow, 1982) that hearing-impaired children, who do not have access to such interpretive parental comments, create systems of meaningful gestures that display crucial language-like properties argues against this claim. It is conceivable that parents facilitate their children's pragmatic development by interpreting their children's behaviors as communicative. For example, such parental behavior may help children recognize that their behavior can have an effect on the behavior of other people. However, even this claim is speculative. Despite these problems, researchers have begun to examine the extent to which the parents of prelinguistic children with mental retardation make attributions of communicative intent, on the assumption that this plays a causal role in the language and communication problems of these children.

One such study is that of Yoder and Feagans (1988). The infants in this investigation averaged slightly less than 1 year of age and included those with mental and physical handicaps of varying degree. Each mother–infant dyad was videotaped as they engaged in free play. Each mother then reviewed her videotape for the purpose of identifying instances of communication on her child's part. Mothers were given only minimal instructions about what constituted communication. Trained observers also scored the videotapes for instances of intentional communication using criteria that have become standard in the field of child-language research (e.g., Sugarman, 1984). It was found that mothers of the infants with the most severe handicaps tended to be more liberal in their identification of communicative behaviors than were the trained observers. This may reflect an overly optimistic picture of the infant on the part of these mothers. It may also reflect, however, their greater familiarity (compared to the trained observers) with the subtle communicative cues produced by severely impaired infants. Moreover, even if mothers of children with severe handicaps are seeing communication where there is none, it is difficult to interpret these results in the absence of any theory or data concerning how such parental judgments could affect the children's development and which aspects of linguistic and communicative competence, if any, would be affected.

TAKING TURNS

The interactions of nondisabled children as young as 1 year of age and their mothers display turn-taking organization, with only one member of the dyad vocalizing at a time (Snow, 1972). Initially, this organization reflects accommodations made by the mothers to their children's limited comprehension and response capabilities, rather than any sophisticated knowledge about turn-taking on the part of their children (Snow, 1984). However, the turn-taking organization imposed by mothers may play an important role in children's acquisition of communicative competence. Maternal modeling of appropriate turn-taking behavior may facilitate children's acquisition of the pragmatic rules governing turn-taking. Additionally, mothers who are especially adept at organizing these dyadic interactions into orderly sequences of turns may increase the likelihood that their children can process and thus learn about the discourse-level regularities (e.g., anaphora, topic maintenance) displayed in maternal utterances. Because of the presumed importance of turn-taking to developmental progress in the area of pragmatics, several researchers have examined the turn-taking organization of dyadic interactions involving parents and their children with mental retardation.

In one study, Berger and Cunningham (1983) found that the interactions of mothers and their prelinguistic infants with Down syndrome were less synchronous as regards turn-taking than is typical during the prelinguistic period. In fact, the proportional frequency of vocal clashes (i.e., of both partners vocalizing simultaneously) increased as the children in these dyads got older. This increase seemed to be due to an increase in vocalization rate for both mothers and children. Interestingly, nondisabled infants and their parents show a decline in vocal clashes over this same age period. It is not clear, however, to what extent Berger and Cunningham's results reflect the difficulty that parents have in adjusting to the behavioral characteristics of children with mental retardation or the problems that the latter have in sharing responsibility for turn-taking organization.

The results of a study by Tannock (1988) are similar to those of Berger and Cunningham (1983). Tannock examined parent–child interactions for children with and without mental retardation. The former children had Down syndrome and ranged from the prelinguistic level to the level of early multiword expressive language. The nondisabled children were matched to the children with Down syndrome on measures of cognitive ability and receptive and expressive language. The dyads were observed in a free-play situation. Maternal age and education was similar across the groups.

Among other things, Tannock (1988) found that the dyads that included a child with Down syndrome were involved in a higher proportion of turn-taking errors (i.e., both members of the dyad speaking simultaneously) than were the other dyads. Whether this difference in error rate reflected problematic behaviors on the part of the children with Down syndrome, their mothers, or both, cannot be determined from the Tannock investigation. Moreover, even for the dyads that included a child with Down syndrome, the vast majority of speaker changes were managed smoothly.

A question that is not answered by the Berger and Cunningham (1983) and Tannock (1988) studies, of course, is what role, if any, these early vocal clashes play in the subsequent pragmatic development of persons with mental retardation. It is interesting to note that, despite the somewhat elevated rate of vocal clashes early in their development, persons with mental retardation eventually become quite skilled in the area of turn-taking (Abbeduto, 1991; Abbeduto & Rosenberg, 1980; chapter 7). In fact, turn-taking is an area of relative strength for them in the domain of linguistic communication (see chapter 7). This raises the possibility that the early mother–child turn-taking "problems" identified by Berger and Cunningham and Tannock actually have little lasting impact on the development of persons with mental retardation.

Additionally, other researchers have not found that the interactions between children with mental retardation and their mothers are characterized by an unusually high rate of turn-taking errors. For instance, Davis and his colleagues (Davis & Oliver, 1980; Davis, Stroud, & Green, 1988) found no difference between the parent–child interactions of language-matched children with and without mental retardation with regard to the relative rates of interruptions of one speaker by another and overlaps of two or more speakers. This may be due to the fact that the children were, on the average, older and more developmentally advanced in the Davis studies than were the subjects in the Berger and Cunningham and Tannock studies.

FOLLOWING THE CHILD'S LEAD

When interacting with nondisabled children, adults typically talk about those objects and events that are the focus of the child's attention and their utterances usually continue the topic of the child's previous utterance (Snow, 1984, 1986).

The extent to which parents follow the child's lead, or produce *semantically contingent language*, is positively correlated with the rate at which nondisabled children progress in some areas of syntax and in vocabulary (Akhtar, Dunham, & Dunham, 1991; Harris, Jones, Brookes, & Grant, 1986; Tomasello & Todd, 1983). Many in the social-interactionist camp have taken this correlation to indicate a causal connection between such adult behavior and the child's language development (e.g., Bohannon & Warren-Leubecker, 1989; Hoff-Ginsberg & Shatz, 1982; Menyuk, 1988; Snow, 1984, 1986). These researchers speculate that such parental behavior facilitates language learning because it allows children to limit the number of hypotheses they must entertain about the meanings and uses of the linguistic forms that they hear their parents produce (e.g., Snow, 1984). Even many of those who believe that there are strong, specifically linguistic constraints on the acquisition of linguistic competence believe that children engage in semantic bootstrapping and that following the child's lead, therefore, may facilitate syntactic development (e.g., Pinker, 1990). As a result, it is not surprising that many researchers have been interested in the extent to which parents of children with mental retardation produce semantically contingent language on the assumption that a failure to do so will contribute to the language and communication problems of these children. However, Gleitman and Wanner (1982), among others, have argued that semantic bootstrapping may be of limited utility to the language-learning child. Other interpretations of the correlation between the tendency of parents to follow their children's lead and their children's subsequent progress in language besides those offered by the social interactionists are also possible (Gleitman, Newport, & Gleitman, 1984). For example, certain child characteristics may mediate both the parent's behavior and the child's subsequent rate of developmental progress (Yoder & Kaiser, 1989). In reviewing the following studies, therefore, one must be cautious in concluding that if the parents of children with mental retardation do not follow their child's lead, they have somehow contributed to their child's language and communication problems.

In an investigation by Petersen and Sherrod (1982), the relation between parent and child utterances was examined for children with Down syndrome and for nondisabled children. The two groups of children were matched in terms of MLU and their mothers were similar in terms of CA and years of education. Language samples were collected during dyadic free play. It was found that the two groups of mothers did not differ in the rates at which they produced utterances that were semantically related to their children's behavior. The interpretation that Petersen and Sherrod offered is that this aspect of the linguistic input is well designed for the needs of the child with Down syndrome; that is, these parents do not contribute to the language and communication problems of their children. Again, it should be kept in mind that it is not clear precisely what role this aspect of maternal behavior plays in the development of language and communication for either children with mental retardation or those without.

Moreover, as we stated earlier, the finding of no difference between these two groups of parents does not imply that a change in the linguistic or social environment of persons with mental retardation will be without benefit for them.

In contrast to Petersen and Sherrod, Tannock (1988) found that mothers of 1- to 4-year-olds with Down syndrome were more likely to produce utterances that did not share their children's attentional focus than were mothers of developmental-level-matched, nondisabled children. Tannock also found, however, that many of the noncontingent utterances of the mothers of the children with Down syndrome were designed to re-engage an inactive child. Together with the Petersen and Sherrod (1982) findings, these results suggest that parents of children with Down syndrome are as inclined to match the semantic content of their language to their children's focus of attention as are the parents of nondisabled children, although this is sometimes made difficult by the unusually low activity levels of children with mental retardation. However, the precise role that this parental behavior plays in promoting or inhibiting the development of linguistic and communicative competence in these children was not illuminated by these studies.

Research has also demonstrated that, as is true for the parents of nondisabled children (Hoff-Ginsberg & Shatz, 1982), some parents of children with organically based forms of mental retardation (e.g., Down syndrome) are more likely than others to follow the attentional focus of their children. This tendency is positively correlated with concurrent measures of verbal productivity in their children (Mahoney, 1988). Although such data are consistent with the social-interactionist claim that the extent to which a parent follows a child's lead affects the latter's rate of developmental progress, other interpretations are possible as well. The simple fact remains that a causal role for parental semantic contingency requires an experimental demonstration that variations in such behavior are associated with variations in subsequent child progress in the acquisition of linguistic and/or pragmatic competence.

We now turn to the area of greatest research activity on parental behavior and mental retardation—parental directiveness. As the reader shall see, parental directiveness is closely related to a number of parental behaviors already considered.

PARENTAL DIRECTIVENESS

Research has indicated that some adult caregivers are more directive than others in their interactions with their typically developing children (Akhtar, Dunham, & Dunham, 1991; Della Corte, Benedict, & Klein, 1983; Harris et al., 1986; Jones & Adamson, 1987; McDonald & Pien, 1982; Newport et al., 1977; Tomasello, Mannle, & Kruger, 1986; Tomasello & Todd, 1983). This directiveness is reflected in a number of parental behaviors, most notably the tendency to use directives to act (especially in an imperative form) and lack of responsiveness to the child's interests, activities, needs, and utterances. Many researchers have claimed that this directive style of interaction inhibits nondisabled children's vocabulary learning and perhaps other aspects of their language development (e.g., Menyuk, 1988). From the social-interactionist perspective, this parental style is thought to be detrimental because it is associated with a frequent failure on the part of parents to: (a) follow the child's lead or produce semantically contingent language, and (b) provide linguistically informative feedback following immature utterances from the child (e.g., in the form of expansions, recasts, and repetitions). It is also claimed that highly directive parents may make interaction uninteresting and lead their children to withdraw from or avoid such interactions. As support for the causal role of parental directiveness in nondisabled children's development, social-interactionists point to the many studies that have uncovered a relation between degree of directiveness and these children's subsequent rate of progress in various areas of language and communication (Della Corte et al., 1983; Harris et al., 1986; Jones & Adamson, 1987; Newport et al., 1977; Tomasello et al., 1986; Tomasello & Todd, 1983). It is important to keep in mind, however, that other explanations also fit the observed correlations between parental directiveness and subsequent child progress (Yoder & Kaiser, 1989); thus, the causal connection between the two remains to be demonstrated. Nevertheless, the claims made concerning a possible causal role for a directive style in typical development have led many researchers to examine the hypothesis that part of the delay in language and communicative development seen in children with mental retardation is due to the adoption of this style of interaction by their parents.

Much of this research has focused on the frequency (or rate) with which parents address directives to act (e.g., *Put that away, Could you move over there?*) to their children with mental retardation. Several of these studies (e.g., Hanzlik & Stevenson, 1986; Maurer & Sherrod, 1987) demonstrated that parents address proportionally more directives to their children with mental retardation than is typically seen in interactions between parents and nondisabled children of the same CA (but see Gunn, Clark, & Berry, 1980, for an exception). However, we cannot rule out the possibility in studies involving CA matching that differences between the two groups of parents reflect the fact that each is adjusting their behavior to their children's very different levels of competence in language, communication, and other areas of psychological functioning.

In studies involving developmentally matched groups of children and their parents, the rate of parental directives has sometimes, but not always, been higher for the parents of children with mental retardation than for the parents of the nondisabled matches. On the one hand, Cardoso-Martins and Mervis (1985) found that mothers of prelinguistic 2- to 3-year-olds with Down syndrome produced imperative requests at a higher rate than did: (a) parents of prelinguistic, nondisabled children, (b) parents of nondisabled children matched to the children with Down syndrome on MA, and (c) parents of nondisabled 2- to 3-year-olds. On the other hand, Rondal (1978b) found no difference between the rates of parental directives for children with Down syndrome and nondisabled children who were matched to them on MLU. This difference may be due to the fact that Rondal's subjects were all speaking and were older, on the average, than the children in the Cardoso-Martins and Mervis study. In another study, Gutman and Rondal (1979) examined parental language directed to children with Down syndrome and to nondisabled children matched to them on MLU during dyadic free play. Among the parental behaviors scored was the *mand* (Skinner, 1957), which is equivalent to the category of directives. Gutman and Rondal found that the two groups of parents did not differ in their rates of mand use. Again, these children were more developmentally advanced than those in the Cardoso-Martins and Mervis investigation. Together, these studies suggest that, despite their unusually high rate of directives early in their children's development, the parents of children with Down syndrome come to produce directives at a rate more similar to that of other parents as their children age and mature.

Maurer and Sherrod (1987) were interested not only in the rate at which the parents of children with mental retardation produced directives but also in the conditions under which these parents used directives. These investigators conducted a 2-year, longitudinal study of the dyadic free play of children with Down syndrome and their parents and of nondisabled children and their parents. The children with Down syndrome were 12 months old at the start of the study. The observations were timed so that the comparisons between the groups sometimes involved verbal-age-matched children and sometimes MA-matched children.

Maurer and Sherrod (1987) found that when the children with Down syndrome were 12 months old, their mothers were more likely than the mothers of the nondisabled, MA matches to use directives when the children: (a) engaged in nonstandard toy play, (b) were not attending to them, and (c) failed to comply with a previous directive. By the time the children with Down syndrome were 3 years of age, their mothers were more likely than the mothers of the nondisabled, verbal-age-matched children to issue directives after their children failed to comply. On the basis of these results, Maurer and Sherrod suggested that mothers of children with Down syndrome use directives to make their children conform to CA expectations. What this study cannot tell us is whether this pattern of maternal behavior has any effect on the children's development of linguistic and communicative competence. Moreover, it is important to keep in mind that Maurer and Sherrod made numerous comparisons among the different groups of mothers, with most comparisons revealing no difference. Thus, the differences between mothers of developmentally matched, nondisabled children and children with Down syndrome are not particularly dramatic. This conclusion is supported as well by Tannock's (1988) finding that mothers of children with Down syndrome used directives in response to the same child behaviors as did the mothers of nondisabled children who were matched to the handicapped children in terms of language and cognitive functioning. It is important to recognize that such results in no way demonstrate that parental directives facilitate or inhibit the growth of language and communication in individuals with mental retardation.

It is interesting to note that the Maurer and Sherrod study is one of the few to include fathers as well as mothers. Maurer and Sherrod observed no differences in the directive behavior of the fathers of children with Down syndrome and the fathers of the developmentally matched, nondisabled children. This, too, supports the notion that the linguistic environment of the child with Down syndrome is not very different with regard to parental directives from that of a nondisabled child who is functioning at a similar developmental level.

Parental responsiveness to, and synchrony with, the child is another dimension of directiveness that has been investigated by researchers in the field of mental retardation. The basic assumption of this work has been that directive parents are more interested in imposing their will on, rather than in being attuned to, their children and, as a result, these parents often ignore their children's initiations or fail to adjust their behavior in a way that makes for a good, give-and-take conversation.

One of the earliest studies on parental responsiveness and synchrony was that of Buckhalt et al. (1978), which we described previously. These investigators found that mothers of 9- to 19-month-olds with Down syndrome were less responsive to their children than mothers of CA-matched, nondisabled children were to their children. The index of responsiveness was the frequency of smiling at and vocalizing to the infant. Again, because the two groups of children were matched on CA rather than on developmental level, we do not know whether the parents of the children with Down syndrome were being as responsive as any parents who have children functioning at the developmental level of the children with Down syndrome.

In fact, studies that have included developmental-level-matched groups of children with and without mental retardation have yielded few differences between their parents in terms of responsiveness and synchrony. Petersen and Sherrod (1982) found no difference between the parents of children with Down syndrome and the parents of MLU-matched, nondisabled 1- to 2-year-olds in terms of the frequencies and rates of parental approval, disapproval, and nonjudgmental responses (e.g., imitations, expansions) in parent–child free play. Similarly, Davis, Stroud, and Green (1988) found that the parents of 1½- to 5-year-olds with mental retardation and the parents of language-matched, nondisabled children did not differ in their rates of immediate (i.e., within 1 second) responses to child utterances. This was true in both free play and parental instructional activities in the Davis et al. study. These results strongly suggest that the responsiveness of parents of children with mental retardation is linked to their children's level of linguistic functioning in much the same way as in typically developing populations.

This conclusion is also supported by the results of a recent investigation by Mahoney (1988). In a study of 1- to 3-year-olds with organic forms of mental retardation, Mahoney found differences among the mothers of these children in terms of their tendency to attend and respond to their children's verbal and nonverbal behaviors. These differences were related to concurrent differences in the children's language skills, conversational participation, and physical health. Such findings are consistent with the claim that the mothers of children with mental retardation are responding on the basis of the unique characteristics of their children. What role, if any, parental responsiveness and synchrony play in promoting or inhibiting the development of language and communication in children with mental retardation is not elucidated, however, by any of the studies we have considered.

Other dimensions of parental directiveness have also been investigated by researchers in the field of mental retardation. In a study described previously, Cardoso-Martins and Mervis (1985) examined the possibility that the directiveness of parents of children with mental retardation would also be manifested as a reluctance to use child-centered labeling strategies (e.g., calling a tiger *cat*). These investigators argued that child-centered labeling strategies reflect a parent's attempt to facilitate conversation by talking about the world in a manner that is closer to the child's conception of the world than to the adult's. Their subjects, it will be recalled, were prelinguistic children with Down syndrome and their mothers, as well as nondisabled CA matches, MA matches, and language matches and their mothers. The mother–child dyads engaged in free play with experimenter-provided toys drawn from categories such as cat and ball. One toy from each category was a "true" (i.e., adult) exemplar from the category, another was a "child" exemplar (i.e., an object that children but not adults were likely to include in the category), and another was a nonmember of the category. For the category of *ball*, for example, a rubber ball served as a true exemplar, a round candle as child exemplar, and a frisbee as the nonmember.

Cardoso-Martins and Mervis (1985) found that the mothers of the children with Down syndrome were more similar in their use of child-centered labeling to the mothers of the chronological age-matched children than to either of the other groups of mothers. Although this result is consistent with the view that parents of children with mental retardation are highly directive, Cardoso-Martins and Mervis suggested that the directiveness may reflect an adjustment that is appropriate to the special characteristics of the child with Down syndrome; for example, it may increase the child's participation in the interaction. Moreover, as we have repeatedly seen, this type of study is simply not designed to establish a causal link between the parental behaviors under investigation and children's progress (or lack of progress) in the areas of language and communication.

What accounts for the greater directiveness of parents of children with mental retardation seen in studies such as that of Cardoso-Martins and Mervis? Davis, Stroud, and Green (1988) tested the hypothesis that the directiveness demonstrated by the parents of many children with mental retardation is a manifestation of their adoption of a teaching strategy when interacting with their children. That is, these parents may see their interactions with their children not as a time for play, but rather as an opportunity to instruct their children about objects and events in the world. The subjects in the Davis et al. investigation were a group of 1- to 5-year-olds with mental retardation and their parents and two groups of nondisabled children and their parents. The children with mental retardation were matched on CA to the children in one nondisabled group, and on expressive- and receptive-language levels to the children in the other nondisabled group. The three groups of parents were matched in terms of socioeconomic status, family size, and maternal age. Each parent–child dyad was observed in free play and in an instructional condition in which the parent taught the child how to solve a match-to-sample problem. Various measures of parental language were calculated, including several that were thought to reflect a directive style of interaction (e.g., interruptions of a child utterance, commands to the child, responsiveness to child utterances).

Davis et al. (1988) found that the parents of the children with mental retardation behaved similarly in the free play and instructional settings, whereas the parents of the nondisabled children were less directive in free play than in the instructional condition. As a result, the differences between the parents of the children with mental retardation and the parents of the nondisabled, language-matched children were greater in free play than in the instructional condition. Similar results were reported in a case study by Gunn et al. (1980). Davis et al. interpreted these results as support for their hypothesis.

The work of Mahoney, Fors, and Wood (1990) also supports the hypothesis that the interactional style of highly directive parents is based on the parents' desire to teach their children with mental retardation. Mahoney et al. included two groups of 30-month-olds with Down syndrome and their parents and a group of nondisabled 15-month-olds and their parents. The children in each group were matched on MA and expressive- and receptive-language levels. The two groups of children with Down syndrome differed only in the proportion of conversational turns they took in a dyadic free-play interaction with their mothers; one group took fewer turns than their mothers (the *turn-imbalanced* group), and the other took the same number of turns as their mothers (the *turn-balanced* group). The groups did not differ in terms of maternal age, but the mothers of the nondisabled children were better educated than the other mothers, which, of course, complicates interpretation of any group differences that were observed.

Mahoney et al. (1990) found that the mothers of the children with Down syndrome, especially the turn-imbalanced children, produced directives at a higher rate than did the mothers of the nondisabled children. The rate of parental directives, however, was not related to any measure of the children's interactional behaviors (e.g., response rate, interactive rate). Moreover, the mothers of the children with Down syndrome requested more developmentally advanced actions from their children than the mothers of the nondisabled children did of theirs. Mahoney et al. interpreted this pattern of results as indicating that the directiveness of mothers of children with Down syndrome is not the result of maternal adjustments to the unique characteristics of children with Down syndrome. Instead, this directiveness reflects the parents' desire to push their children with Down syndrome to attempt behaviors that are chronological-age-appropriate. It should be kept in mind, however, that the mothers in this study may have been adjusting their directiveness to child characteristics not measured by the researchers. At the same time, we must stress that the Mahoney et al. data do not address the question of the causal role of directiveness in the development of persons with mental retardation.

There is little doubt that, on the average, the parents of children with mental retardation are more directive than the parents of these children's nondisabled, CA matches. It is also clear that, as a group, the parents of children with mental retardation, at least those children who are prelinguistic, are even more directive than the parents of nondisabled children at the same developmental levels. As mentioned previously, however, demonstrating that the parents of children with mental retardation are more directive than the parents of nondisabled children is not, in and of itself, sufficient to demonstrate that the former contribute to their children's problems in language and communication. Establishing a negative, causal role for excessive parental directives will require an experimental demonstration that variations in such behavior are associated with variations in subsequent child progress in the acquisition of linguistic and/or communicative competence. On many theories (e.g., the theory of parameters described in chapters 2 and 5), evidence of an inhibitory effect of parental directiveness, at least as regards children's acquisition of linguistic competence, is not likely to be forthcoming. It also is worth noting that until the requisite experimental work is done, we cannot rule out the possibility that a highly directive style of parenting will actually turn out to be beneficial for children with mental retardation (even if it turns out to play a negative role, or no role, in the development of nondisabled children).

Another issue unresolved by the studies is whether excessive parental directiveness also characterizes the naturally occurring interactions of parents and their children with mental retardation. That is, because these parents are no doubt sensitive to the special status of their children, they may be directive as a way of getting their children to look their best (i.e., most capable) for the researchers. In addition, these parents may want to demonstrate to the researchers that their children's retardation is not due to poor parenting. In this case, their directiveness would be an attempt to demonstrate that they are able teachers who are highly involved in their children's activities. At the same time, the parents of nondisabled children have nothing to prove and they may not change their behavior when they are observed by a team of researchers. Thus, it is possible that the parents of children with mental retardation are not unusually directive in their typical, daily interactions with their children. Such reactive effects of observation pose a considerable methodological problem for researchers in mental retardation. However, such effects must be considered before we suggest that the parents of children with mental retardation are part of their children's language and communication problems.

In closing this section, it is important to recognize that, despite the emphasis placed on parental directiveness by researchers in mental retardation, directiveness is but one dimension along which the interactive styles of parents can be described. For example, in a factor-analytic study conducted by Mahoney, Finger, and Powell (1985), ratings of 10-minute segments of videotaped dyadic free-play interactions involving 1- to 3-year-olds with organically based mental retardation and their mothers yielded not only a factor of maternal directiveness but also one that reflected the amount of stimulation the mother provided her child and another that reflected her sensitivity to child-state variables. In more recent work, Mahoney (1988) identified additional factors that describe the behavior of mothers of children with mental retardation and showed that different factors are correlated with different child behaviors and characteristics.

Crawley and Spiker (1983) recognized the many facets of parental-interactional style and made the important additional point that parental directiveness in and of itself may not be detrimental to the developmental progress of children with mental retardation. Consistent with this claim, Crawley and Spiker found that some mothers were rated by observers as highly directive and highly responsive when interacting with their 2-year-olds with Down syndrome during free play, and these mothers actually had the most competent children. These directive-plus-responsive mothers also received high ratings for the amount of stimulation they provided for their children and for their expression of positive affect. Although Crawley and Spiker's results do not establish a causal link between the parental and child behaviors observed, they call into question the claim that directiveness per se will be associated with negative outcomes for children with mental retardation. Recent results in the literature on typical development (e.g., Akhtar et al., 1991), have also failed to find a correlation between overall parental directives and the rate of children's language development.

PARENTAL SPEECH ACTS

The parents of children with mental retardation, even those parents who are highly directive, do more with language than simply direct the behavior of their children. A number of researchers have sought to determine whether parents of children with mental retardation perform the same types of speech acts, at the same relative rates, when interacting with their children as do parents of nondisabled children. Unfortunately, this research is difficult to interpret because it has not been based on any explicit hypothesis about which aspects of language and communication development should be affected by such parental behavior. One could speculate that, very early in children's development, they learn about the range of speech acts their language codes, partly as a function of parental input. Later, perhaps, they learn the particular linguistic means whereby speech acts are performed, also partly through their observations of parental speech-act behavior. Although plausible, it is important to keep in mind when reviewing the following studies that there is no convincing evidence that parental behavior plays such a role in nondisabled children's pragmatic development (Abbeduto & Benson, 1992).

Among the several published reports on the speech-act usage of the parents of children with mental retardation is that of Hanzlik and Stevenson (1986). This study included an examination of the speech acts of the mothers of three groups of 1- to 2-year-olds who were matched in terms of CA. The three groups of children were comprised of children with mental retardation, children with mental retardation and cerebral palsy, and typically developing children. No differences were found across the mothers of the three groups of children in terms of their proportional use of the nondirective speech-act categories of praise and verbal interaction. Hanzlik and Stevenson also found no differences between the three groups of mothers in terms of the rate of information-seeking questions. These results are difficult to interpret because, among other things, it is not clear whether the maternal behaviors studied should be expected to vary as a function of the children's capabilities in areas such as language and communication. That is, the nondisabled children, as a group, were more capable—linguistically and communicatively—than were the children with disabilities. Should we have expected the speech-act behavior of these three groups of mothers to reflect the differences in their children? Without an answer to this question, it is simply unclear what we are to make of this study.

In studies in which the children with mental retardation were matched on measures of cognitive or linguistic maturity, no differences in parents' use of questions or nondirective speech acts has emerged. For example, Leifer and Lewis (1983) examined the question-asking of mothers of children with Down syndrome. Two groups of children with Down syndrome and their mothers were included: One group of children was prelinguistic with a CA range of 18 to 23 months; the other had MLUs ranging from 1 to 1.5 and CAs ranging from 42 to 54 months. Also included was a group of nondisabled children and their mothers. The nondisabled children were matched to the younger group of children with Down syndrome on CA and to the older group with Down syndrome in terms of MLU.

The mother–child dyads were videotaped during free play, with maternal questions categorized into five types: (a) test questions (e.g., *What's this?*), (b) requests for information the mother lacked (e.g., *Are you hungry?*), (c) requests for clarification (e.g., *Huh?*), (d) requests for confirmation (e.g., *A ball?* following the child's *A ball*), and (e) directive questions (e.g., *Can you move it?*). Leifer and Lewis found that, although some differences emerged between the CA-matched groups, the parents of the MLU-matched groups of children did not differ on the frequencies or proportions of each question type. Moreover, Leifer and Lewis argued that the differences in maternal question-asking for the age-matched groups reflected maternal adjustments to the very different language abilities of the children in these two groups.

In the previously described study by Tannock (1988), no differences were observed between the mothers of developmental-level matched children with and without Down syndrome in terms of the proportional use of: (a) speech acts that obligated a response from the child, and (b) speech acts that carried no such obligation. Moreover, the two groups of mothers used obligating speech acts under similar conditions. In particular, they were equally likely to produce such acts when their children were not involved in any activity during free play.

The results of the Leifer and Lewis (1983) and Tannock (1988) investigations were also supported by the work of other researchers (e.g., Davis & Oliver, 1980; Mahoney, 1988; Petersen & Sherrod, 1982). Together, these studies strongly suggest that parents of children with mental retardation provide their children exemplars of many types of questions and nondirective speech acts at rates that are typical for the children's linguistic competence and cognitive capabilities. Which aspects of the children's competence and/or performance in these domains affect parent speech-act usage, however, is not clear from these studies. Moreover, it is surprising that no attempt has been made to examine the relation between parental speech-act behavior and various aspects of children's functioning in the pragmatic domain, because one would expect that parental adjustments in this area would be most closely tied to child pragmatic knowledge and skill. Finally, whether these adjustments in parental speech-act usage are facilitative of, or necessary for, any particular pragmatic or linguistic developments cannot be determined, given the designs employed in the studies we have considered.

VERBAL ROUTINES

Social-interactionists (e.g., Conti-Ramsden & Friel-Patti, 1987; Snow, Perlmann, & Nathan, 1987) have proposed that the acquisition of linguistic and communicative competence by nondisabled children is facilitated by their participation in highly routinized activities with their parents (e.g., the repeated reading of a favorite book, games such as peek-a-boo). For instance, these researchers suggested that the children can devote more of their limited information-processing capacities to the linguistic analysis of parental utterances because they need attend only minimally to the highly familiar, nonverbal aspects of the interaction. On the strength of such claims, researchers have begun to examine the routine verbal interactions of children with mental retardation and their parents. It is important to note that the social-interactionists' claims about verbal routines are at odds with theories of development that allot only a minimal role to general information-processing and learning strategies (e.g., the theory of parameters discussed in chapter 2). Moreover, it should be kept in mind that there is no experimental evidence demonstrating a causal role for participation in verbal routines in the acquisition of linguistic or communicative competence. Once again, therefore, we must be cautious in concluding that verbal routines hold the key to explaining, even in part, the occurrence of language and communication problems in individuals with mental retardation.

One of the more interesting studies in this area is that of Yoder and Davies (1992). These investigators tested the hypothesis that children with mental retardation, many of whom produce speech low in intelligibility because of various articulatory difficulties, would be more intelligible in routine interactions with their parents than in nonroutines. Such a result could arise, it has been argued (e.g., Conti-Ramsden & Friel-Patti, 1987), because children can devote more of their limited attentional resources to planning their utterances (rather than to processing nonverbal information) in a familiar context than in an unfamiliar one. The subjects in the Yoder and Davies investigation were children with mental retardation who ranged in CA from 36 to 76 months and who had MLUs between 1.01 and 2.0. The subjects were videotaped while engaged in dyadic free play with their mothers. Verbal routines were identified from the videotape and the proportions of child utterances that were intelligible to a naive transcriber of the tapes for the routine and nonroutine portions of each interaction were compared. Yoder and Davies defined routines as "conversations that (a) recur frequently, (b) have a predictable and recognizable sequence, (c) have at least one spoken turn for each interlocutor, (d) have content that is limited to a small set of variations" (p. 78). Examples included recitations of the ABCs and question–answer sequences such as *What's this?*

In fact, Yoder and Davies found that child utterances were more likely to be intelligible to the transcriber when they occurred in routines than when they occurred in nonroutine interactions. However, in subsequent work, they discovered that the children's articulation was no better in the routine than in the nonroutine interactions. Instead, the greater intelligibility observed in the former interactions was due to the fact that the transcribers had more contextual cues available for deciphering the children's utterances in those situations than in the nonroutine situations. Of course, this finding does not support the social-interactionist claim that routine interactions allow children to direct their cognitive resources to the most difficult or important aspects of the communicative interaction.

QUANTITY OF PARENTAL TALK

In several of the studies discussed previously (Davis & Oliver, 1980; Davis et al., 1988; Rondal, 1978b), the possibility was examined that the parents of children with mental retardation talk less to their children than the parents of typically developing children talk to their children. The assumption in these investigations is that a lower frequency of parental talk contributes to the language and communication difficulties of children with mental retardation. However, this assumption is highly questionable. Although children must certainly have some exposure to their native language to be able to acquire competence in it, there is no evidence that variations in frequency of parental talk have an effect on the development of nondisabled children, with the exception of nearly complete deprivation of input (see chapter 2). In the studies involving individuals with mental retardation and their parents, the frequency of talk for these parents, as a group, is far from complete deprivation. In fact, most of these parents appear to be within the normal range of variation for frequency of child-directed talk. As a result, it is not clear what these studies tell us about the language and communication problems of this population.

Davis and Oliver (1980) compared the dyadic free play of children with mental retardation and their mothers to that of nondisabled children and their mothers. The children in both groups were prelinguistic or at the one-word stage. Several etiologies were represented in the group with mental retardation. Davis and Oliver found that the mothers of the children with mental retardation produced vocalizations (i.e., language and nonlanguage utterances) more often and at a faster rate than did the other mothers. Davis and Oliver interpreted this to indicate that mothers of children with mental retardation are intrusive and present their children with a processing task that is more difficult than necessary. This conclusion is not warranted, however, given our previous remarks.

In contrast to the Davis and Oliver (1980) study, other investigators have not found that mothers of children with mental retardation differ from mothers of nondisabled children in terms of the quantity of their talk. For instance, Rondal (1978b) found no difference in terms of the number of words produced in a 30-minute free-play session for mothers of children with Down syndrome and mothers of language-matched, nondisabled children. Davis et al. (1988) also failed to find a difference between mothers of language-matched children with and without mental retardation on several measures of the quantity of their talk.

SUMMARY

The linguistic and communicative environments that parents provide their children with mental retardation differ in many respects from what is typical for nondisabled children of the same CAs. This, no doubt, is due to the fact that these parents are trying to communicate with children whose linguistic and communicative competencies are, on the average, significantly below CA expectations. Thus, the parents of children with mental retardation display many of the features of CDL that are claimed by social-interactionists to simplify for the child the task of becoming linguistically and communicatively competent. Moreover, these features of CDL are linked to the same dimensions of child competence and developmental status for the parents of children with mental retardation as they are for the parents of nondisabled children. Many of the discourse and interactional behaviors displayed by the parents of children with mental retardation are also linked more closely to their children's current level of competence than to their CA.

Nevertheless, differences have been observed on occasion between the parents of children with and without mental retardation who are matched on some measure of linguistic or cognitive functioning. These differences have typically been interpreted as evidence that parents contribute to the language or communicative delays that characterize children with mental retardation. Differences in parental directiveness have been the source of the most speculation in this regard. It is important to keep in mind, however, that even when differences have been found between parents of developmentally matched children, they have been small in magnitude. Further, the number of studies in which differences were found between the parents of developmentally matched groups of children are balanced by studies in which no differences were found. In summary, the linguistic and communicative environment of the child with mental retardation, at least within the context of the family, is more similar to (than different from) that of the typically developing child.

Whether one focuses on the typical or on the unique aspects of the linguistic and communicative environment provided by the parents of children with mental retardation, the simple fact remains that there is no evidence that parental behavior matters; that is, that it inhibits or promotes the development of these children. In no study that we considered was the design appropriate for establishing any relation, let alone a causal relation, between the parental behavior of interest and the children's subsequent progress (or lack of progress) in acquiring further linguistic or communicative competence. Researchers in this area must move to the use of experimental and longitudinal designs if they hope to establish the existence of such causal relations. Moreover, we argue that their selection of parental and child behaviors for study needs to be better justified in terms of an adequate theory of typical development and explicit hypotheses about the precise nature of the language and communication problems of persons with mental retardation.

9

*Language and
Communication Intervention*

We have shown that most persons with mental retardation experience problems in acquiring and using nearly every facet of language, although their problems are often greater in some areas than in others. In this chapter, we discuss the effectiveness of various attempts to treat these language and communication problems. We begin by outlining decisions that must be made when planning these interventions. These decisions concern: (a) the assessment process, (b) the skills and knowledge to be imparted to the subjects, (c) the approach taken to instruction, and (d) the criteria for evaluating the success of the intervention. Next, we describe recent research on the treatment of problems in mastering the linguistic system. We then consider interventions that have focused less on promoting the acquisition of the linguistic system and more on improving the pragmatic knowledge and/or linguistic communication of individuals with mental retardation. In the final section, we consider some issues that have not received adequate attention from researchers concerned with treating the language and communication problems of persons with mental retardation.

DECISIONS INVOLVED IN PLANNING
AN INTERVENTION

Assessment

An adequate intervention requires a comprehensive assessment of the subject's strengths and weaknesses in all areas relevant to functioning in the domain of language (Miller, 1983). This requires a description of the subject's progress in each of the components of language (i.e., phonology, semantics, syntax, and morphology). It is only through such a comprehensive assessment that one can determine the nature of the subject's language problems and, thus, the type of intervention likely to be effective. To illustrate, suppose that two children are producing largely two-word utterances when, on the basis of their chronological ages, they should be producing longer, more complex utterances. Despite the superficial similarity in these children's problems, they may have different sources. For one child, the problems may reflect difficulties in the area of acquiring the linguistic means of encoding three-element or longer propositions. The other child, in contrast, may have the linguistic wherewithal needed to produce longer utterances but may avoid them because of the low intelligibility of his or her speech (i.e., the shorter the utterance, the less the chance that a syllable will be unintelligible to a listener). Clearly, these two children would require very different interventions (Fey, 1986). Thus, even an intervention designed to improve performance in one component of language (e.g., syntax) requires information about strengths and weaknesses in other facets of language functioning.

A comprehensive language assessment also needs to target pragmatic deficits (Fey, 1986; Leonard & Fey, 1991). That is, although developments in the pragmatic domain do not appear to function as prerequisites for acquisitions in grammar (Curtiss, 1988b; Yamada, 1990; chapter 5), children can only make appropriate communicative use of acquired linguistic forms if they possess the requisite pragmatic knowledge (Leonard & Fey, 1991). Moreover, pragmatic deficits may sometimes impede the treatment of problems in syntax or in other components of language (Fey, 1986; Leonard & Fey, 1991). For example, many individuals with mental retardation talk infrequently (Yoder & Davies, 1990, 1992). This reticence may reflect their limited (for their CA) knowledge of, or interest in, the social uses of language. Individuals who talk infrequently make it difficult to use syntax-teaching techniques that involve the provision of contingent feedback from a clinician, teacher, or parent (Warren & Kaiser, 1986). For reticent individuals, then, the frequency of talking will need to be increased before a meaningful, syntactically based intervention can be begun (Fey, 1986).

A comprehensive assessment must also tap both expressive and receptive language because of the possibility of asynchrony between the two modalities (Miller, 1983). For example, Miller and Chapman (e.g., Chapman, 1981a; Miller, 1987; Miller & Chapman, 1984) argued: (a) that some persons with mental retardation exhibit delays of equivalent magnitude in the two modalities, whereas others evidence more severe impairments in expressive language than in receptive language, and (b) that the two profiles dictate different types of interventions (Chapman, 1981a; Miller, 1987; Miller & Chapman, 1984). Although the data needed to prove the existence of these two profiles are lacking (see our comments in chapter 5), these profiles are consistent with the notion that the skills involved in using grammatical knowledge for speaking and listening are different and that individuals may differ in these performance skills.

For persons with mental retardation, a comprehensive assessment must extend far beyond the domain of language to domains such as cognition and social functioning (Abbeduto & Nuccio, 1989; Abbeduto & Rosenberg, 1992; Gallagher, 1991a; Miller, 1983; Rusch & Karlan, 1983). For example, there are cognitive prerequisites for the acquisition of the nonargument aspects of word meaning (Connell, 1987; Curtiss, 1988a; Rice, 1984; Yamada, 1990). Such prerequisites need to be in place before the relevant lexical–semantic targets can be taught. Moreover, there are likely to be cognitive and social skills that, if they are deficient, will prevent a subject from using trained linguistic forms in pragmatically appropriate ways (Abbeduto & Rosenberg, 1992; Leonard & Fey, 1991). In fact, there is evidence, albeit from typically developing children, that intervention-induced gains in certain cognitive skills sometimes lead to gains in nontargeted pragmatic skills (e.g., Steckol & Leonard, 1981). At the same time, however, there is substantial evidence (see chapters 2 and 5) that many cognitive abilities (assessed by Piagetian, standardized IQ, and information-processing measures) "are neither sufficient nor necessary for the emergence and development of grammar" (Yamada, 1990, pp. 109–110). Thus, grammatical targets can be attacked directly in intervention, that is, without prior training in the cognitive domain.

Unfortunately, comprehensive, multidomain assessments of the type we are advocating are seldom conducted in published intervention studies (Rusch & Karlan, 1983). As a result, it is probably the case that the approach to treatment and/or the aspects of language targeted for treatment are inappropriate for at least some of the subjects. This means that the effectiveness of many interventions is evaluated under less than optimal conditions. Moreover, assessments in the grammatical domain should be based on viable theories of mature, linguistic competence such as that of Chomsky (see chapter 2). In practice, however, language assessments prior to and following an intervention are seldom informed by relevant work in linguistics, which makes it difficult to interpret the importance of any gains in performance associated with the intervention.

Targets of Intervention

After assessment, the next step in planning an intervention is to decide which skills or knowledge to target for improvement. That is, an individual with mental retardation who comes to the intervention will probably lack many of the skills and much of the knowledge acquired by his or her typically developing peers. Assuming that it is impractical to target all of these areas of weakness, which should be the focus of the intervention? Moreover, for any language skill that is targeted, there may be earlier steps along the path to acquisition. Do these earlier steps need to be targeted before tackling the language skills of real interest?

There have been two basic approaches to selecting the targets of language intervention: (a) the developmental, and (b) the remedial (Fey, 1986). According to Fey (1986), a developmental logic dictates that the "normal sequence of development should serve as the basis for specific goal selection" (p. 101). For example, typically developing children do not master grammatical morphemes such as the plural -s until after they have begun to produce combinations of content words (e.g., *more milk*). A developmental logic, therefore, would dictate that a child at the single-word stage be trained on multiword combinations prior to the introduction of grammatical morphemes as training targets. As another example, children who are developing language normally usually acquire the present progressive marker -ing (e.g., as in *he is running*) before the past tense marker -ed (e.g., as in *he walked*). A developmental logic would dictate targeting the former morpheme for work first with the latter being introduced only at some later point in the intervention. This developmental approach is based on the assumption that the process by which language is acquired is the same for persons with and without mental retardation. In light of this assumption, it is argued that a training sequence that recapitulates typical development is the simplest and most natural relative to the way in which learners approach the task of acquiring their language (e.g., Bloom & Lahey, 1978; Bricker & Bricker, 1974; Miller & Yoder, 1974).

In contrast, a remedial logic dictates that targets should be selected so as to have the greatest, quickest impact on communication (e.g., Caro & Snell, 1989; Guess, Keogh, & Sailor, 1978). In the remedial approach, for example, clinicians might analyze the subject's daily routines and target those skills that are required in the greatest number of interactions or in those interactions that are deemed the most important to his or her adaptive functioning.

Both the developmental and the remedial approaches have their limitations. For example, Connell (1987) argued that a strong reliance on typical development when selecting targets may be misguided because, although for many linguistic forms we know when typically developing children reach a level of complete mastery, we know little about when they begin the process of acquiring any particular form. According to Connell, the latter data, if available, would provide a better basis for selecting the targets of intervention than would the data on when mastery is reached.

A limitation of the remedial approach is that there are few theoretically motivated criteria for deciding in advance which targets will have the quickest, greatest impact on the communicative performance and adaptive functioning of individuals with mental retardation (Fey, 1986). As a result, target selection on this approach is often based on trial and error and the clinician's intuition, although recent work on the pragmatic aspects of language use may eventually provide a more rational basis for the selection of targets (Gallagher, 1991a;

Leonard & Fey, 1991). In particular, work in pragmatics may eventually lead to the identification of those pragmatic skills which, if deficient, have the most pervasive negative effects on communicative performance or lead to the most negative evaluations by communicative partners (Gallagher, 1991a; Leonard & Fey, 1991).

Interestingly, there have been few direct comparisons of the effectiveness of interventions differing only in their approaches to the selection of targets. As a result, there is no evidence that one approach leads to faster acquisition of targets or to a greater and more rapid improvement in communication than the other (Fey, 1986). In practice, clinicians probably rely on a combination of developmental and remedial approaches (Leonard & Fey, 1991; Warren & Kaiser, 1988).

Instructional Approaches

Language interventions can be classified as *didactically oriented* or *milieu oriented* (Fey, 1986; Kaiser, Yoder, & Keetz, 1992; Leonard & Fey, 1991; Schwartz, 1987; Warren & Kaiser, 1986, 1988). In the didactic approach, the course of the interaction is controlled largely by the therapist (e.g., speech-language clinicians, teachers). For example, the therapist might show the subject pictures of objects and elicit an imitation of the label for each picture by saying something like *This is an apple. Say "apple."* In addition to the high degree of control exerted by the therapist, didactic approaches (Warren & Kaiser, 1988) typically involve: (a) reliance on massed trials (i.e., numerous, consecutive trials on a small set of linguistic targets), (b) a high rate of differential rewards (i.e., desirable behaviors are rewarded at a rate approaching 100%, whereas undesirable behaviors seldom if ever receive rewards), and (c) administration of the intervention procedures within the context of a dyadic interaction involving the therapist and the subject in a therapy room (as opposed to the subject's classroom, work place, or home).

Most didactic interventions have been based on operant or social-learning theory (Rusch & Karlan, 1983; Warren, 1987; Warren & Kaiser, 1986). Operant theory is most closely associated with Skinner (1974) and is based on the notion that behaviors that are followed consistently by positive events, or reinforcement, will become part of a person's behavior repertoire, whereas those behaviors that are not reinforced or that lead to negative events will be eliminated from the person's repertoire. Social-learning theory is most closely associated with Bandura (e.g., Bandura, 1977) and differs from operant theory in claiming that much of what is learned is acquired through observation of other people. Reinforcement is also important in social-learning theory in that it is thought that people incorporate into their repertoires those behaviors for which they are reinforced or for which they see other people being reinforced.

A number of factors have led to a decline in the popularity of the didactic approach, especially in its operant variants, and the rise of milieu approaches to language intervention. One such factor is the obvious failure of operant theory and related learning theories to account for the phenomena of language acquisition in typically developing children. Work on Child Directed Language (CDL) (see chapter 8), although stressing possible environmental influences on language acquisition, has also played a role. In particular, this work led interventionists to abandon the concept of reinforcement contingencies in favor of a search for the presumably special, pedagogical characteristics of the linguistic and social environment. Perhaps the most important factor has been the finding that although didactic interventions lead to substantial gains in performance on the targeted aspects of language within the therapeutic context, they have little impact on: (a) the subject's language performance in everyday interactions, (b) other nontargeted aspects of the linguistic system, and (c) the subject's ability to acquire new linguistic knowledge and skills (Kaiser, Yoder, & Keetz, 1992; Leonard & Fey, 1991; Warren & Kaiser, 1986, 1988; Warren & Rogers-Warren, 1983).

In large measure, milieu approaches represent an extension of work on CDL (see chapter 8). In milieu approaches, the intervention procedures are implemented within contexts in which the subject normally spends a substantial portion of his or her day, such as the classroom, and the agents of change are often those people with whom the child interacts on a daily basis, such as teachers (Hart & Rogers-Warren, 1978; Kaiser et al., 1992; Schwartz, 1987; Warren & Kaiser, 1988; Warren & Rogers-Warren, 1986). This reflects the belief that children normally learn language during the course of social interaction (Fey, 1986). In addition, claims that certain features of CDL play a causal role in typically developing children's acquisition of language (see chapter 8) led to the notion that an intervention should display these features as well (Hart & Rogers-Warren, 1978; Schwartz, 1987; Warren & Kaiser, 1988). For example, it has been claimed that CDL is sensitive to the interests of the child; that is, adults talk about what children are interested in and attending to (Hoff-Ginsberg & Shatz, 1982; Snow, 1984). Thus, a number of milieu approaches use the subject's spontaneously occurring attempts to communicate an idea as an opportunity to teach him or her more sophisticated means of expressing the same idea. We consider research on milieu approaches in detail later. It is worth noting here, however, that the role of social interaction and CDL appears to be minimal for many achievements in language (see chapters 2, 5, and 8) and, thus, it is unlikely that milieu-oriented interventions will be a panacea for the language and communication problems characteristic of persons with mental retardation.

Although the milieu approaches emerged because of what was considered the failure of didactic interventions, there have been few direct comparisons of the effectiveness of the two approaches (Schwartz, 1987). One comparison is that of Yoder, Kaiser, and Alpert (1989), who compared the effectiveness of a milieu technique (i.e., incidental teaching, which will be described in a subsequent section) with a popular didactic intervention program, the Communication Training Program of Waryas and Stremel-Campbell (1982). The subjects, who were forty 2- to 7-year-olds with mental retardation ranging from borderline to severe and MLUs from 1 to 4.72, were randomly assigned to the two interventions. Various measures of productive and receptive language were taken before, during, and after the 60-session intervention. The intervention sessions were conducted every school day with about 10 minutes of intervention devoted to each child per session.

Yoder et al. (1989) found that both interventions led to improvements on many of the language measures; there were no overall differences at the end of treatment between the groups receiving the different interventions. However, when the developmental status of the subjects was taken into account, an interesting difference between the two interventions emerged; namely, the children who were most linguistically advanced benefitted more from the didactic approach than from the milieu approach, whereas the reverse was true for the children who were the least linguistically advanced. It is not entirely clear why this pattern of results should have emerged and, therefore, these results should be replicated before any definitive conclusions are reached. Nevertheless, it is important to keep in mind that there may be no one best approach to language intervention. Instead, different approaches may be needed for different types of subjects or to teach different aspects of language.

Evaluating the Effectiveness of an Intervention

The ultimate goal of intervention is not simply to have the subjects learn the specific exemplars included in training or improve in speaking and listening only in the context in which the intervention is conducted (Caro & Snell, 1989). Instead, most interventionists are interested in promoting generalized change, or simply generalization (Fey, 1986). In fact, most intervention studies involving persons with mental retardation include specific procedures to promote generalization, or at least measure whether generalization has occurred (Rusch & Karlan, 1983; Stokes & Baer, 1977; Warren, 1987).

But what is generalization? For most interventionists, especially those working within an operant framework, there are two types of generalization: (a) *stimulus* generalization, and (b) *response* generalization (Rusch & Karlan, 1983). The former refers to the use of a trained language skill under conditions different from training. For example, the use of a trained word or phrase with a partner other than the therapist, within the context of an activity different from that of training, or in a physical setting other than the location in which the intervention was conducted all reflect stimulus generalization. In contrast, response generalization refers to the use of a language behavior that is structurally or functionally similar but not identical to a trained behavior. If, for example, a child was trained to produce the agent–action sentences *baby cry*, *dog run*, and *man jump*, the child's production of the novel (i.e., nontrained) *girl drink* would be an instance of response generalization. Promoting these two types of generalization is thought by many to be simply a matter of introducing sufficient variability into the training. It is assumed, for example, that stimulus generalization can be promoted by having more than one trainer or by embedding training in multiple activities, and so on, whereas response generalization can be promoted by presenting a large number of exemplars of the rule or concept of interest (e.g., Courtright & Courtright, 1976; Goldstein, 1983; Hedge & Geirut, 1979; Spradlin & Siegel, 1982; Stremel-Campbell & Campbell, 1985).

In recent years, a number of researchers (e.g., Connell, 1987) have argued that response and stimulus generalization, as typically defined, represent rather meager goals for language intervention. The occurrence of response generalization, for instance, often means only that the subject is not simply reproducing—in rote fashion—utterances modeled by the therapist. Similarly, the occurrence of stimulus generalization often means only that the subject has recognized that targets of intervention have some applicability outside of the specifics of the intervention setting. Many researchers believe that an intervention should have a greater impact on the subject's knowledge of language and ability to acquire new linguistic knowledge and skills.

Johnston (1988) has been a particularly outspoken critic of the way in which generalization has traditionally been measured and promoted. In fact, Johnston did not accept as generalization the mere production of a novel utterance or a trained utterance in a novel context. She argued that generalization has occurred if and only if there has been a broadening or extension of the rules or categories underlying the subject's linguistic performances. The following are examples of generalization in this sense:

1. A pattern that is first tied to a specific lexical item comes to be used with a variety of words. This form of generalization has occurred if, for example, a child who uses *is* as his or her only auxiliary or copular verb comes to abstract a category that includes other forms of the word *be*.

2. A category is redefined. This form of generalization has occurred if, for instance, a child who uses the grammatical morpheme for past tense only with change-of-state verbs comes to recognize that this marker provides a means of marking other types of predicates as well.

3. A linguistic element is assigned to a category. This form of generalization has occurred if a child who uses a particular word (e.g., *chase*) comes to recognize the category to which the word belongs (e.g., verb) and, as a result, extends to it all the distributional privileges of that category (e.g., tense marking).

It is important to recognize that not every instance of novel language use would qualify as generalization in Johnston's view; for example:

> Given that a child (a) has said *Mommy go, kitty eat,* and *Daddy run,* (b) has produced these utterances via an Agent + Action rule, and (c) has an Agent category that includes *birdie* and an action category that includes *drink,* the utterances *Mommy run* or *birdie drink* are not remarkable. They represent no developmental change at all, merely the application of available schemes to a new communicative task. (1988, pp. 320-321)

Johnston (1988) also argued that generalization, in her sense, can occur only if the experiences provided by the interventionist are matched to the subject's current state of knowledge. The finding that the effectiveness of many interventions depends on the developmental level of the subject (e.g., Friedman & Friedman, 1980; Warren & Rogers-Warren, 1983; Yoder, Kaiser, & Alpert, 1989) is consistent with this claim. Unfortunately, implementation of Johnston's approach to the promotion of generalization is difficult because we lack data about the types of input that are important for producing particular changes in language knowledge. As we have seen, however, the work on parameter setting conducted by Chomsky and others (e.g., Lightfoot, 1991) offers the promise of such data.

Warren and Kaiser (1986) have also been critical of the limited way in which generalization has been conceptualized in language interventions involving persons with mental retardation. In particular, they argued that language interventions should have generalized effects in the sense of leading the subject to employ more effective strategies for acquiring new linguistic knowledge. In this case, generalization would be manifested as an increased rate of developmental progress after the intervention. In terms of improving mastery of the linguistic system, such generalized effects are likely to occur only if the targets of intervention exemplify the "core" rules of mature grammatical competence (Connell, 1987)—rules that, once acquired, allow other rules to be deduced or work to set parameters (see chapter 2).

In reality, there are few published reports of interventions involving persons with mental retardation that have measured or tried to promote generalization in the ways proposed by Johnston (1988) or Warren and Kaiser (1986). Instead, researchers have usually evaluated the effectiveness of their intervention by focusing on response generalization as it has been defined traditionally—that is, as the use of novel exemplars of the category or rule targeted in the intervention (Rusch & Karlan, 1983; Warren, 1987). In addition, researchers in this area have seldom been concerned with whether intervention-related improvements in the trained modality (e.g., the expressive) transfer to the untrained modality or whether such transfer is limited, instead, by various performance factors (Connell, 1987; Warren, 1987). Further, in most intervention studies, generalization is tested through procedures designed to explicitly elicit or prompt the behaviors of interest, rather than by analyzing the spontaneous occurrence of the behaviors in the subjects' everyday interactions (Warren, 1987). These limitations should be kept in mind as one considers the studies described here.

PROMOTING THE ACQUISITION
OF LINGUISTIC KNOWLEDGE

In this section, we consider research on interventions designed to promote the acquisition of linguistic forms and contents by persons with mental retardation. We begin by examining didactic approaches to training vocabulary and syntactic–semantic mappings. For the most part, these approaches were based on the assumption that linguistic forms and contents can be taught outside of a naturalistic social interaction, without provision of information about the pragmatic functions of those forms and contents (Fey, 1986), an assumption that has been criticized by many researchers (e.g., Hart & Rogers-Warren, 1978; Warren & Kaiser, 1986, 1988).

Research on vocabulary instruction conducted within a didactic framework has been largely concerned with the impact of variations in stimulus conditions on learning and generalization. For example, Welch and Pear (1980) were interested in whether the type of stimuli used to teach labels for concrete objects affected the extent to which persons with mental retardation used the labels to refer to the appropriate objects in their natural environments. Their subjects were children with moderate to severe mental retardation who were functioning at a 2- to 4-year level. Welch and Pear found greater generalization to the natural environment when training involved real objects rather than schematic drawings or photographs of the objects. This is an important finding because of the popularity of two-dimensional representations over real objects in vocabulary instruction (e.g., Biberdorf & Pear, 1977; Olenick & Pear, 1980; Stephens, Pear, Wray, & Jackson, 1975). Notice, however, that Welch and Pear were interested in a rather limited type of generalization (Johnston, 1988). Moreover, for some of their subjects, the nature of the training stimuli had little effect on generalization. The reader interested in other didactic approaches to vocabulary instruction should see Anderson and Spradlin (1980), Garcia, Guess, and Byrnes (1973), Waldo, Guess, and Flanagan (1982), and Zwitman and Sonderman (1979).

Several intervention studies have involved attempts to train persons with mental retardation who exhibit limited production of multiword utterances to produce particular types of multiword, syntactic–semantic patterns. For example, Leonard (1975) used an approach based on social-learning theory (e.g., Bandura, 1977) in an attempt to teach 3- to 4-year-olds with mild mental retardation (of unknown etiology) who were at the one-word stage to express two-word semantic relations such as agent–object. In this study, the experimenter asked an adult model to describe various events that were enacted with people and objects (e.g., a man sitting in a chair, a baby doll falling). The experimenter reinforced the model for correct (i.e., semantically appropriate two-word) descriptions (e.g., *man sit, baby fall*). The subjects were subsequently asked to describe the events and they, too, were reinforced for correct descriptions. Leonard also implemented several variations of the procedure across subjects. For example, some subjects heard only utterances expressing agentive relations, whereas others heard utterances expressing a range of semantic relations (i.e., agentive, dative, instrumental, and objective).

Leonard (1975) found that each variant of the training procedure improved performance relative to a control group in terms of performance on a prompted production test (i.e., *Tell me what's happening here*) involving pictures and enactments of events not involved in training. Leonard also found that the children, regardless of training condition, made the greatest progress in their expression of agentive relations. This suggests that there may be something particularly salient about the agent role or that the expression of the agent role involves linguistic mappings (e.g., its position in the utterance) that are inherently simpler for young children with mental retardation.

What we do not know from the Leonard (1975) study is the extent to which (a) the gains that the children made in the intervention were extended to naturally occurring interactions, and (b) the children expressed the trained relations spontaneously (i.e., without the prompt *Tell me what's happening here*). There is reason to believe, however, that the gains promoted by the type of intervention Leonard conducted may not be limited to prompted performance in the therapeutic context. This is suggested by the results of a study by Prelock and Panagos (1980). These investigators found that modeling of agent–action–object sentences led to the spontaneous production of such sentences outside the laboratory by individuals with severe mental retardation who had MAs similar to those of Leonard's subjects. Further, although Spiegel (1983) did not use a modeling approach, he too found that training two- and three-word semantic relations within a didactic context led to improvements in the productive language (as measured by MLU) of adolescents with severe mental retardation in their daily interactions.

Goldstein, Angelo, and Mousetis (1987) designed an intervention to increase the use of two- and three-word utterances expressing object–location relations by individuals with mental retardation. These investigators were interested in the utility of a *matrix* approach for determining the range and types of exemplars that need to be presented so that a subject can abstract a syntactic rule (Connell, 1987; Leonard & Fey, 1991; Johnston, 1988). In this approach, a matrix is devised to represent all of the utterances of a particular syntactic type that can be formed from some limited pool of linguistic elements. A simple example is provided in Fig. 9.1. If one is targeting mastery of an object–location pattern, as Goldstein et al. did, the matrix in Fig. 9.1 yields a total of nine possible

LOCATIONS

		bed	couch	TV
	balloon	balloon on bed	balloon on couch	balloon on TV
OBJECTS	comb	comb on bed	comb on couch	comb on TV
	key	key on bed	key on couch	key on TV

FIG. 9.1.   An example of a matrix for generating object-location utterances for training.

utterances (e.g., *balloon on bed, balloon on couch, comb on bed*). In Goldstein et al.'s matrix approach, training began with the combination in the upper left cell of the matrix and continued with each cell along the diagonal (e.g., *balloon on bed* followed by *comb on couch*) until the subject demonstrated response generalization. If, for example, a subject said *balloon on couch* or *comb on bed* after being trained only on *balloon bed*, Goldstein et al. would have credited him or her with response generalization. Before proceeding, it is important to recognize that this is a limited type of generalization in that such novel utterances may reflect the acquisition of limited scope formulae rather than true syntactic rules (Johnston, 1988).

The subjects in the Goldstein et al. (1987) investigation were 3 individuals with severe mental retardation whose CAs ranged from 7;5 to 18;11. All were producing some multiword utterances, with their MLUs ranging from 1.07 to 2.23. None of the subjects spontaneously produced object–location (e.g., *balloon bed*) or object–preposition–location (e.g., *balloon on bed*) utterances, which were the targets of training.

Both receptive and expressive training were conducted. The former involved acting out sentences (e.g., the experimenter told the subject to put a toy balloon on a toy bed), whereas the latter involved eliciting a description of an event performed by the experimenter (e.g., after the experimenter put the balloon on the bed, he or she asked the subject *What did I do?*). In both types of training, the correct responses were taught through a combination of modeling and prompted imitation, with massed trials on each training target. The subject's comprehension and production of a large set of nouns were evaluated, and matrices were formed for each subject, including both familiar words (i.e., those on which criterion was met in both a comprehension and a production test) and unfamiliar words (i.e., those on which criterion was not met).

The major results of the Goldstein et al. (1987) investigation were as follows. All of the subjects produced novel (i.e., untrained) combinations of familiar words after training with only a few combinations of familiar words. Moreover, the subjects produced novel combinations composed of unfamiliar words after being trained on only a single word combination involving familiar words and a single combination involving unfamiliar words. As more and more combinations were trained, however, it was necessary to include more and more examples of unfamiliar word combinations. Goldstein et al. demonstrated cross-modal transfer for the subjects; that is, training in expression often led to gains in comprehension, and vice versa, a finding that is consistent with claims (e.g., chapter 2) that a common grammar underlies both performance modes. Goldstein et al. also provided evidence that these improvements transferred to nontraining settings and new trainers.

Despite the apparent success of Goldstein et al.'s (1987) matrix approach, it is important to keep in mind our comments about the limited types of generalization demonstrated. Moreover, the gains that the subjects made came after considerable investment of time and effort on the part of the trainer and subjects; subjects were trained on an individual basis 20 to 30 minutes a day, 4 days a week, for an average of over 7 months.

Warren and Rogers-Warren (1983) were interested in the types of generalization that were prompted by operant-learning-based, didactic approaches to intervention. Their subjects were 6 institutionalized individuals with severe mental retardation, whose CAs ranged from 8.1 to 20.8 years. The approach to training as well as its targets were drawn from a program developed by Guess, Sailor, and Baer (1978). In this program, the trainer presents a stimulus (e.g., an object to be described, a question) and then shapes the correct response through the use of reinforcers (e.g., praise, edibles, the object named in the targeted response) and modeling of the adult form. Warren and Rogers-Warren used the program to train a total of 73 different two-, three-, and four-word forms. These forms included: (a) *I want* + noun, (b) *I want* + verb, (c) *I want you* + verb, (d) *What that?*, and (e) *What doing?*. As is evident from these examples, the Guess et al. program targets formulaic language and limited-scope sentence patterns. Given this rather limited input, it would be surprising if the participants in such a program could make broad syntactic generalizations.

Warren and Rogers-Warren (1983) found that the intervention led to response and stimulus generalization as traditionally defined; that is, the subjects produced novel, nonimitative exemplars in nontraining settings (e.g., mealtime) for 56% of the trained forms. More interesting, however, were Warren and Rogers-Warren's findings concerning the limits of this generalization:

1. The subjects were most likely to generalize the shorter, less linguistically complex forms on which they were trained. This suggests that generalization may be limited by a subject's current level of expertise.

2. No changes in the subjects' MLUs occurred during the course of the study. Warren and Rogers-Warren took this to mean that the subjects had not learned new, more efficient strategies for acquiring linguistic knowledge as a result of the intervention.

3. The subjects came to rely more heavily on the trained forms while abandoning many of the forms that they had used prior to the intervention. These abandoned forms were no less mature than the trained forms; thus, the intervention changed but did not improve the linguistic repertoires of the subjects.

In summary, the impact of this intensive, operant-learning-based, didactic intervention was less than impressive.

Numerous other interventions that can be characterized as didactic have been conducted. Their targets included simple, clausal constructions such as subject–verb–object sentences (Hester & Hendrickson, 1977; Jeffree, Wheldall, & Mittler, 1973; Lutzker & Sherman, 1974), auxiliaries and other verb phrase elements (Hegde, 1980), expansions of the noun phrase (Smeets & Streifel, 1976), and grammatical morphology (Guess, 1969; Guess & Baer, 1973). In general, these interventions have been successful in increasing the frequency of use of the linguistic targets within the training setting (Rusch & Karlan, 1983). They have been less successful, however, in leading to the types of generalization considered important by Johnston (1988) and Warren and Kaiser (1988).

As indicated in a previous section, the failure of didactic approaches to promote meaningful generalization, as well as the increasing popularity of social-interactional views of language acquisition, have led many interventionists to abandon didactic approaches in favor of new milieu approaches to training language contents and forms. This shift has also been fueled by the increased interest in pragmatics that has characterized child-language research since the mid-1970s. In most didactic approaches, linguistic forms and contents are presented in the absence of information about the social uses to which they could be put, and the reinforcers used in training are not those naturally linked to the forms in question (Leonard & Fey, 1991; McLean & Snyder-McLean, 1978; Reichle, Rogers, & Barrett, 1984). For example, a client might be taught the word *juice* without being taught that it can be used to make a comment or a request, and a successful production of the word might be rewarded with a *Good talking* rather than with a topic-continuing utterance or the object named. In milieu approaches, in contrast, the intervention begins with the subject's attempts to communicate; the therapist's task is to provide a more mature linguistic means for expressing the subject's intent.

A number of milieu approaches to intervention have been developed in recent years. We describe some of them here. Additional examples and more detailed discussions of the strengths and limitations of each can be found in Barnett (1987), Caro and Snell (1989), Fey (1986), Kaiser, Yoder, and Keetz (1992), McCormick and Schiefelbusch (1984), Schwartz (1987), and Warren and Kaiser (1986, 1988).

Perhaps the most popular of the milieu approaches has been *incidental teaching* (Hart & Risley, 1968, 1974, 1975, 1980). According to Warren and Kaiser (1986,

1988), the basic premise of incidental teaching is that language learning is facilitated when the adult's talk follows the child's lead. This procedure involves: (a) arranging the environment to increase the likelihood that the subject will initiate a verbal interaction, (b) selecting language targets that are slightly in advance of the child's current level of competence, (c) responding to the subject's utterances with requests for more developmentally advanced versions of his or her utterances, (d) using increasingly more specific prompts to elicit the more advanced productions, and (e) responding to the subject's successful attempts at a target with reinforcers that are naturally linked to the target. This approach is also characterized by distributed trials; that is, several behaviors are targeted for intervention simultaneously. Moreover, the specific targets that are taught at any given time depend on the child's behavior and the situation.

The incidental teaching procedure is illustrated in the following scenario, adapted from Warren and Kaiser (1986). During free play in a classroom, the subject approaches an out-of-reach shelf that is full of art materials. The subject says *color* as he or she stares longingly at a box of crayons. Because one of the targets for this particular subject is an increase in the use of two-word requests, the teacher responds with *What do you want?* and, if *want color* is not forthcoming after one or two prompts, the teacher might try to elicit it through *Say "want color"*. When the subject does produce the target, the teacher provides the requested crayons. Most likely, the teacher would try to ensure that several opportunities for training this request form occurred each day—likewise for the several other behaviors targeted for this particular subject.

Hart and Risley (1968, 1974, 1975, 1980) were among the first to systematically examine the effectiveness of incidental teaching. The subjects in these investigations were economically disadvantaged 3- to 4-year-olds, who were at risk for mental retardation and other developmental problems. The major results of this series of investigations can be summarized as follows:

1. Improvements within the training setting (i.e., the preschool) were seen on several types of linguistic targets (e.g., production of complex sentences, nouns).

2. The subjects extended the more advanced language forms targeted in the intervention to preschool peers and to situations in which the training procedures were not in effect.

3. The gains on target forms engendered by the intervention were maintained after training on the forms ceased.

4. The disadvantaged preschoolers involved in the intervention were observed to increase their rates of language development subsequent to training so that they outdistanced their control disadvantaged peers and, in some areas, approached the level of language proficiency of more economically advantaged preschoolers.

Incidental procedures have also been used with more severely impaired populations of subjects. For example, Cavallaro and Poulson (1985) took this approach in an intervention designed to teach vocabulary to children with moderate to severe mental retardation. Moreover, although the procedure is best suited to teaching the production of language and has been used most often for that purpose (Warren & Kaiser, 1986, 1988), there are published reports in which it has been used in training receptive language skills in a variety of populations (e.g., McGee, Krantz, Mason, & McClannahan, 1983; McGee, Krantz, & McClannahan, 1985). In all of these studies, the procedure has been effective in achieving an increase in the frequency of use of the targeted language behaviors. Generalization of these gains, however, has not always been assessed.

A serious limitation of incidental teaching is that teaching can occur only in response to a limited number of child actions and situations. For example, training on a productive language target must wait until the child makes a verbal initiation that is an immature version of the targeted form. Many children who have language problems, including those with mental retardation, are also infrequent talkers and, thus, they may not initiate at a rate high enough to provide sufficient teaching opportunities (Fey, 1986; Leonard & Fey, 1991; Warren & Kaiser, 1986, 1988). A failure to initiate is especially characteristic of individuals with more severe levels of mental retardation (Barnett, 1987; Caro & Snell, 1989; Rusch & Karlan, 1983). Therefore, incidental teaching in its pure form is probably not the technique of choice for many persons with mental retardation. For this reason, several variants of incidental teaching have emerged, all involving a greater degree of clinician control compared to incidental teaching (e.g., see Alpert & Rogers-Warren, 1984; Cavallaro & Bambara, 1982; Neff, Walters, & Egel, 1984; Oliver & Halle, 1982).

The *mand-model* procedure is one such variant (Schwartz, 1987). In this procedure, the therapist responds to any situation in which the subject has a need to be met (e.g., for materials, assistance) with a prompt for verbalization (e.g., *Tell me what you want*) rather than, as in incidental teaching, waiting for the subject to verbalize. If the targeted form is not forthcoming, the clinician elicits an imitation from the subject (e.g., *Say "juice"*). The adult provides verbal praise and the materials or assistance the subject desires after the subject has produced the target successfully or after two or three failed attempts at that production.

Rogers-Warren and Warren (1980) used the mand-model technique to teach production of new vocabulary and syntactic–semantic patterns to language-delayed preschoolers and observed not only gains on the targets in training but increases in the children's rates of verbalization, the diversity of their productive vocabularies, and the overall syntactic–semantic complexity of their language in a nontraining setting. Similar findings were obtained in a study by Warren, McQuarter, and Rogers-Warren (1984), again involving language-delayed preschoolers. There are, however, no published reports of the use of this technique in interventions involving persons with mental retardation.

Other variants of incidental teaching, such as the time-delay procedure of Halle (Halle, Baer, & Spradlin, 1981; Halle, Marshall, & Spradlin, 1979), are specifically designed to increase the rate of verbalizations in reticent subjects. Although these procedures do not teach new language forms, they may be useful as the first step in an intervention, with incidental teaching as a possible second step. Time delay and other procedures for increasing verbalization rates are discussed later in this chapter when we focus on interventions that have targeted pragmatic rather than linguistic behaviors.

In summarizing the results of numerous interventions involving milieu techniques, Warren and Kaiser (1986, 1988) concluded that such techniques typically led to immediate, dramatic improvements on the targets of training within the training setting and that these improvements were seen for individuals with mental retardation ranging from mild to severe, across different trainers (e.g., teachers, parents, speech-language clinicians) and for a variety of language targets. The language targets included concrete nouns, adjectives, two-word semantic relations, responses to yes–no questions, and conjoined sentences. Warren and Kaiser also pointed out that gains in nontraining settings were documented in several studies, although this form of generalization has not always been measured. There have only been a few studies in which researchers attempted to determine whether the intervention led to changes in nontrained language forms or, more importantly, to changes in the rate at which the subjects acquired new forms. Moreover, Warren and Kaiser pointed out that, because most interventions involving milieu techniques have targeted such limited aspects of the subjects' linguistic repertoires, there is little reason to suppose that they would have more generalized effects on those repertoires. In addition, Warren and Kaiser (1986) suggested that persons with mental retardation are less likely to show such generalized effects in milieu-oriented interventions than are persons with other types of developmental disabilities (e.g., specific language impairment).

Warren and Kaiser (1986) also pointed to a number of other limitations of the milieu approach. They noted that there has been a lack of research on the effectiveness of the approach as a function of factors such as severity of impairment, level of linguistic competence, and etiology (see also Schwartz, 1987). They also claimed that many linguistic forms do not readily lend themselves to the milieu approach (see also Schwartz, 1987). For example, grammatical morphology, which is especially deficient in many persons with Down syndrome (chapters 2 and 5), is difficult to fit into a milieu framework. Similarly, the milieu approach is better suited to training expressive rather than receptive skills. In fact, Warren and Kaiser (1986) believe that milieu techniques are largely useful in improving the expressive repertoires of those individuals with mental retardation who have expressive skills that are more impaired than their receptive skills.

They also suggested that, in most intervention studies, it is not clear which aspects of the milieu approach were important in changing the behavior of the subjects (see also Schwartz, 1987). Further, Warren and Kaiser suggested that milieu techniques are not easy to employ in structured situations such as the elementary or high-school classroom.

We would like to add two items to this list of limitations:

1. It is often difficult to decide from published reports when the intervention has succeeded in teaching a new form or content to the subjects and when it has simply encouraged them to make greater use of a form or content already in their repertoires.

2. Most importantly, there is little in the way of empirical support or theoretical rationale for supposing that all aspects of language (e.g., syntactic rules and categories) must be taught within the context of a social interaction (see chapters 2 and 5). In fact, some researchers have argued that syntactic targets are taught best in didactic interactions that have no social purpose other than to teach those targets (e.g., Connell, 1987; Fey, 1986; see Leonard & Fey, 1991, for a contrasting view).

IMPROVING THE PRAGMATIC ASPECTS OF LANGUAGE PERFORMANCE

We now consider interventions that have focused on performance in the area of linguistic communication rather than on grammatical competence. The goal of these interventions has been to improve the subjects' use of their existing linguistic repertoires to fulfill various communicative ends. We first consider those studies that have targeted a single dimension of communicative performance before turning to studies that have focused on multiple dimensions. Most of these interventions have been didactic in their approach. This is probably because most of the subjects have been adolescents and adults in structured classroom or workshop environments. As already mentioned, milieu approaches are more difficult to conduct in these settings.

As already noted, a problem frequently faced by those involved in intervention is the unwillingness or inability of people with language problems, including those with mental retardation, to initiate talk. That is, many intervention procedures serve to correct or alter a subject's productions, and such procedures are of limited utility with a reticent subject (Fey, 1986). It is often necessary, therefore, that the rate of verbal initiations by the participants in an intervention be increased. Several investigations involving persons with mental retardation have been designed to evaluate various procedures for doing this.

Halle and his colleagues (Halle, Baer, & Spradlin, 1981; Halle, Marshall, & Spradlin, 1979) examined the utility of *time delay* in increasing the use of spoken language by persons with mental retardation. In the time-delay procedure, the agent of change (e.g., teacher, clinician) demonstrates that he or she is available for, and expecting, social interaction. In addition, the agent of change does not talk for some specified time period. For instance, in the Halle et al. (1981) study, preschool teachers were instructed to refrain from talking to their developmentally delayed students for 5 seconds (or until the students vocalized) when (a) the teacher was physically close to the student, (b) the teacher's head was oriented toward the student, and (c) the student was oriented toward the teacher.

Halle et al. (1981) found that training the teachers to use the time-delay procedure increased the frequency of contextually appropriate verbal initiations by the children. However, this change in the children's behavior did not reflect a greater propensity on their part to initiate verbal exchanges. Instead, the children were simply responding to the teacher's time-delay prompt; thus, the more prompts the teacher provided, the more often the children produced a verbal initiation. It does not appear, therefore, that the children in this study acquired any new or even sharpened any existing pragmatic skill. Moreover, Halle et al. (1981) found—in this study and in a second study involving older children with mental retardation—that teachers often failed to use time delays even after extensive training. In contrast to claims to the contrary (e.g., Schwartz, 1987), then, time delay does not appear to be an effective means of increasing the verbal assertiveness of children with mental retardation.

As we noted in our discussion of linguistic communication (chapter 6), the talk of competent speakers is determined in part by various listener characteristics. For example, we talk differently to babies than to other adults, and to high status listeners than to low status listeners. This variation due to listener differences is evident in the choices that speakers make about, among other things, topics, vocabulary, syntactic form, intonation, and speech acts. We also pointed out (chapter 7) that speakers with mental retardation demonstrate sensitivity to such listener characteristics at a later age than do typically developing children. Therefore, there is a need for interventions that will establish links between linguistic elements in the repertoires of persons with mental retardation and categories of listeners (e.g., adult vs. child, familiar vs. unfamiliar, high vs. low social status).

A study designed to address this need was conducted by Silverman, Anderson, Marshall, and Baer (1986). The subjects were 2 adolescent males who had MAs of 5;6 and 9;2. A *match-to-sample* procedure employing puppets as listeners was employed. In this procedure, the subjects were first taught, using operant techniques (i.e., prompting and reinforcement of correct responses), that there were two categories of listeners, each containing two exemplars (i.e., Puppet A went with, or matched, Puppet B, whereas Puppet C matched Puppet D). One puppet from each category, the teacher, then taught the subject, again using operant techniques, a unique response to a question about word opposites.

For example, Puppet A taught the subject to respond to *What's the opposite of good?* with *bad*, whereas Puppet C taught the subject to respond to the same question with *evil*. The next step was to determine if the subjects had simply learned to associate a response with an individual teacher puppet or whether they had learned to associate a response with a category of puppets. To do this, Silverman et al. used the nonteacher puppets to ask the questions. The basic idea was that if a link had been established between a response and a category of puppet, then the trained response should be made to the teacher as well as to the nonteacher from that category.

Silverman et al. (1986) found that the subjects virtually always responded to the nonteacher puppet's question with the response taught by the teacher puppet from the same category as the nonteacher. Moreover, in the few instances in which the subject erred, the responses were from other questions taught by the teacher puppet from the same category as the nonteacher puppet. Thus, Silverman et al. concluded that adolescents with mental retardation can be trained to associate different linguistic elements from their repertoires with different categories of listeners.

The reader should note that in the Silverman et al. (1986) study, the listener categories were defined arbitrarily (i.e., there was nothing inherent in the puppets that led to their category assignment). Pragmatic rules, in contrast, involve meaningful categories (e.g., those based on social status or familiarity). Moreover, the linguistic elements targeted by Silverman et al. are typically not subject to alternation as a function of listener characteristics in the real world. For example, it is unlikely that our response to a question about word opposites would differ depending on whether the questioner was of high or low social status. Future work along these lines should involve naturally occurring categories of listeners as well as linguistic elements that are actually linked to listener variables in the repertoires of competent speakers.

The requesting behavior of individuals with mental retardation was the focus of an intervention study conducted by McCook, Cipiani, Madigan, and La Campagne (1988). These researchers used what they termed a *mand-model plus correction* procedure with older adults (i.e., chronological age over 50) with moderate to profound mental retardation. The trainer presented a visual stimulus (e.g., a cup of juice) and waited for the subject to make the desired verbal response (e.g., *juice*). If the response was not forthcoming, the trainer provided prompts which were at first quite explicit (e.g., *Say juice*) and eventually less so (e.g., simply pointing to the juice while looking at the subject).

It is important to note that correct responses were reinforced with praise (e.g., *Good asking*). This is very different from the reinforcement that the subject would receive for this response in most real-world interactions. That is, uttering *juice* in most situations like that employed by McCook et al. would get the speaker some juice. This is a common problem in studies conducted within an operant-learning framework and no doubt accounts, in part, for the fact that gains observed in the operant-training setting seldom generalize to naturalistic situations (Reichle, Rogers, & Barrett, 1984).

McCook et al. (1988) were able to increase the frequency with which 2 female subjects used the word *juice*, which was already in their vocabularies, to make a request of an experimenter who held a cup of juice near the subject. They also demonstrated that their procedures were effective in decreasing the latency of the subjects' verbal requests. McCook et al. also found that the intervention led the subjects to use the word *juice* to make requests even when there was no juice present. That is, there was some evidence for stimulus generalization. However, the addressee in these generalization assessments was the same individual who had done the training and, thus, we have no way of knowing whether the subjects recognized the utility of the word *juice* for dealing with other people in their world.

A mand-model approach has been used by other investigators to improve the requesting behaviors of persons with mental retardation. For example, Cavallaro and Bambara (1982) used it to increase the use of: (a) *want* + noun, (b) *need* + noun, and (c) *please* + noun by individuals with severe to moderate retardation within the context of free-play activities.

Topic-related pragmatic skills were the focus of an intervention study conducted by Haring, Roger, Lee, Breen, and Gaylord-Ross (1986). The subjects were 3 adolescents with moderate mental retardation (CAs between 10 and 13 and IQs between 40 and 57). Haring et al. interviewed typically developing fifth graders about techniques they used to (a) initiate a conversation, and (b) expand on a partner's conversational topic. The techniques identified in these interviews were then taught to the subjects with mental retardation through a combination of time delay, prompting, and modeling of the techniques during the course of a dyadic interaction with an experimenter.

To assess the impact of the training, each subject was observed during dyadic interactions with a typically developing peer during and after the intervention. All subjects showed improvement over baseline in terms of topic initiation and expansion rates. However, Haring et al. (1986) did not determine whether the subjects had acquired new discourse skills or had simply learned how to use their existing skills.

In many intervention studies involving persons with mental retardation, several very different pragmatic behaviors have been simultaneously targeted for improvement. For example, Wildman, Wildman, and Kelly (1986) took an approach based largely on social-learning theory (e.g., Bandura, 1977) in their attempt to improve several aspects of the conversational performance of adults with mild to moderate mental retardation. Their 7 subjects ranged in CA from 27 to 55 and in IQ from 45 to 70. Baseline measurements of the conversational behaviors of interest were taken during sessions in which dyads of subjects were instructed to "get to know each other better." In the initial treatment sessions, the subjects first watched videotaped and live performances of the targeted behaviors by nondisabled adult models. In later sessions, the subjects practiced the targeted behaviors and received feedback during conversations with each other. Throughout treatment, as well as immediately and 6 months after treatment, each subject engaged in dyadic conversations with another subject and with an unfamiliar nondisabled adult. Measurements of the behaviors of interest were taken during these post-intervention dyadic interactions.

The intervention was designed to increase the frequency of questions and compliments directed to the partner and, at the same time, to decrease the frequency of self-disclosure statements (e.g., *I work at the downtown workshop*). The rationale for this was that good conversationalists should be interested in their partners and should not simply talk about themselves. Although this seems to be a sound rationale at first glance, a good conversation is not likely to consist of, for example, all questions or to contain no self-disclosure. Moreover, a speaker who uses an excessive number of compliments might seem patronizing or insincere. A more appropriate goal would have been to achieve a balance among these different categories of behavior.

Problems in treatment goals notwithstanding, Wildman et al.'s (1986) treatment did appear to improve the conversational performance of the subjects. During dyadic interactions with a peer, the frequencies of question-asking and complimenting of the partner increased, whereas self-disclosure decreased throughout the treatment sessions. These gains were maintained for the most part at the 6-month follow-up and, moreover, they generalized to the interactions involving nondisabled adults. In addition, Wildman et al. assessed the "social validity" of the treatment by asking nondisabled adults to rate pre- and posttreatment tapes of the subjects' conversations in terms of the subjects' conversational skill. Higher ratings were given to tapes of the posttreatment sessions.

In recent years, a number of programs for improving social (including conversational) behaviors have been developed. Many of these programs depend heavily on *self-monitoring* techniques; that is, subjects monitor their own progress toward various intervention goals. The motivation for this approach is that self-instruction is more time- and cost-efficient than the more typical clinician/ teacher-guided intervention. In an examination of their self-monitoring program, Matson and Adkins (1980) supplied their adult subjects with audiotapes of conversational behaviors that were appropriate for various trainer prompts. For example, in response to the prompt *Say something nice about someone*, the audiotape portrayed *That's a nice shirt you're wearing* as an appropriate response. It should be noted, however, that this self-instructional component of training was supplemented by some instruction from a trainer. Moreover, the extent of the trainer's supplemental instructions is not clear, which makes evaluation of the self-monitoring technique difficult at best. Nevertheless, the subjects, who were 2 adults in their twenties with moderate mental retardation, showed improvement in the targeted conversational behaviors as determined by the ratings of staff members who observed them outside of the training setting.

Other investigators have shown that the method by which subjects monitor their progress determines the effectiveness of the self-monitoring approach. For example, Schloss and Wood (1990) found that self-monitoring was more effective when the subjects kept a running tally of the frequency of their appropriate conversational behaviors instead of simply noting whether such a behavior occurred.

Although self-monitoring frequently leads to improvements not only in the training setting but in generalization settings as well (i.e., stimulus generalization has sometimes been observed), two limitations of this method are worth noting:

1. Self-monitoring works best when combined with clinician-guided instruction. How much and what type of clinician-guided instruction is most effective with self-monitoring, however, has not been determined.
2. Self-monitoring has been used most often with adults with mental retardation. An important question, therefore, is whether this procedure is limited in its effectiveness by subject age or level of functioning.

In addition to interventions that have targeted various conversational skills, researchers in the field of mental retardation have focused on improving performance in specialized communication tasks. For instance, Karen, Astin-Smith, and Creasey (1985) analyzed the task of answering a telephone and taking a message into its component behaviors and designed an intervention that led to improvement in all of the component behaviors for 6 adolescents and adults (CAs from 17 to 45 years) with moderate to mild mental retardation.

In summary, intervention research has focused on a number of pragmatic skills, largely in adolescents and adults with mental retardation. This research, however, has been characterized by a number of methodological and conceptual limitations. As for methodology, many interventions involved the use of multiple-instructional procedures (e.g., self-monitoring and clinician-guided instruction); thus, it is often impossible to determine which aspects of the intervention were responsible for the improved communicative performance of the subjects. As for conceptualization, in many interventions the pragmatic skills taught often bear little resemblance to the pragmatic skills involved in real-world communicative interactions. For example, instruction in listener-based language alternations has involved arbitrary, meaningless types of listener characteristics as well as aspects of language not normally subject to listener-based alternation. As another example, researchers have often attempted to increase or decrease the rates of various communicative behaviors to levels that are not representative of the rates seen in real-world communicative exchanges. Moreover, research in this area has seldom involved any attempt to compare the effectiveness of different approaches to teaching pragmatic skills, nor has the evaluation of treatment effectiveness involved more than the assessment of stimulus and response generalization as traditionally defined.

CONCLUSION

When planning an intervention, one faces decisions about the assessment process, the skills and knowledge to be imparted to the subjects, the approach to be taken to instruction, and the criteria to be employed in evaluating the success of the intervention. We have argued that one can hope to intervene effectively only if the nature of a subject's language problems has been adequately described. Such description requires a comprehensive assessment, that is, an assessment that targets all domains of language (including the pragmatic domain), receptive and expressive language performance, and the relevant social and cognitive prerequisites. In most intervention research, however, comprehensive assessments seldom precede implementation of the treatment; thus, the treatment is probably inappropriate (in terms of content and/or approach) for at least some of the subjects included. Moreover, any assessment must be based on an adequate characterization of mature linguistic and communicative competence and on what is known about the process of language development in persons with and without mental retardation. This is seldom the case in intervention research and this, too, may have limited the success of many intervention efforts. In deciding on the behaviors to be targeted for improvement, researchers have argued for following either a developmental or a remedial approach. Both approaches suffer from a number of limitations in conceptualization and implementation, and direct comparisons of the effectiveness of the two approaches have not been conducted. In terms of the approach to instruction, researchers have adopted either a didactic or a milieu approach. The former grew out of learning theory, the latter out of social-interactional perspectives on normal language acquisition. Direct comparisons of the effectiveness of the two approaches have seldom been made. However, some researchers (e.g., Yoder et al., 1989) have suggested that the two approaches may be appropriate for teaching individuals at different levels of language development or for teaching different aspects of language. In terms of evaluating the effectiveness of any single intervention, researchers are in agreement that the criteria must include more than the simple imitation of trained behaviors within the therapeutic context. There is disagreement, however, as to the type of generalized behavior toward which interventionists should strive. In practice, most researchers have been satisfied if their intervention leads a subject to use a behavior that is in some way novel in comparison to the behavior explicitly trained. Some researchers, in contrast, have argued that language and communication interventions should lead to broader changes in subject behavior.

Interventions that have targeted aspects of the linguistic system (e.g., vocabulary, syntax) have been based on either a didactic or a milieu approach. The former have been successful in that they have led to improvement in the aspects of language targeted, at least within the therapeutic context. These approaches have not always led to meaningful changes in the linguistic skills of persons with mental retardation, however. In many studies, it has been demonstrated that, after intervention, the subjects can be prompted to produce novel exemplars of the language targets, but no evidence is provided that they do so spontaneously. Moreover, sometimes these interventions simply alter rather than improve the linguistic repertoires of persons with mental retardation.

Interventions that have targeted pragmatic skills and knowledge have also involved didactic and/or milieu approaches. Therefore, studies examining the effectiveness of these interventions suffer from many of the same limitations described for linguistically oriented interventions. In addition, the former have seldom been based on any model of mature communicative performance and, as a result, the targets of intervention often bear little resemblance to the skills that are needed to communicate effectively in real-world social interactions.

In addition to the problems mentioned to this point, research on language and communication intervention involving persons with mental retardation has been limited in several other important respects:

1. Most of the research has involved older children or adults as the targets of intervention; thus, we know little about the effectiveness of various interventions for children with mental retardation who are younger than 6 years of age (Warren, 1987). This is especially true in research on the treatment of pragmatic problems.

2. Researchers have seldom attended to differences in the effectiveness of their intervention across subjects. This is reflected both in the failure to conduct comprehensive assessments prior to intervention and in the analysis of outcome data (e.g., generalization). In this regard, Rice (1986) identified a number of dimensions of individual differences that may interact with the nature of the intervention to determine a subject's progress. She suggested that culture is one such dimension. That is, there are cultural differences in how language is used in social interaction, and this fact needs to be appreciated when selecting language and communication targets for the intervention. Moreover, Rice suggested that there may be a need to teach subjects to switch to different registers according to the cultural context in which they find themselves. As another example, Rice pointed out that interventionists must consider the subject's motivation and attitude toward intervention. It is possible, for example, that for adolescents with mild mental retardation the first step in an intervention will be to demonstrate the value of improved language and communication skills. Otherwise, the interventionist may be struggling to teach something to an unwilling student. (The reader is referred to Rice's original paper for a more complete discussion of individual differences and intervention; see also Miller, 1983.)

3. Another limitation of existing research involving persons with mental retardation has been the heavy reliance on adults as the agents of change. That is, the person responsible for carrying out most intervention procedures is an adult, typically a teacher or speech–language clinician, although recently parents have been recruited for this role (Cheseldine & McConkey, 1979; McConkey & O'Connor, 1982; Rosenberg & Robinson, 1985; Slater, 1986; Tannock & Girolametto, 1992). Rice (1986) pointed out that, under normal circumstances, children probably acquire information about language and its social uses from peers as well as from adults. Therefore, she suggested that language interventions would be more effective if they included peer trainers in addition to the speech-language clinician or other adult. The few peer-based interventions that have been conducted (e.g., Ezell & Goldstein, 1991; Goldstein & Kaczmarek, 1992) confirm Rice's hypothesis.

4. The exclusive focus on the utterance as the unit of intervention is also a limitation; that is, targets have involved various formal or functional properties of an utterance and interventions have been evaluated with reference to utterance-level properties of language. It is important to keep in mind, however, that most naturally occurring communicative exchanges involve the production of talk over a number of turns. For example, the participants in a conversation contribute to a topic one turn at a time and in such a way as to move the topic toward a logical end (Dorval & Eckerman, 1984). There is a need, therefore, for interventions that focus on supra-utterance language behaviors such as those involved in topic control and discourse cohesion.

5. It is probably the case in many interventions that the exemplars included in training are not sufficient to illustrate the breadth and limits of the rule, category, or concept being taught. Consider, for example, a subject who is reinforced through operant procedures for producing two-word agent–action constructions in response to some stimulus. How is the subject to know whether the reinforcement is contingent on the production of a semantic relation, a noun–verb relation, a subject–predicate relation, a prosodic pattern, a phonological string, a pragmatic pattern, or some combination of these? Some of these possibilities may be ruled out by various constraints on the subject's processing of the input such as those hypothesized by Chomsky (see chapters 2 and 5). Other possibilities will need to be ruled out by the provision of stimuli that make clear that the reinforcement is contingent on the production of an agent–action relation rather than simply a noun–verb string, a subject–predicate relation, and so on. There is little evidence in most intervention research involving individuals with mental retardation, however, that the stimulus conditions and reinforcement schedules have been structured in this way. This may account for the limited generalization seen in so many interventions with this population.

6. Most approaches to intervention have targeted only narrowly defined areas of linguistic competence and/or communication and have failed to recognize the interdependencies that sometimes exist between achievements in different do-

mains. For example, because prelexical phonological development has an impact on the phonological structure of the early lexicon of nondisabled children (see chapter 2), it may be necessary to target (to whatever extent is possible) the former prior to initiation of lexical training. This has seldom been done in intervention research involving persons with mental retardation. As another example, the lexical entries of mature language users are marked not only for conceptual content but also for phonological structure, prosody, the semantic argument structures that impact on syntax, and various pragmatic functions. Nondisabled children do not necessarily acquire these different aspects of a lexical entry independently (e.g., knowledge of a word's argument structure may often help them make decisions about the word's conceptual content). Lexical interventions that aim only to establish links between labels and concepts, as do many interventions involving persons with mental retardation, therefore, are not structured to be consistent with the way that the subjects typically learn. Moreover, the rather narrow set of targets involved in most interventions has made it impossible to determine whether some aspects of grammar or communication are easier to teach to persons with mental retardation than others or whether training in some domains of language (e.g., lexical-semantics) leads to improvements in other, nontargeted domains (e.g., phonology) for these individuals.

The effectiveness of language and communication intervention is also limited by the many gaps in our knowledge about development in persons with and without mental retardation. As we saw in the previous chapters, there is nothing to suggest that the process of language acquisition is different in persons with mental retardation and in nondisabled children. Nevertheless, it is not clear precisely what factors slow down the process in the former, although it is likely to be factors that are linguistic rather than cognitive in the grammatical domain. Similarly, we have suggested (chapter 7) that cognitive factors may play a greater role in many developments in the pragmatic domain than do linguistic factors, but here too we do not know the precise cognitive factors involved (Abbeduto, 1991; Abbeduto & Rosenberg, 1992). As another example, identification of the parameters of Universal Grammar and the input that serves to set them has not progressed far. This means that we do not know which exemplars of the language serve to bring a learner's grammar more in line with that of a mature language user and, thus, which exemplars should form the core of any intervention effort.

In closing, we note that an important goal of language intervention must be to improve the subject's ability to participate in social interaction (Abbeduto, 1991; Abbeduto & Rosenberg, 1992). For many individuals with mental retardation, particularly those with severe to profound impairments, this often means forgoing training in spoken language in favor of manual or other nonspoken communication systems (Barnett, 1987). Even for less severely impaired persons, it may sometimes be useful to train in a nonspoken system prior to targeting spoken language (Reichle, Mirenda, Locke, Piche, & Johnston, 1992). We have not considered research on such alternative communication systems. The reader interested in this topic can turn to Barnett (1987), Calculator and Bedrosian (1988), Romski and Sevcik (1992), and Reichle et al. (1992) for more information.

References

Abbeduto, L. (1984). Situational influences on mentally retarded and nonretarded children's production of directives. *Applied Psycholinguistics, 5,* 147–166.

Abbeduto, L. (1991). The development of linguistic communication in persons with mild to moderate mental retardation. In N. Bray (Ed.), *International review of research in mental retardation* (pp. 91–115). New York: Academic.

Abbeduto, L., & Benson, G. (1992). Speech act development in nondisabled children and individuals with mental retardation. In R. Chapman (Ed.), *Processes in language acquisition and disorders* (pp. 257–278). Chicago: Mosby-Year Book.

Abbeduto, L., Davies, B., & Furman, L. (1988). The development of speech act comprehension in mentally retarded individuals and nonretarded children. *Child Development, 59,* 1460–1472.

Abbeduto, L., Davies, B., Solesby, S., & Furman, L. (1991). Identifying the referents of spoken messages: The use of context and clarification requests by children with mental retardation and by nonretarded children. *American Journal on Mental Retardation, 95,* 551–562.

Abbeduto, L., Furman. L., & Davies, B. (1989a). Identifying speech acts from contextual and linguistic information. *Language and Speech, 32,* 189–203.

Abbeduto, L., Furman, L., & Davies, B. (1989b). Relation between the receptive language and mental age of persons with mental retardation. *American Journal on Mental Retardation, 93,* 535–543.

Abbeduto, L., & Nuccio, J. (1989). Evaluating the pragmatic aspects of communication in school-age children and adolescents: Insights from research on atypical development. *School Psychology Review, 18,* 502–512.

Abbeduto, L., Nuccio, J. B., Al-Mabuk, R., Rotto, P., & Maas, F. (1992). Interpreting and responding to spoken language: Children's recognition and use of a speaker's goal. *Journal of Child Language, 19,* 677–693.

Abbeduto, L., Nuccio, J. B., Short, K., & Benson, G. (1992, March). *Interpreting and responding to spoken language: Recognition and use of a speaker's goal by persons with mental retardation.* Paper presented at the Gatlinburg Conference on Mental Retardation, Gatlinburg, TN.

Abbeduto, L., & Rosenberg, S. (1980). The communicative competence of mildly retarded adults. *Applied Psycholinguistics, 1,* 405–426.

Abbeduto, L., & Rosenberg, S. (1985). Children's knowledge of the presuppositions of know and other cognitive verbs. *Journal of Child Language, 12,* 621-641.

Abbeduto, L., & Rosenberg, S. (1987). Linguistic communication and mental retardation. In S. Rosenberg (Ed.), *Advances in applied psycholinguistics: Vol. 1. Disorders of first language development* (pp. 76-125). Cambridge, England: Cambridge University Press.

Abbeduto, L., & Rosenberg, S. (1992). The development of linguistic communication in persons with mental retardation. In S. Warren & J. Reichle (Eds.), *Perspectives on communication and language intervention* (pp. 331-359). Baltimore, MD: Brookes.

Ackerman, B. P. (1978). Children's understanding of speech acts in unconventional directive frames. *Child Development, 49,* 311-318.

Ackerman, B. P. (1981). Performative bias in children's interpretations of ambiguous referential communications. *Child Development, 52,* 1224-1230.

Ackerman, B. P., Szymanski, J., & Silver, D. (1990). Children's use of the common ground in interpreting ambiguous referential expression. *Developmental Psychology, 26,* 234-245.

Aitchison, J. (1987). *Words in the mind: An introduction to the mental lexicon.* Oxford: Blackwell.

Akhtar, N., Dunham, F., & Dunham, P. J. (1991). Directive interactions and early vocabulary development: The role of joint attentional focus. *Journal of Child Language, 18,* 41-49.

Alpert, C. L., & Rogers-Warren, A. K. (1984). *Mothers as incidental language trainers of their language-disordered children.* Unpublished manuscript, University of Kansas, Lawrence.

Anderson, B. J., Vietze, P., & Dokecki, P. R. (1977). Reciprocity in vocal interactions of mothers and infants. *Child Development, 48,* 1676-1681.

Anderson, S. R., & Spradlin, J. E. (1980). The generalized effects of productive labeling training involving common object classes. *Journal of Association for the Severely Handicapped, 5,* 143-157.

Andrews, R. J., & Andrews, J. G. (1977). A study of the spontaneous oral language of Down's syndrome children. *Exceptional Child, 24,* 86-94.

Anisfeld, M. (1984). *Language development from birth to three.* Hillsdale, NJ: Lawrence Erlbaum Associates.

Anselmi, D., Tomasello, M., & Acunzo, M. (1986). Young children's responses to neutral and specific contingent queries. *Journal of Child Language, 13,* 135-144.

Ashman, A. F. (1982). Coding, strategic behavior, and language performance of institutionalized mentally retarded young adults. *American Journal of Mental Deficiency, 86,* 627-636.

Aslin, R. N., Pisoni, D. B., & Jusczyk, P. W. (1983). Auditory development and speech perception in infancy. In M. M. Haith & J. J. Campos (Eds.), *Handbook of child psychology: Vol. 2. Infancy and developmental psychobiology.* New York: Wiley.

Astington, J. (1988). Promises: Words or deeds? *First Language, 3,* 259-270.

Astington, J. (1990). Metapragmatics: Children's conception of promising. In G. Conti-Ramsden & C. Snow (Eds.), *Children's language* (Vol. 7, pp. 223-244). Hillsdale, NJ: Lawrence Erlbaum Associates.

Astington, J. W., Harris, P. L., & Olson, D. R. (1988). *Developing theories of mind.* New York: Cambridge University Press.

Au, T. K. F., & Glusman, M. (1990). The principle of mutual exclusivity in word learning: To honor or not to honor? *Child Development, 61,* 1474-1490.

Austin, J. L. (1962). *How to do things with words.* Oxford: Oxford University Press.

Axia, G., & Baroni, M. R. (1985). Linguistic politeness at different age levels. *Child Development, 56,* 918-927.

Bach, K., & Harnish, R. M. (1979). *Linguistic communication and speech acts.* Cambridge, MA: MIT Press.

Bandura, A. (1977). *Social learning theory.* Englewood Cliffs, NJ: Prentice-Hall.

Barnes, S. B., Gutfreund, M., Satterly, D. J., & Wells, C. G. (1983). Characteristics of adult speech which predict children's language development. *Journal of Child Language, 10,* 65-84.

Barnett, J. (1987). Research on language and communication in children who have severe handicaps: A review and some implications for intervention. *Educational Psychology, 7,* 117-128.

Baroni, M. R., & Axia, G. (1989). Children's meta-pragmatic abilities and the identification of polite and impolite requests. *First Language, 9,* 285-297.

Barrett, M. D., & Diniz, A. (1989). Lexical development in mentally handicapped children. In M. Beveridge, G. Conti-Ramsden, & I. Leudar (Eds.), *Language and communication in mentally handicapped people* (pp. 2-32). London: Chapman & Hall.

Bartel, N. R., Bryen, D., & Keehn, S. (1973). Language comprehension in the mentally retarded child. *Exceptional Children, 39,* 375-382.

Bates, E. (1976). *Language and context: The acquisition of pragmatics.* New York: Academic.

Bates, E., Bretherton, I., & Snyder, L. (1988). *From first words to grammar: Individual differences and dissociable mechanisms.* Cambridge, England: Cambridge University Press.

Bates, E., Camaioni, L., & Volterra, V. (1975). The acquisition of performatives prior to speech. *Merrill-Palmer Quarterly, 21,* 205-226.

Bates, E., & Snyder, L. (1987). The cognitive hypothesis in language development. In I. Uzgiris & J. M. Hunt (Eds.), *Research with scales of psychological development.* Champaign-Urbana: University of Illinois Press.

Bateson, M. (1969). *The interpersonal context of infant vocalizations* (Quarterly Progress Report No. 100, pp. 170-176). Cambridge, MA: MIT Research Laboratory of Electronics.

Baumeister, A. (1967). Problems in comparative studies of mental retardates and normals. *American Journal of Mental Deficiency, 71,* 869-875.

Beal, C. R. (1987). Repairing the message: Children's monitoring and revision skills. *Child Development, 58,* 401-408.

Beal, C. R., & Flavell, J. H. (1983). Young speaker's evaluations of their listener's comprehension in a referential task. *Child Development, 54,* 148-153.

Beal, C. R., & Flavell, J. H. (1984). Development of the ability to distinguish communicative intention and literal message meaning. *Child Development, 55,* 920-928.

Beattie, G. W. (1980). The role of language production processes in the organization of behavior in face-to-face interaction. In B. Butterworth (Ed.), *Language production: Vol. 1. Speech and talk* (pp. 69-107). New York: Academic.

Becker, J. A. (1986). Bossy and nice requests: Children's production and interpretation. *Merrill-Palmer Quarterly, 32,* 393-413.

Becker, J. A. (1988). The success of parents' indirect techniques for teaching their preschoolers pragmatic skills. *First Language, 8,* 173-181.

Becker, J. A. (1990). Processes in the acquisition of pragmatic competence. In G. Conti-Ramsden & C. Snow (Eds.), *Children's language* (Vol. 7, pp. 7-24). Hillsdale, NJ: Lawrence Erlbaum Associates.

Bedrosian, J. L. (1988). Adults who are mildly to moderately mentally retarded: Communicative performance, assessment, and intervention. In S. N. Calculator & J. L. Bedrosian (Eds.), *Communication assessment and intervention for adults with mental retardation* (pp. 265-307). Boston: College-Hill Press.

Bedrosian, J. L., Wanska, S., Sykes, K. M., Smith, A. J., & Dalton, B. M. (1988). Conversational turn-taking violations in mother-child interactions. *Journal of Speech and Hearing Research, 31,* 81-86.

Bellugi, U. (1988). The acquisition of a spatial language. In F. S. Kessel (Ed.), *The development of language and language researchers* (pp. 153-185). Hillsdale, NJ: Lawrence Erlbaum Associates.

Benedict, H. (1979). Early lexical development: Comprehension and production. *Journal of Child Language, 6,* 183-200.

Berger, J., & Cunningham, C. C. (1983). Development of early vocal behaviors and interactions in Down syndrome and nonhandicapped infant-mother pairs. *Developmental Psychology, 19,* 322-331.

Berko, J. (1958). The child's learning of English morphology. *Word, 14,* 150-177.

Berman, R. A. (1986). A cross-linguistic perspective: Morphology and syntax. In P. Fletcher & M. Garman (Eds.), *Language acquisition* (2nd ed., pp. 429-447). Cambridge, England: Cambridge University Press.

Bernicot, J., & Legros, S. (1987). Direct and indirect directives: What do young children understand? *Journal of Experimental Child Psychology, 43*, 346–358.

Beveridge, M. C., Spencer, J., & Mittler, P. (1979). Self-blame and communication failure in retarded adolescents. *Journal of Child Psychology and Psychiatry and Allied Disciplines, 20*, 129–138.

Beveridge, M. C., & Tatham, A. (1976). Communication in retarded adolescents: Utilization of known language skills. *American Journal of Mental Deficiency, 81*, 96–99.

Biberdorf, J. R, & Pear, J. J. (1977). Two-to-one versus one-to-one student–teacher ratios in the operant verbal training of retarded children. *Journal of Applied Behavior Analysis, 10*, 506.

Bickerton, D. (1990). *Language and species.* Chicago: University of Chicago Press.

Bishop, D. V. M. (1982). *Test for reception of grammar.* Unpublished test, available from Department of Psychology, University of Manchester, England.

Bishop, D. V. M., & Adams, C. (1991). What do referential communication tasks measure? A study of children with specific language impairment. *Applied Psycholinguistics, 12*, 199–215.

Black, B., & Hazen, N. L. (1990). Social status and patterns of communication in acquainted and unacquainted preschool children. *Developmental Psychology, 26*, 388–397.

Blank, M. (1974). Cognitive functions of language in the preschool years. *Developmental Psychology, 10*, 229–245.

Blank, M. (1975). Mastering the intangible through language. In D. Aaronson & R. W. Rieber (Eds.), *Developmental psycholinguistics and language disorders* (pp. 44–58). New York: New York Academy of Sciences.

Blank, M., Gessner, M., & Esposito, A. (1979). Language without communication: A case study. *Journal of Child Language, 6*, 329–352.

Bleile, K. (1982). Consonant ordering in Down's syndrome phonology. *Journal of Communication Disorders, 15*, 275–285.

Bliss, L. S. (1985). The development of persuasive strategies by mentally retarded children. *Applied Research in Mental Retardation, 6*, 437–447.

Bliss, L. S., Allen, D. V., & Walker, G. (1978). Sentence structures of trainable and educable mentally retarded subjects. *Journal of Speech and Hearing Research, 21*, 722–731.

Bloom, L. (1970). *Language development: Form and function in emerging grammars.* Cambridge, MA: MIT Press.

Bloom, L., & Lahey, M. (1978). *Language development and language disorders.* New York: Wiley.

Bloom, L., Lahey, M., Hood, L., Lifter, K., & Fiess, K. (1980). Complex sentences: Acquisition of syntactic connectives and the meaning relations they encode. *Journal of Child Language, 7*, 235–261.

Bloom, L., Rispoli, M., Gartner, B., & Hafitz, J. (1989). Acquisition of complementation. *Journal of Child Language, 16*, 101–120.

Bloom, L., Rocissano, L., & Hood, L. (1976). Adult–child discourse: Developmental interaction between information processing and linguistic knowledge. *Cognitive Psychology, 8*, 521–552.

Bloom, P. (1990). Syntactic distinctions in child language. *Journal of Child Language, 17*, 343–355.

Bock, J. K., & Hornsby, M. E. (1981). The development of directives: How children ask and tell. *Journal of Child Language, 8*, 151–163.

Bohannon, J. N., III, MacWhinney, B., & Snow, C. E. (1990). No negative evidence revisited: Beyond learnability or who has to prove what to whom. *Developmental Psychology, 26*, 221–226.

Bohannon, J. N., III, & Marquis, A. (1977). Children's control of adult speech. *Child Development, 48*, 1002–1008.

Bohannon, J. N., III, & Stanowicz, L. (1988). The issue of negative evidence: Adult responses to children's language errors. *Developmental Psychology, 24*, 684–689.

Bohannon, J. N., III, & Warren-Leubecker, A. (1989). Theoretical approaches to language acquisition. In J. B. Gleason (Ed.), *The development of language* (pp. 167–225). Columbus, OH: Merrill.

Boskey, M., & Nelson, K. (1980, October). *Answering unanswerable questions: The role of imitation.* Paper presented at the Boston University Conference on Language Development, Boston, MA.

Bowerman, M. (1973). *Early syntactic development: A cross-linguistic study with special reference to Finnish.* Cambridge, England: Cambridge University Press.

Bowerman, M. (1975). Cross-linguistic similarities at two stages of syntactic development. In E. H. Lenneberg & E. Lenneberg (Eds.), *Foundations of language development* (Vol. 1, pp. 267–282). New York: Academic.

Bowerman, M. (1978). Semantic and syntactic development. In R. L. Schiefelbusch (Ed.), *Bases of language intervention* (pp. 97–189). Baltimore: University Park Press.

Bowerman, M. (1979). The acquisition of complex sentences. In P. Fletcher & M. Garman (Eds.), *Language acquisition* (pp. 285–305). Cambridge, England: Cambridge University Press.

Bowerman, M. (1982). Reorganizational processes in lexical and syntactic development. In E. Wanner & L. R. Gleitman (Eds.), *Language acquisition: The state of the art* (pp. 319–346). New York: Cambridge University Press.

Bowerman, M. (1987). Commentary. In B. MacWhinney (Ed.), *Mechanisms of language acquisition* (pp. 443–466). Hillsdale, NJ: Lawrence Erlbaum Associates.

Bowerman, M. (1988). Inducing the latent structure of language. In F. S. Kessel (Ed.), *The development of language and language researchers* (pp. 23–49). Hillsdale, NJ: Lawrence Erlbaum Associates.

Bowler, D. M., Cuffin, J., & Kiernan, C. (1985). Dichotic listening of verbal and nonverbal material by Down's syndrome children and children of normal intelligence. *Cortex, 21,* 637–644.

Braine, M. D. S. (1976). Children's first word combinations. *Monographs of the Society for Research in Child Development, 41*(1, Serial No. 164).

Brainerd, C. J. (1978). The stage question in cognitive-developmental theory. *Behavioral and Brain Sciences, 2,* 173–213.

Bray, N. W., Biasini, F. J., & Thrasher, K. A. (1983). The effect of communicative demands on request-making in the moderately and severely mentally retarded. *Applied Research in Mental Retardation, 4,* 13–27.

Bredart, S. (1984). Children's interpretation of referential ambiguities and pragmatic inference. *Journal of Child Language, 11,* 665–672.

Bretherton, I., Bates, E., Benigni, L., Camaioni, L., & Volterra, V. (1979). Relationships between cognition, communication, and quality of attachment. In E. Bates, L. Benigni, I. Bretherton, L. Camaioni, & V. Volterra (Eds.), *The emergence of symbols* (pp. 223–269). New York: Academic.

Bretherton, I., McNew, S., Snyder, L., & Bates, E. (1983). Individual differences at 20 months: Analytic and holistic strategies in language acquisition. *Journal of Child Language, 10,* 293–320.

Bricker, W., & Bricker, D. (1974). An early language training strategy. In R. Schiefelbusch & L. Lloyd (Eds.), *Language perspectives: Acquisition, retardation, and intervention* (pp. 431–468). Baltimore: University Park Press.

Bridges, A., & Smith, J. V. (1984). Syntactic comprehension in Down's syndrome children. *British Journal of Psychology, 75,* 187–196.

Brinton, B., & Fujiki, M. (1984). Development of topic manipulation skills in discourse. *Journal of Speech and Hearing Research, 27,* 350–358.

Brinton, B., Fujiki, M., Loeb, D., & Winkler, E. (1986). The development of conversational repair strategies in response to requests for clarification. *Journal of Speech and Hearing Research, 29,* 75–81.

Brooks, P., McCauley, C., & Merrill, E. C. (1987). Cognition and mental retardation. In F. Mendolascino & J. A. Stark (Eds.), *Preventive and curative intervention in mental retardation.* Baltimore: Brookes Publishing.

Brooks, P., Sperber, R., & McCauley, C. (Eds.). (1984). *Learning and cognition in the mentally retarded.* Hillsdale, NJ: Lawrence Erlbaum Associates.

Browman, S., Nichols, P. L., Shaughnessy, P., & Kennedy, W. (1987). *Retardation in young children.* Hillsdale, NJ: Lawrence Erlbaum Associates.

Brown, A. L., Bransford, J. D., Ferrara, R. A., & Campione, J. C. (1983). Learning, remembering, and understanding. In J. H. Flavell & E. M. Markman (Eds.), *Handbook of child psychology* (Vol. 3, pp. 77–166). New York: Wiley.

Brown, C. (1970). *Down all the days*. Greenwich, CT: Fawcett.

Brown, P., & Levinson, S. (1978). Universals in language usage: Politeness phenomena. In E. Goody (Ed.), *Questions and politeness* (pp. 256–289). Cambridge, England: Cambridge University Press.

Brown, P., & Levinson, S. C. (1987). *Politeness: Some universals in language usage*. Cambridge: Cambridge University Press.

Brown, R. (1973). *A first language*. Cambridge, MA: Harvard University Press.

Brown, R. (1977). Introduction. In C. E. Snow & C. Ferguson (Eds.), *Talking to children: Language input and language acquisition* (pp. 1–27). Cambridge, England: Cambridge University Press.

Brown, R., & Hanlon, C. (1970). Derivational complexity and the order of acquisition in child speech. In R. Brown (Ed.), *Psycholinguistics* (pp. 155–207). New York: The Free Press.

Brownell, M. D., & Whiteley, J. (1992). Development and training of referential communication in children with mental retardation. *American Journal on Mental Retardation, 97*, 161–172.

Bruner, J. (1981). The social context of language acquisition. *Language and Communication, 1*, 155–178.

Buckhalt, J. A., Rutherford, R. B., & Goldberg, K. E. (1978). Verbal and nonverbal interaction of mothers with their Down's syndrome and nonretarded infants. *American Journal of Mental Deficiency, 82*, 337–343.

Buium, N., Rynders, J., & Turnure, J. (1974). Early maternal linguistic environment of normal and Down's syndrome language-learning children. *American Journal of Mental Deficiency, 79*, 52–58.

Burr, D. B., & Rohr, A. (1978). Patterns of psycholinguistic development in the severely retarded: A hypothesis. *Social Biology, 25*, 15–22.

Calculator, S. N., & Bedrosian, J. L. (Eds.). (1988). *Communication assessment and intervention for adults with mental retardation*. Boston, MA: Little, Brown & Company.

Campione, J. C., Brown, A. L., & Ferrara, R. A. (1982). Mental retardation and intelligence. In R. J. Sternberg (Ed.), *Handbook of human intelligence* (pp. 392–490). New York: Cambridge University Press.

Campione, J. C., Brown, A. L., Ferrara, R. A., Jones, R. S., & Steinberg, E. (1985). Breakdowns in flexible use of information: Intelligence-related differences in transfer following equivalent learning performance. *Intelligence, 9*, 297–315.

Camras, L. A., Pristo, T. M., & Brown, M. J. K. (1985). Directive choice by children and adults: Affect, situation, and linguistic politeness. *Merrill-Palmer Quarterly, 31*, 19–31.

Caplan, D. (1988). The biological basis for language. In F. J. Newmeyer (Ed.), *Linguistics: The Cambridge survey* (Vol. 3, pp. 237–255). Cambridge, England: Cambridge University Press.

Cardoso-Martins, C., & Mervis, C. B. (1985). Maternal speech to prelinguistic children with Down syndrome. *American Journal of Mental Deficiency, 89*, 451–458.

Cardoso-Martins, C., & Mervis, C. B. (1990). Mothers' use of substantive diexis and nouns with their children with Down syndrome: Some discrepant findings. *American Journal on Mental Retardation, 94*, 633–637.

Cardoso-Martins, C., Mervis, C. B., & Mervis, C. A. (1985). Early vocabulary acquisition by children with Down syndrome. *American Journal of Mental Deficiency, 90*, 177–184.

Carey, S. (1982). Semantic development: The state of the art. In E. Wanner & L. R. Gleitman (Eds.), *Language acquisition: The state of the art* (pp. 347–389). New York: Cambridge University Press.

Caro, P., & Snell, M. E. (1989). Characteristics of teaching communication to people with moderate and severe disabilities. *Education and Training of the Mentally Retarded, 23*, 63–77.

Carrell, P. L. (1981). Children's understanding of indirect requests: Comparing child and adult comprehension. *Journal of Child Language, 8*, 329–345.

Carroll, D. W. (1986). *Psychology of language*. Monterey, CA: Brooks/Cole.

Carrow, M. A. (1968). The development of auditory comprehension of language structure in children. *Journal of Speech and Hearing Disorders, 33*, 99–111.

Cartwright, P. G., Cartwright, C. A., & Ward, M. E. (1984). *Educating special learners* (2nd ed.). Belmont, CA: Wadsworth.

Cattell, R. B. (1971). *Abilities: Their structure, growth, and action.* Boston: Houghton Mifflin.

Cavallaro, C. C., & Bambara, L. M. (1982). Two strategies for teaching language during free play. *Journal of the Association for the Severely Handicapped, 7*, 80–92.

Cavallaro, C. C., & Poulson, C. L. (1985). Two strategies for teaching language during free play. *Education and Treatment of Children, 8*, 1–25.

Chapman, D. L., & Nation, J. E. (1981). Patterns of learning performance in educable mentally retarded children. *Journal of Communication Disorders, 14*, 245–254.

Chapman, R. (1981a, April). *A clinical perspective on individual differences in language acquisition among mentally retarded children.* Paper presented at the biennial meeting of the Society for Research in Child Development, Boston, MA.

Chapman, R. (1981b). Exploring children's communicative intents. In J. Miller (Ed.), *Assessing language production in children* (pp. 111–136). Baltimore, MD: University Park Press.

Chapman, R., Miller, J. F., MacKenzie, H., & Bedrosian, J. (1981, August). *The development of discourse skills in the second year of life.* Paper presented at the 2nd International Congress for the Study of Child Language, University of British Columbia, Vancouver, BC, Canada.

Cheseldine, S., & McConkey, R. (1979). Parental speech to young Down's syndrome children: An intervention study. *American Journal of Mental Deficiency, 83*, 612–620.

Chien, Y. C., & Lust, B. (1985). The concepts of topic and subject in first language acquisition of Mandarin Chinese. *Child Development, 56*, 1359–1375.

Chien, Y. C., & Wexler, K. (1990). Children's knowledge of locality conditions in binding as evidence for the modularity of syntax and pragmatics. *Language Acquisition, 1*, 225–295.

Chomsky, N. (1957). *Syntactic structures.* The Hague, Netherlands: Mouton.

Chomsky, N. (1965). *Aspects of the theory of syntax.* Cambridge, MA: MIT Press.

Chomsky, N. (1980). *Rules and representations.* New York: Columbia University Press.

Chomsky, N. (1981). *Lectures on government and binding.* Dordrecht, Holland: Foris.

Chomsky, N. (1986). *Knowledge of language: Its nature, origin, and use.* Westport, CT: Praeger.

Chomsky, N. (1988). *Language and problems of knowledge: The Managua lectures.* Cambridge, MA: MIT Press.

Chomsky, N. (1990). On the nature, use, and acquisition of language. In W. G. Lycan (Ed.), *Mind and cognition* (pp. 627–646). Oxford, England: Blackwell.

Clahsen, H. (1990–1991). Constraints on parameter setting: A grammatical analysis of some acquisition stages in German child language. *Language Acquisition, 1*, 361–391.

Clark, H. H. (1979). Responding to indirect speech acts. *Cognitive Psychology, 11*, 430–477.

Clark, H. H., Schreuder, R., & Buttrick, S. (1983). Common ground and the understanding of demonstrative reference. *Journal of Verbal Learning and Verbal Behavior, 22*, 245–258.

Clark, H. H., & Schunk, D. H. (1980). Polite responses to polite requests. *Cognition, 8*, 111–143.

Clark, H. H., & Wilkes-Gibbs, D. (1990). Referring as a collaborative process. In P. R. Cohen, J. Morgan, & M. E. Pollack (Eds.), *Intentions in communication* (pp. 463–493). Cambridge, MA: MIT Press.

Coates, J. (1988). The acquisition of the meanings of modality in children aged 8 and 12. *Journal of Child Language, 15*, 425–434.

Coggins, T. E. (1979). Relational meaning encoded in the two-word utterances of Stage I Down's syndrome children. *Journal of Speech and Hearing Research, 22*, 166–178.

Coggins, T. E., & Carpenter, R. L. (1981). The communicative intention inventory: A system for observing and coding children's early intentional communication. *Applied Psycholinguistics, 2*, 235–251.

Coggins, T. E., Carpenter, R. L., & Owings, N. O. (1983). Examining early intentional communication in Down's syndrome and nonretarded children. *British Journal of Disorders of Communication, 18*, 99–107.

Coggins, T. E., & Stoel-Gammon, C. (1982). Clarification strategies used by four Down's syndrome children for maintaining normal conversational interaction. *Education and Training of the Mentally Retarded, 16,* 65-67.

Cohen, P., Morgan, J., & Pollack, M. (Eds.). (1990). *Intentions in communication.* Cambridge, MA: MIT Press.

Comrie, B. (1981). *Language universal and linguistic typology: Syntax and morphology.* Oxford, England: Blackwell.

Comrie, B. (1988). Linguistic typology. In F. J. Newmeyer (Ed.), *Linguistics: The Cambridge survey* (pp. 447-461). New York: Cambridge University Press.

Connell, P. J. (1987). Teaching language form, meaning, and function to specific-language-impaired children. In S. Rosenberg (Ed.), *Advances in applied psycholinguistics: Vol. 1. Disorders of first-language development* (pp. 40-76). Cambridge, England: Cambridge University Press.

Conti, D. J., & Camras, L. A. (1984). Children's understanding of conversational principles. *Journal of Experimental Child Psychology, 38,* 456-463.

Conti-Ramsden, G., & Friel-Patti, S. (1987). Scriptedness: A factor in children's variation in language use? In K. Nelson & A. van Kleeck (Eds.), *Children's language* (Vol. 6, pp. 197-222). Hillsdale, NJ: Lawrence Erlbaum Associates.

Cook, V. J. (1988). *Chomsky's universal grammar: An introduction.* Oxford, England: Blackwell.

Cooper, R. P., & Aslin, R. N. (1990). Preference for infant-directed speech in the first month after birth. *Child Development, 61,* 1584-1595.

Cornwell, A. C. (1974). Development of language, abstraction, and numerical concept formation in Down's syndrome children. *American Journal of Mental Deficiency, 79,* 179-190.

Corrigan, R. (1978). Language development as related to Stage 6 object permanence development. *Journal of Child Language, 5,* 173-190.

Cosgrove, J. M., & Patterson, C. J. (1977). Plans and the development of listener skills. *Developmental Psychology, 13,* 557-564.

Courtright, J., & Courtright, I. (1976). Imitative modeling as a theoretical base for instructing language-disordered children. *Journal of Speech and Hearing Research, 19,* 655-663.

Crawley, S. B., & Spiker, D. (1983). Mother-child interactions involving 2-year-olds with Down syndrome: A look at individual differences. *Child Development, 54,* 1312-1323.

Cromer, R. F. (1975). Are subnormals linguistic adults? In N. O'Connor (Ed.), *Language, cognitive deficits, and retardation* (pp. 169-187). London: Butterworths.

Cromer, R. F. (1987). Word knowledge acquisition in retarded children: A longitudinal study of acquisition of a complex linguistic structure. *Journal of Speech and Hearing Disorders, 52,* 324-334.

Cromer, R. F. (1988). The cognition hypothesis revisited. In F. S. Kessel (Ed.), *The development of language and language researchers* (pp. 223-248). Hillsdale, NJ: Lawrence Erlbaum Associates.

Cromer, R. F. (1991). *Language and thought in normal and handicapped children.* Oxford, England: Blackwell.

Cross, T. G. (1977). Mothers' speech adjustments: The contribution of selected child listener variables. In C. E. Snow & C. A. Ferguson (Eds.), *Talking to children: Language input and acquisition* (pp. 151-188). New York: Cambridge University Press.

Crystal, D. (1987). *Cambridge encyclopedia of language.* Cambridge, England: Cambridge University Press.

Cunningham, C. C., Glenn, S. M., Wilkinson, P., & Sloper, P. (1985). Mental ability, symbolic play, and receptive and expressive language of young children with Down's syndrome. *Journal of Child Psychology and Psychiatry, 26,* 255-265.

Cunningham, C. C., & Sloper, P. (1984). The relationship between maternal ratings of first word vocabulary and Reynell language scores. *British Journal of Educational Psychology, 54,* 160-167.

Curtiss, S. (1979). Genie: Language and cognition. *UCLA Working Papers in Cognitive Linguistics, 1,* 15-62.

Curtiss, S. (1980). The critical period and feral children. *UCLA Working Papers in Cognitive Linguistics, 2,* 21-36.

Curtiss, S. (1988a). Abnormal language acquisition and the modularity of language. In F. E. Newmeyer (Ed.), *Linguistics: The Cambridge survey: Vol. II. Linguistic theory: Extensions and implication* (pp. 96–116). Cambridge, England: Cambridge University Press.

Curtiss, S. (1988b). The special talent of grammar acquisition. In L. Obler & D. Fein (Eds.), *The neuropsychology of talent and special abilities*. New York: Guilford.

Dale, P. S. (1980). Is early pragmatic development measurable? *Journal of Child Language, 7*, 1–12.

Davies, D., Sperber, R. D., & McCauley, C. (1981). Intelligence-related differences in semantic processing speed. *Journal of Experimental Child Psychology, 31*, 387–402.

Davis, H., & Oliver, B. (1980). A comparison of aspects of the maternal speech environment of retarded and nonretarded children. *Child: Care, Health, and Development, 6*, 135–145.

Davis, H., Stroud, A., & Green, L. (1988). Maternal language environment of children with mental retardation. *American Journal on Mental Retardation, 93*, 144–153.

de Boysson-Bardies, B., Halle, P., Sagart, L., & Durand, C. (1989). A crosslinguistic investigation of vowel formants in babbling. *Journal of Child Language, 16*, 1–18.

de Boysson-Bardies, B., Sagart, L., & Bacri, N. (1981). Phonetic analysis of late babbling: A case study of a French child. *Journal of Child Language, 8*, 511–524.

Della Corte, M., Benedict, H., & Klein, D. (1983). The relationship of pragmatic dimensions of mothers' speech to the referential-expressive distinction. *Journal of Child Language, 10*, 35–43.

Demetras, M., Post, K., & Snow, C. (1986). Feedback to first language learners: The role of repetitions and clarification questions. *Journal of Child Language, 13*, 275–292.

Deutsch, W. (1979). The conceptual impact of linguistic input: A comparison of German family children's and orphan's acquisition of kinship terms. *Journal of Child Language, 6*, 313–352.

Deutsch, W., & Pechmann, T. (1982). Social interaction and the development of definite descriptions. *Cognition, 11*, 159–184.

Dever, R. (1972). A comparison of the results of a revised version of Berko's test of morphology with the free speech of mentally retarded children. *Journal of Speech and Hearing Research, 15*, 169–178.

Dever, R., & Gardner, W. I. (1970). Performance of normal and retarded boys on Berko's test of morphology. *Language and Speech, 13*, 162–181.

Dewart, M. H. (1979). Language comprehension processes of mentally retarded children. *American Journal of Mental Deficiency, 84*, 177–183.

Dickson, W. P. (Ed.). (1981). *Children's oral communication skills*. New York: Academic.

Dickson, W. P. (1982). Two decades of referential communication research: A review and meta-analysis. In C. J. Brainerd & M. Pressley (Eds.), *Progress in cognitive development research* (Vol. 2, pp. 1–33). New York: Springer-Verlag.

Dodd, B. J. (1972). Comparison of babbling patterns in normal and Down-syndrome infants. *Journal of Mental Deficiency Research, 16*, 35–40.

Dodd, B. J. (1976). A comparison of the phonological systems of mental-age-matched normal, severely subnormal, and Down's syndrome children. *British Journal of Disorders of Communication, 11*, 27–42.

Dooley, J. F. (1976). *Language acquisition and Down's syndrome: A study of early semantics and syntax*. Unpublished doctoral dissertation. Harvard University, Cambridge, MA.

Dore, J. (1975). Holophrases, speech acts, and language universals. *Journal of Child Language, 2*, 21–41.

Dore, J. (1976). Children's illocutionary acts. In R. Freedle (Ed.), *Discourse relations: Comprehension and production*. Hillsdale, NJ: Lawrence Erlbaum Associates.

Dore, J. (1977). Children's illocutionary acts. In R. O. Freedle (Ed.), *Discourse production and comprehension* (Vol. 1, pp. 227–244). Norwood, NJ: Ablex.

Dorval, B., & Eckerman, C. O. (1984). Developmental trends in the quality of conversation achieved by small groups of acquainted peers. *Monographs of the Society for Research in Child Development, 49*(2, Serial No. 206).

Duchan, J. F., & Erickson, J. G. (1976). Normal and retarded children's understanding of semantic relations in different verbal contexts. *Journal of Speech and Hearing Research, 19*, 767–776.

Duncan, S., Jr., & Fiske, D. W. (1977). *Face-to-face interaction: Research methods and theory.* Hillsdale, NJ: Lawrence Erlbaum Associates.

Eco, U., Santambrogio, M., & Violi, P. (1988). *Meaning and mental representations.* Bloomington, IN: Indiana University Press.

Eimas, P. D. (1974). Auditory and linguistic processing of cues for place of articulation by infants. *Perception and Psychophysics, 16*, 513–521.

Eimas, P. D., Siqueland, E. R., Jusczyk, K. P., & Vigorito, J. (1971). Speech perception in infants. *Science, 171*, 303–306.

Elliott, C. (1978). Factors influencing the response latencies of subnormal children in naming pictures. *British Journal of Psychology, 69*, 295–303.

Elliott, D., Edwards, J. M., Weeks, D. J., Lindley, S., & Carnahan, H. (1987). Cerebral specialization in young adults with Down syndrome. *American Journal of Mental Deficiency, 91*, 480–485.

Elliott, D., Weeks, D. J., & Elliott, C. L. (1987). Cerebral specialization in individuals with Down syndrome. *American Journal of Mental Deficiency, 92*, 263–271.

Ellis, N. R., & Cavalier, A. R. (1982). Research perspectives in mental retardation. In I. E. Zigler & D. Balla (Eds.), *Mental retardation: The developmental-difference controversy.* Hillsdale, NJ: Lawrence Erlbaum Associates.

Elrod, M. M. (1983). Young children's responses to direct and indirect directives. *The Journal of Genetic Psychology, 143*, 217–227.

Emmorey, K. D., & Fromkin, V. A. (1988). The mental lexicon. In F. J. Newmeyer (Ed.), *Linguistics: The Cambridge survey* (Vol. 3, pp. 124–149). Cambridge, England: Cambridge University Press.

Ervin-Tripp, S. (1977). "Wait for me, rollerskate!" In C. Mitchell-Kernan & S. Ervin-Tripp (Eds.), *Child discourse* (pp. 165–188). New York: Academic.

Ervin-Tripp, S. (1984). The art of conversation: Commentary on "Developmental trends in the quality of conversation achieved by small groups of acquainted peers" by B. Dorval & C. O. Eckerman. *Monographs of the Society for Research in Child Development, 49*(2, Serial No. 206).

Ervin-Tripp, S., & Gordon, D. (1986). The development of requests. In R. L. Schiefelbusch (Ed.), *Communicative competence: Assessment and intervention* (pp. 61–95). Baltimore, MD: University Park Press.

Ervin-Tripp, S., Guo, J., & Lampert, M. (1990). Politeness and persuasion in children's control acts. *Journal of Pragmatics, 14*, 307–331.

Eson, M. E., & Shapiro, A. S. (1982). When "don't" means "do": Pragmatic and cognitive development in understanding an indirect imperative. *First Language, 3*, 83–91.

Ezell, H. K., & Goldstein, H. (1991). Observational learning of comprehension monitoring skills in children who exhibit mental retardation. *Journal of Speech and Hearing Research, 34*, 141–154.

Fay, D., & Mermelstein, R. (1982). Language in infantile autism. In S. Rosenberg (Ed.), *Handbook of applied psycholinguistics: Major thrusts of research and theory* (pp. 393–428). Hillsdale, NJ: Lawrence Erlbaum Associates.

Feagans, L., & Applebaum, M. I. (1986). Validation of language subtypes in learning disabled children. *Journal of Educational Psychology, 78*, 358–364.

Feldman, H., Goldin-Meadow, S., & Gleitman, L. R. (1978). Beyond Herodotus: The creation of language by linguistically deprived deaf children. In A. Lock (Ed.), *Action, symbol, and gesture: The emergence of language* (pp. 351–413). New York: Academic.

Fernald, A., Taeschner, T., Dunn, J., Papousek, M., de Boysson-Bardies, B., & Fukui, I. (1989). A cross-language study of prosodic modifications in mothers' and fathers' speech to preverbal infants. *Journal of Child Language, 16*, 477–502.

Ferrara, R. A., Brown, A. L., & Campione, J. C. (1986). Children's learning and transfer of inductive reasoning rules: Studies of proximal development. *Child Development, 57*, 1087–1099.

Fey, M. E. (1986). *Language intervention with young children*. Boston, MA: College-Hill Press.

Flavell, J. H. (1985). *Cognitive development* (2nd ed.). Englewood Cliffs, NJ: Prentice-Hall.

Flavell, J. H., Speer, J. R., Green, F. L., & August, D. L. (1981). The development of comprehension monitoring and knowledge about communication. *Monographs of the Society for Research in Child Development, 46*(5, Serial No. 192).

Fletcher, P., & Garman, M. (Eds.). (1986). *Language acquisition* (2nd ed.). Cambridge, England: Cambridge University Press.

Fodor, J. A. (1980). Fixation of belief and concept acquisition. In M. Piattelli-Palmarini (Ed.), *Language and learning* (pp. 142-162). Cambridge, MA: Harvard University Press.

Fodor, J. A. (1983). *The modularity of mind*. Cambridge, MA: MIT Press.

Fodor, J. A. (1989). Modules, frames, fridgeons, sleeping dogs, and the music of the spheres. In J. L. Garfield (Ed.), *Modularity in knowledge representation and natural-language understanding* (pp. 25-36). Cambridge, MA: MIT Press.

Fodor, J. A., & Pylyshyn, Z. W. (1988). Connectionism and cognitive architecture: A critical analysis. In S. Pinker & J. Mehler (Eds.), *Connections and symbols* (pp. 3-71). Cambridge, MA: MIT Press.

Folger, J. P., & Chapman, R. S. (1978). A pragmatic analysis of spontaneous imitation. *Journal of Child Language, 5*, 25-38.

Foss, D. J., & Hakes, D. T. (1978). *Psycholinguistics: An introduction to the psychology of language*. Englewood Cliffs, NJ: Prentice-Hall.

Fourcin, A. J. (1975). Language development in the absence of expressive speech. In E. H. Lenneberg & E. Lenneberg (Eds.), *Foundations of language development* (Vol. 2, pp. 263-268). New York: Academic.

Fowler, A. E. (1988). Determinants of rate of language growth in children with Down syndrome. In L. Nadel (Ed.), *The psychobiology of Down syndrome* (pp. 217-245). Cambridge, MA: MIT Press.

Fowler, A. E., Gelman, R., & Gleitman, L. R. (1980, October). *A comparison of normal and retardate language equated on MLU*. Paper presented at the Fifth Annual Boston University Conference on Child Language Development, Boston, MA.

Friedman, P., & Friedman, K. (1980). Accounting for individual differences when comparing the effectiveness of remedial language teaching methods. *Applied Psycholinguistics, 1*, 151-171.

Fromkin, V. A., & Rodman, R. (1988). *An introduction to language* (4th ed.). New York: Holt, Rinehart & Winston.

Fujiki, M., Brinton, B., & Sonnenberg, E. A. (1990). Repair of overlapping speech in the conversations of specifically language-impaired and normally developing children. *Applied Psycholinguistics, 11*, 201-215.

Furman, L. N., & Walden, T. A. (1990). Effect of script knowledge on preschool children's communicative interactions. *Developmental Psychology, 26*, 227-233.

Furrow, D., & Nelson, K. (1986). A further look at the motherese hypothesis: A reply to Gleitman, Newport, and Gleitman. *Journal of Child Language, 13*, 163-176.

Gallagher, T. M. (1977). Revision behaviors in the speech of normal children developing language. *Journal of Speech and Hearing Research, 20*, 303-318.

Gallagher, T. M. (1981). Contingent query sequences within adult-child discourse. *Journal of Child Language, 8*, 51-62.

Gallagher, T. M. (1991a). Language and social skills: Implications for assessment and intervention with school-age children. In T. Gallagher (Ed.), *Pragmatics of language: Clinical practice issues* (pp. 11-41). San Diego: Singular Publishing Group.

Gallagher, T. M. (Ed.). (1991b). *Pragmatics of language: Clinical practice issues*. San Diego, CA: Singular Publishing Group.

Garcia, E., Guess, D., & Byrnes, J. (1973). Development of syntax in a retarded girl using procedures of imitation, reinforcement, and modeling. *Journal of Applied Behavior Analysis, 6*, 299-318.

Garfield, J. L. (1987). Introduction: Carving the mind at its joints. In J. L. Garfield (Ed.), *Modularity in knowledge representation and natural-language understanding* (pp. 1-13). Cambridge, MA: MIT Press.

Garvey, C. (1975). Requests and responses in children's speech. *Journal of Child Language, 2*, 41-60.

Garvey, C. (1977). The contingent query: A dependent act in conversation. In M. Lewis & L. A. Rosenblum (Eds.), *Interaction, conversation, and the development of language* (pp. 63-93). New York: Wiley.

Garvey, C., & BenDebba, M. (1978). An experimental investigation of contingent query sequences. *Discourse Processes, 1*, 36-50.

Garvey, C., & Berninger, G. (1981). Timing and turn-taking in children's conversation. *Discourse Processes, 4*, 27-58.

Gelman, R., & Baillargeon, R. (1983). A review of some Piagetian concepts. In J. H. Flavell & E. M. Markman (Eds.), *Cognitive development* (pp. 167-230). New York: Wiley.

Gibson, D. (1966). Early developmental staging as a prophesy index in Down's syndrome. *American Journal of Mental Deficiency, 70*, 825-828.

Gillham, B. (1979). *The first words language programme.* London: George Allen & Unwin.

Gilmore, P., & Glatthorn, A. A. (1982). *Children in and out of school.* Washington, DC: Center for Applied Linguistics.

Gleason, J. B. (1989). *The development of language* (2nd ed.). Columbus, OH: Merrill.

Gleason, J. B., Perlmann, R. Y., & Greif, E. B. (1984). What's the magic word: Learning language through politeness routines. *Discourse Processes, 7*, 493-502.

Gleitman, L. R. (1990). The structural sources of verb meanings. *Language Acquisition, 1*, 3-55.

Gleitman, L. R., Gleitman, H., Landau, B., & Wanner, E. (1988). Where learning begins: Initial representations for language learning. In F. J. Newmeyer (Ed.), *Linguistics: The Cambridge survey* (Vol. 3, pp. 150-193). Cambridge, England: Cambridge University Press.

Gleitman, L. R., Newport, E. L., & Gleitman, H. (1984). The current state of the motherese hypothesis. *Journal of Child Language, 11*, 43-70.

Gleitman, L. R., & Wanner, E. (1982). Language acquisition: The state of the art. In E. Wanner & L. R. Gleitman (Eds.), *Language acquisition: The state of the art* (pp. 3-48). Cambridge: Cambridge University Press.

Glenn, S. M., & Cunningham, C. C. (1983). What do babies listen to most? A developmental study of auditory preferences in nonhandicapped infants and infants with Down's syndrome. *Developmental Psychology, 19*, 332-337.

Glidden, L. M., & Mar, H. H. (1978). Availability and accessibility of information in the semantic memory of retarded and nonretarded adolescents. *Journal of Experimental Child Psychology, 25*, 33-40.

Glucksberg, S., & Krauss, R. M. (1967). What do people say after they have learned how to talk? Studies of the development of referential communication. *Merrill-Palmer Quarterly, 13*, 309-316.

Glucksberg, S., Krauss, R. M., & Higgins, E. T. (1975). The development of referential communication skills. In F. D. Horowitz (Ed.), *Review of child development research* (Vol. 4, pp. 305-345). Chicago: University of Chicago Press.

Goldfield, B. A., & Reznick, J. S. (1990). Early lexical acquisition: Rate, content, and the vocabulary spurt. *Journal of Child Language, 17*, 171-183.

Goldfield, B. A., & Snow, C. E. (1989). Individual differences in language acquisition. In J. B. Gleason (Ed.), *The development of language* (2nd ed., pp. 303-325). Columbus, OH: Merrill.

Goldin-Meadow, S. (1982). The resilience of recursion: A study of a communication system developed without a conventional language model. In E. Wanner & L. R. Gleitman (Eds.), *Language acquisition: The state of the art* (pp. 51-77). Cambridge, England: Cambridge University Press.

Goldin-Meadow, S., & Feldman, H. (1977). The development of language-like communication without a language model. *Science, 197*, 401-403.

Goldin-Meadow, S., & Mylander, C. (1990a). Beyond the input given: The child's role in the acquisition of language. *Language, 66*, 323-355.

Goldin-Meadow, S., & Mylander, C. (1990b). The role of parental input in the development of a morphological system. *Journal of Child Language, 17*, 527-564.

Goldstein, H. (1983). Recombinative generalization: Relationship between environmental conditions and the linguistic repertoires of language learners. *Analysis and Intervention in Developmental Disabilities, 3*, 279-293.

Goldstein, H., Angelo, D., & Mousetis, L. (1987). Acquisition and extension of syntactic repertoires by severely mentally retarded youth. *Research in Developmental Disabilities, 8*, 549-574.

Goldstein, H., & Kaczmarek, L. (1992). Promoting communicative interaction among children in integrated intervention settings. In S. F. Warren & J. Reichle (Eds.), *Causes and effects in communication and language intervention* (pp. 81-111). Baltimore, MD: Brookes.

Golinkoff, R. M. (1983). The preverbal negotiation of failed messages: Insights into the transition period. In R. M. Golinkoff (Ed.), *The transition from prelinguistic to linguistic communication.* Hillsdale, NJ: Lawrence Erlbaum Associates.

Golinkoff, R. M. (1986). "I beg your pardon?": The preverbal negotiation of failed messages. *Journal of Child Language, 13*, 455-476.

Golinkoff, R. M., & Hirsh-Pasek, K. (1987, October). *A new picture of language development: Evidence from comprehension.* Paper presented at the 12th Annual Boston University Conference on Language Development, Boston, MA.

Goodluck, H. (1986). Language acquisition and linguistic theory. In P. Fletcher & M. Garman (Eds.), *Language acquisition* (2nd ed., pp. 49-68). Cambridge, England: Cambridge University Press.

Gopnik, A. (1987, July). *Language before stage 6.* Paper presented at the Fourth International Congress for the Study of Child Language, Lund, Sweden.

Gopnik, A., & Meltzoff, A. N. (1987). The development of categorization in the second year and its relation to other cognitive and linguistic development. *Child Development, 58*, 1523-1531.

Gopnik, A., & Meltzoff, A. N. (1986). Relating between semantic and cognitive development in the one-word stage: The specificity hypothesis. *Child Development, 57*, 1040-1053.

Gopnik, M. (1990). Feature blindness: A case study. *Language Acquisition, 1*, 136-164.

Gopnik, M. (1992). When language is a problem. In R. Campbell (Ed.), *Mental lies: Case studies in cognition* (pp. 61-83). Oxford: Blackwell.

Gordon, D., & Ervin-Tripp, S. (1984). The structure of children's requests. In R. L. Schiefelbusch & J. Pickar (Eds.), *The acquisition of communicative competence* (pp. 295-321). Baltimore: University Park Press.

Gordon, D. P., Budwig, N., Strage, A., & Carrell, P. (1980, October). *Children's requests to unfamiliar adults: Form, social function, age variations.* Paper presented at the Boston University Conference on Language Development, Boston, MA.

Gordon, P. (1990). Learnability and feedback. *Developmental Psychology, 26*, 215-218.

Green, G. M. (1989). *Pragmatics and natural language understanding.* Hillsdale, NJ: Lawrence Erlbaum Associates.

Greenfield, P. M., & Smith, J. (1976). *The structure of communication in early language.* New York: Academic.

Greenwald, C. A., & Leonard, L. B. (1979). Communicative and sensorimotor development of Down's syndrome children. *American Journal of Mental Deficiency, 84*, 296-303.

Grice, H. P. (1975). Logic and conversation. The William James Lectures at Harvard University, Lesson II, 1967. In P. Cole & J. L. Morgan (Eds.), *Syntax and semantics—Speech acts* (pp. 41-58). New York: Academic.

Greif, E. B., & Gleason, J. B. (1980). Hi, thanks, and goodbye: More routine information. *Language in Society, 9*, 159-166.

Grieser, D. L., & Kuhl, P. K. (1988). Maternal speech to infants in a tonal language: Support for universal prosodic features in motherese. *Developmental Psychology, 24*, 14-20.

Griffiths, P. (1986). Early vocabulary. In P. Fletcher & M. Garman (Eds.), *Language acquisition* (2nd ed., pp. 279-306). Cambridge, England: Cambridge University Press.

Grodzinsky, Y. (1990). *Theoretical perspectives on language deficits*. Cambridge, MA: MIT Press.

Groff, M. G., & Linden, K. W. (1982). The WISC-R factor score profiles of cultural-familial mentally retarded and nonretarded youth. *American Journal of Mental Deficiency, 87*, 147–152.

Grossman, H. J. (Ed.). (1983). *Manual on terminology and classification in mental retardation* (3rd rev. ed.). Washington, DC: American Association on Mental Deficiency.

Guess, D. (1969). A functional analysis of receptive language and productive speech: Acquisition of the plural morpheme. *Journal of Applied Behavior Analysis, 2*, 55–64.

Guess, D., & Baer, D. M. (1973). An analysis of individual differences in generalization between receptive and productive language in retarded children. *Journal of Applied Behavior Analysis, 6*, 311–329.

Guess, D., Keogh, W., & Sailor, W. (1978). Generalization of speech and language behavior. In R. Schiefelbusch (Ed.), *Bases of language intervention* (pp. 373–395). Baltimore: University Park Press.

Guess, D., Sailor, W., & Baer, D. M. (1978). *Functional speech and language training for the severely handicapped* (Part I). Lawrence, KS: H & H Enterprises.

Gunn, P., Clark, D., & Berry, P. (1980). Maternal speech during play with a Down's syndrome infant. *Mental Retardation, 18*, 15–18.

Gutmann, A. J., & Rondal, J. A. (1979). Verbal operants in mothers' speech to nonretarded and Down's syndrome children matched for linguistic level. *American Journal of Mental Deficiency, 83*, 446–452.

Haegeman, L. (1991). *Introduction to government and binding theory*. Oxford: Blackwell.

Hagtvet, B. (1979). *Prestandardization edition of the Reynell Developmental Language Scales*. Hosle, Baerum, Norway: Statens spesiallaererhoyskole.

Hahn, W. K. (1987). Cerebral lateralization of function: From infancy through childhood. *Psychological Bulletin, 101*, 376–392.

Halle, J. W., Baer, D. M., & Spradlin, J. E. (1981). Teachers' generalized use of delay as a stimulus control procedure to increase language use in handicapped children. *Journal of Applied Behavior Analysis, 14*, 389–409.

Halle, J. W., Marshall, A., & Spradlin, J. (1979). Time delay: A technique to increase language use and facilitate generalization in retarded children. *Journal of Applied Behavior Analysis, 12*, 431–439.

Hanzlik, J. R., & Stevenson, M. B. (1986). Interaction of mothers with their infants who are mentally retarded, retarded with cerebral palsy, or nonretarded. *American Journal of Mental Deficiency, 90*, 513–520.

Harding, C. (1983). Setting the stage for language acquisition: Communication development in the first year. In R. M. Golinkoff (Ed.), *The transition from prelinguistic to linguistic communication*. Hillsdale, NJ: Lawrence Erlbaum Associates.

Haring, T. G., Roger, B., Lee, M., Breen, C., & Gaylord-Ross, R. (1986). Teaching social language to moderately handicapped students. *Journal of Applied Behavior Analysis, 19*, 159–171.

Harkness, S. (1977). Aspects of social environment and first language acquisition in rural Africa. In C. E. Snow & C. Ferguson (Eds.), *Talking to children: Language input and language acquisition*. Cambridge, England: Cambridge University Press.

Harris, M., Jones, D., Brookes, S., & Grant, J. (1986). Relations between non-verbal context of maternal speech and rate of language development. *British Journal of Developmental Psychology, 4*, 261–268.

Hart, B., & Risley, T. (1968). Establishing use of descriptive adjectives in the spontaneous speech of disadvantaged preschool children. *Journal of Applied Behavior Analysis, 1*, 109–120.

Hart, B., & Risley, T. (1974). Using preschool materials to modify the language of disadvantaged children. *Journal of Applied Behavior Analysis, 7*, 243–256.

Hart, B., & Risley, T. (1975). Incidental teaching of language in the preschool. *Journal of Applied Behavior Analysis, 8*, 411–420.

Hart, B., & Risley, T. (1980). In vivo language intervention: Unanticipated general effects. *Journal of Applied Behavior Analysis, 13*, 407–432.

Hart, B., & Rogers-Warren, A. (1978). A milieu approach to teaching language. In R. Schiefel-busch (Ed.), *Language intervention strategies* (pp. 193–235). Baltimore: University Park Press.

Hartley, X. Y. (1985). Receptive language processing and ear advantage of Down's syndrome children. *Journal of Mental Deficiency Research, 29,* 197–205.

Hawkins, J. A. (Ed.). (1988). *Explaining language universals.* Oxford: Blackwell.

Hegde, M. (1980). An experimental–clinical analysis of grammatical and behavioral distinctions between verbal auxiliary and copula. *Journal of Speech and Hearing Research, 23,* 864–877.

Hegde, M., & Geirut, J. (1979). The operant training and generalization of pronouns and a verb form in a language delayed child. *Journal of Speech and Hearing Disorders, 12,* 23–34.

Heibeck, T. H., & Markman, E. M. (1987). Word learning in children: An examination of fast mapping. *Child Development, 58,* 1021–1034.

Hemphill, L., Picardi, N., & Tager-Flusberg, H. (1991). Narrative as an index of communicative competence in mildly mentally retarded children. *Applied Psycholinguistics, 12,* 263–279.

Hemphill, L., & Siperstein, G. N. (1990). Conversational competence and peer response to mildly retarded children. *Journal of Educational Psychology, 82,* 128–134.

Hester, P., & Hendrickson, J. (1977). Training functional expressive language: The acquisition and generalization of five-element syntactic responses. *Journal of Applied Behavior Analysis, 10,* 316.

Hirsh-Pasek, K., Treiman, R., & Schneiderman, M. (1984). Brown and Hanlon revisited: Mothers' sensitivity to ungrammatical forms. *Journal of Child Language, 11,* 81–88.

Hoff-Ginsberg, E. (1985). Some contributions of mothers' speech to their children's syntactic growth. *Journal of Child Language, 12,* 367–385.

Hoff-Ginsberg, E. (1990). Maternal speech and the child's development of syntax: A further look. *Journal of Child Language, 17,* 85–99.

Hoff-Ginsberg, E., & Shatz, M. (1982). Linguistic input and the child's acquisition of language. *Psychological Bulletin, 92,* 3–26.

Horn, J. L. (1976). Human abilities: A review of research and theory in the early 1970s. *Annual Review of Psychology, 27,* 437–485.

Huttenlocher, J. (1974). The origins of language comprehension. In R. Solso (Ed.), *Theories in cognitive psychology* (pp. 331–368). Hillsdale, NJ: Lawrence Erlbaum Associates.

Huttenlocher, J., & Smiley, P. (1987). Early word meanings: The case of object names. *Cognitive Psychology, 19,* 63–89.

Huttenlocher, P. R. (1975). Synaptic and dendritic development and mental deficits. In N. A. Buchwald & M. A. Brazier (Eds.), *Brain mechanisms in mental retardation* (pp. 123–140). New York: Academic.

Hyams, N. M. (1986). *Language acquisition and the theory of parameters.* Dordrecht, Holland: Reidel.

Ingram, D. (1976). *Phonological disability in children.* New York: Elsevier.

Ingram, D. (1986). Phonological development: Production. In P. Fletcher & M. Garman (Eds.), *Language acquisition* (2nd ed., pp. 223–239). Cambridge, England: Cambridge University Press.

Ingram, D. (1989). *First language acquisition.* Cambridge, England: Cambridge University Press.

Inhelder, B. (1968). *The diagnosis of reasoning in the mentally retarded.* New York: John Day.

Ironsmith, M., & Whitehurst, G. J. (1978). The development of listener abilities in communication: How children deal with ambiguous information. *Child Development, 49,* 348–352.

Jackendoff, R. C. (1987). *Consciousness and the computational mind.* Cambridge, MA: MIT Press.

Jackson, S., & Jacobs, S. (1982). Ambiguity and implications in children's discourse comprehension. *Journal of Child Language, 9,* 209–216.

Jacobs, R. A., & Rosenbaum, P. S. (1968). *English transformational grammar.* Waltham, MA: Blaisdell.

James, S. (1978). The effect of listener age and situation on the politeness of children's directives. *Journal of Psycholinguistic Research, 7,* 307–317.

Jeffree, D., Wheldall, K., & Mittler, P. (1973). Facilitating two-word utterances in two Down's syndrome boys. *American Journal of Mental Deficiency, 78,* 117–122.

Jellinger, J. (1972). Neuropsychological features in unclassified mental retardation. In J. B. Cavanaugh (Ed.), *The brain in unclassified mental retardation* (pp. 293–306). Baltimore: Williams & Wilkins.

Johnson, J. S., & Newport, E. L. (1989). Critical period effects in second language learning: The influence of maturational state on the acquisition of English as a second language. *Cognitive Psychology, 21,* 60–99.

Johnson-Laird, P. N. (1975). Commentary. In N. O'Connor (Ed.), *Language, cognitive deficits, and retardation* (pp. 188–192). London: Butterworths.

Johnston, J. R. (1985). Cognitive prerequisites: The evidence from children learning English. In D. I. Slobin (Ed.), *The crosslinguistic study of language acquisition: Vol. 2. Theoretical issues* (pp. 961–1004). Hillsdale, NJ: Lawrence Erlbaum Associates.

Johnston, J. R. (1988). Generalization: The nature of change. *Language, Speech, and Hearing Services in Schools, 19,* 314–329.

Jones, C. P., & Adamson, L. B. (1987). Language use in mother–child and child–sibling interactions. *Child Development, 58,* 356–366.

Kahn, J. V. (1975). Relationship of Piaget's sensorimotor period to language acquisition of profoundly retarded children. *American Journal of Mental Deficiency, 79,* 640–643.

Kaiser, A. P., Yoder, P. J., & Keetz, A. (1992). Evaluating milieu teaching. In S. F. Warren & J. Reichle (Eds.), *Causes and effects in communication and language intervention* (pp. 9–47). Baltimore, MD: Brookes.

Kamhi, A. G., & Johnston, J. R. (1982). Toward an understanding of retarded children's linguistic deficiencies. *Journal of Speech and Hearing Research, 25,* 435–445.

Kamhi, A. G., & Masterson, J. J. (1989). Language and cognition in mentally handicapped people: Last rites for the difference–delay controversy. In M. Beveridge, G. Conti-Ramsden, & I. Leudar (Eds.), *Language and communication in mentally handicapped people* (pp. 83–111). London: Chapman & Hall.

Karen, R. L., Astin-Smith, S., & Creasey, D. (1985). Teaching telephone-answering skills to mentally retarded adults. *American Journal of Mental Deficiency, 89,* 595–609.

Karmiloff-Smith, A. (1986). Some fundamental aspects of language development after age 5. In P. Fletcher & M. Garman (Eds.), *Language acquisition* (pp. 455–474). Cambridge, England: Cambridge University Press.

Keenan, E. O. (1974). Conversational competence in children. *Journal of Child Language, 1,* 163–185.

Keenan, E. O., & Schieffelin, B. B. (1976). Topic as a discourse notion: A study of topic in the conversations of children and adults. In C. Li (Ed.), *Subject and topic.* New York: Academic.

Kemler Nelson, D. G., Hirsh-Pasek, K., Jusczyk, P. W., & Wright Cassidy, K. (1989). How prosodic cues in motherese might assist language learning. *Journal of Child Language, 16,* 55–68.

Kempson, R. M. (1975). *Presupposition and the delimitation of semantics.* New York: Cambridge University Press.

Kernan, K. T. (1990). Comprehension of syntactically indicated sequence by Down's syndrome and other mentally retarded adults. *Journal of Mental Deficiency Research, 34,* 169–178.

Kernan, K. T., & Sabsay, S. (1987). Referential first mention in narratives by mildly mentally retarded adults. *Research in Developmental Disabilities, 8,* 361–369.

Kitano, M. K. (1987). Piagetian approach to special education. In C. R. Reynolds & L. Mann (Eds.), *Encyclopedia of special education* (Vol. 2, pp. 1202–1209). New York: Wiley.

Klein, N. K., & Safford, P. L. (1977). Application of Piaget's theory to the study of thinking of the mentally retarded: A review of research. *Journal of Special Education, 11,* 201–216.

Klink, M., Gerstman, L., Raphael, L., Schlanger, B. B., & Newsome, L. (1986). Phonological process usage by young EMR children and nonretarded preschool children. *American Journal of Mental Deficiency, 91,* 190–195.

Kuhl, P., & Miller, J. D. (1975). Speech perception by the chinchilla: Voiced–voiceless distinction in alveolar plosive consonants. *Science, 190,* 69–72.

Kuhl, P., & Padden, D. M. (1982). Enhanced discrimination at the phonetic boundaries for the voicing feature in macaques. *Perception and Psychophysics, 32,* 542–550.

Lackner, J. R. (1968). A developmental study of language behavior in retarded children. *Neuropsychologia, 6,* 301–320.

Layton, T. L., & Sharifi, H. (1979). Meaning and structure of Down's syndrome and nonretarded children's spontaneous speech. *American Journal of Mental Deficiency, 83,* 439–445.

Ledbetter, P. J., & Dent, C. H. (1988). Young children's sensitivity to direct and indirect request structure. *First Language, 8,* 227–246.

Leifer, J. S., & Lewis, M. (1983). Maternal speech to normal and handicapped children: A look at question-asking behavior. *Infant Behavior and Development, 6,* 175–187.

Leifer, J. S., & Lewis, M. (1984). Acquisition of conversational response skills by young Down syndrome and nonretarded young children. *American Journal of Mental Deficiency, 88,* 610–618.

Lempers, J. D., & Elrod, M. M. (1983). Children's appraisal of different sources of referential communicative inadequacies. *Child Development, 54,* 509–515.

Leonard, L. B. (1975). Relational meaning and the facilitation of slow-learning children's language. *American Journal of Mental Deficiency, 80,* 180–185.

Leonard, L. B. (1982). The nature of specific language impairment in children. In S. Rosenberg (Ed.), *Handbook of applied psycholinguistics: Major thrusts of research and theory* (pp. 295–327). Hillsdale, NJ: Lawrence Erlbaum Associates.

Leonard, L. B. (1987). Is specific language impairment a useful construct? In S. Rosenberg (Ed.), *Advances in applied psycholinguistics* (Vol. 1, pp. 1–29). New York: Cambridge University Press.

Leonard, L. B., & Fey, M. E. (1991). Facilitating grammatical development: The contribution of pragmatics. In T. M. Gallagher (Ed.), *Pragmatics of language: Clinical practice issues* (pp. 333–355). San Diego, CA: Singular Press.

Leonard, L. B., Wilcox, M. J., Fulmer, K. C., & Davis, G. A. (1978). An investigation of children's comprehension of pragmatic meanings. *Journal of Speech and Hearing Research, 21,* 528–537.

Levinson, S. C. (1983). *Pragmatics.* Cambridge, England: Cambridge University Press.

Levy, Y. (1988). On the early learning of formal grammatical systems: Evidence from studies of the acquisition of gender and countability. *Journal of Child Language, 15,* 179–187.

Lightfoot, D. (1991). *How to set parameters.* Cambridge, MA: MIT Press.

Limber, J. (1973). The genesis of complex sentences. In T. E. Moore (Ed.), *Cognitive development and the acquisition of language* (pp. 169–185). New York: Academic.

Limber, J. (1976). Unraveling competence, performance and pragmatics in the speech of young children. *Journal of Child Language, 3,* 309–318.

Lincoln, A. J., Courchesne, E., Kilman, B. A., & Galambos, R. (1985). Neuropsychological correlates of information-processing by children with Down syndrome. *American Journal of Mental Deficiency, 84,* 403–414.

Lipsky, D., & Gartner, A. (Eds.). (1989). *Beyond separate education: Quality education for all.* Baltimore, MD: Paul H. Brookes Publishing.

Lobato, D., Barrera, R. D., & Feldman, R. S. (1981). Sensorimotor functioning and prelinguistic communication of severely and profoundly retarded individuals. *American Journal of Mental Deficiency, 85,* 489–496.

Locke, J. L. (1983). *Phonological acquisition and change.* New York: Academic.

Locke, J. L. (1986). Speech perception and the emergent lexicon: An ethological approach. In P. Fletcher & M. Garman (Eds.), *Language acquisition* (2nd ed., pp. 240–250). Cambridge, England: Cambridge University Press.

Locke, J. L. (1988). The sound shape of early lexical representations. In M. D. Smith & J. L. Locke (Eds.), *The emergent lexicon* (pp. 3–22). San Diego: Academic.

Locke, J. L., & Mather, P. L. (1989). Genetic factors in the ontogeny of spoken language: Evidence from monozygotic and dizygotic twins. *Journal of Child Language, 16,* 553–560.

Locke, J. L., & Pearson, D. M. (1990). Linguistic significance of babbling: Evidence from a tracheotomized infant. *Journal of Child Language, 17,* 1–16.

Longhurst, T. M. (1974). Communication in retarded adolescents: Sex and intelligence level. *American Journal of Mental Deficiency, 78*, 607-618.

Longhurst, T. M., & Berry, G. W. (1975). Communication in retarded adolescents: Response to listener feedback. *American Journal of Mental Deficiency, 80*, 158-164.

Loveland, K. A., Tunali, B., McEvoy, R., & Kelly, M. L. (1989). Referential communication and response adequacy in autism and Down's syndrome. *Applied Psycholinguistics, 10*, 301-313.

Lovell, K., & Bradbury, B. (1967). The learning of English morphology in educationally subnormal special school children. *American Journal of Mental Deficiency, 72*, 609-615.

Lust, B., & Mazuka, R. (1989). Cross-linguistic studies of directionality in first language acquisition: The Japanese data—A response to O'Grady, Suzukiwei & Cho (1986). *Journal of Child Language, 16*, 665-684.

Lutzker, J., & Sherman, J. (1974). Producing generative sentence usage by imitation and reinforcement procedures. *Journal of Applied Behavior Analysis, 7*, 447-460.

MacKain, K. S. (1988). Filling the gap between speech and language. In M. D. Smith & J. L. Locke (Eds.), *The emergent lexicon* (pp. 51-74). San Diego: Academic.

MacWhinney, B. (1989). Competition and lexical categorization. In R. Corrigan, F. Eckman, & M. Noonan (Eds.), *Linguistic categorization* (pp. 195-241). Amsterdam: John Benjamins.

MacWhinney, B., & Leinbach, J. (1991). Implementations are not conceptualizations: Revising the verb learning model. *Cognition, 40*, 121-157.

MacWhinney, B., Leinbach, J., Taraban, R., & McDonald, J. (1989). Language learning: Cues or rules? *Journal of Memory and Language, 28*, 255-277.

Madison, L. S., George, C., & Moeschler, J. B. (1986). Cognitive functioning in the fragile-X syndrome: A study of intellectual, memory and communication skills. *Journal of Mental Deficiency Research, 30*, 129-148.

Mahoney, G. (1988). Maternal communication style with mentally retarded children. *American Journal on Mental Retardation, 92*, 352-359.

Mahoney, G., Finger, I., & Powell, A. (1985). Relationship of maternal behavioral style to the development of organically impaired mentally retarded infants. *American Journal of Mental Deficiency, 90*, 296-302.

Mahoney, G., Fors, S., & Woods, S. (1990). Maternal directive behavior revisited. *American Journal on Mental Retardation, 94*, 398-406.

Mahoney, G., Glover, A., & Finger, I. (1981). Relationship between language and sensorimotor development of Down syndrome and nonretarded children. *American Journal of Mental Deficiency, 86*, 21-27.

Maratsos, M. (1988). Crosslinguistic analysis, universals, and language acquisition. In F. S. Kessel (Ed.), *The development of language and language researchers* (pp. 121-152). Hillsdale, NJ: Lawrence Erlbaum Associates.

Marcell, M. M., & Armstrong, V. (1982). Auditory and visual sequential memory of Down syndrome and nonretarded children. *American Journal of Mental Deficiency, 87*, 86-95.

Marcell, M. M., & Weeks, S. L. (1988). Short-term memory difficulties and Down's syndrome. *Journal of Mental Deficiency Research, 32*, 153-162.

Markman, E. M., & Wachtel, G. F. (1988). Children's use of mutual exclusivity to constrain the meanings of words. *Cognitive Psychology, 20*, 121-157.

Marshall, J. C. (1990). Foreword. In J. E. Yamada, *Laura: A case for the modularity of language* (pp. vii-xi). Cambridge, MA: MIT Press.

Matson, J. L., & Adkins, J. (1980). A self-instructional social skills training program for mentally retarded persons. *Mental Retardation, 18*, 245-248.

Matthei, E. H. (1989). Crossing boundaries: More evidence for phonological constraints on early multi-word utterances. *Journal of Child Language, 16*, 41-54.

Maurer, H., & Sherrod, K. B. (1987). Context of directives given to young children with Down syndrome and nonretarded children: Development over two years. *American Journal of Mental Deficiency, 91*, 579-590.

McCauley, C., Sperber, R. D., & Roaden, S. K. (1978). Verification of property statements by retarded and nonretarded adolescents. *American Journal of Mental Deficiency, 83,* 276–282.

McConkey, R., & O'Connor, M. (1982). A new approach to parental involvement in language intervention programmes. *Child: Care, Health, and Development, 8,* 163–176.

McCook, B., Cipiani, E., Madigan, K., & La Campagne, J. (1988). Developing requesting behavior: Acquisition, fluency, and generality. *Mental Retardation, 26,* 137–143.

McCormick, L., & Schiefelbusch, R. (Eds.). (1984). *Early language intervention.* Columbus, OH: Merrill.

McDaniel, D., Cairns, H. S., & Hsu, J. R. (1990–1991). Control principles in the grammars of young children. *Language Acquisition, 1,* 297–335.

McDonald, L., & Pien, D. (1982). Mother conversational behavior as a function of interactional intent. *Journal of Child Language, 9,* 337–358.

McGee, G., Krantz, P. J., Mason, D., & McClannahan, L. E. (1983). A modified incidental teaching procedure for autistic youth: Acquisition and generalization of receptive object labels. *Journal of Applied Behavior Analysis, 16,* 329–338.

McGee, G. G., Krantz, P. J., & McClannahan, L. E. (1985). The facilitative effects of incidental teaching on preposition use by autistic children. *Journal of Applied Behavior Analysis, 18,* 17–31.

McLaren, J., & Bryson, S. E. (1987). Review of recent epidemiological studies of mental retardation: Prevalence, associated disorders and etiology. *American Journal on Mental Retardation, 92,* 243–254.

McLean, J., & Snyder-McLean, L. (1978). *A transaction approach to early language training.* Columbus, OH: Merrill.

McTear, M. F., & Conti-Ramsden, G. (1992). *Pragmatic disability in children.* London: Whurr Publishers.

Mein, R., & O'Connor, N. (1960). A study of the oral vocabulary of severely subnormal patients. *Journal of Mental Deficiency Research, 4,* 130.

Menig-Peterson, C. L. (1975). The modification of communicative behavior in preschool-aged children as a function of the listener's perspective. *Child Development, 46,* 1015–1018.

Menn, L. (1989). Phonological development: Learning sounds and sound patterns. In J. B. Gleason (Ed.), *The development of language* (2nd ed., pp. 59–100). Columbus, OH: Merrill.

Menyuk, P. (1988). *Language development: Knowledge and use.* Glenview, IL: Scott Foresman.

Menyuk, P., Menn, L., & Silber, R. (1986). Early strategies for the perception and production of words and sounds. In P. Fletcher & M. Garman (Eds.), *Language acquisition* (2nd ed., pp. 198–222). Cambridge, England: Cambridge University Press.

Merrill, E. C. (1985). Differences in semantic processing speed of mentally retarded and nonretarded persons. *American Journal of Mental Deficiency, 90,* 71–80.

Merrill, E. C., & Mar, H. H. (1987). Differences between mentally retarded and nonretarded persons' efficiency of auditory processing. *American Journal of Mental Deficiency, 91,* 406–414.

Mervis, C. B. (1983). Acquisition of a lexicon. *Contemporary Educational Psychology, 8,* 210–236.

Mervis, C. B. (1988). Early lexical development: Theory and application. In L. Nadel (Ed.), *The psychobiology of Down syndrome* (pp. 101–143). Cambridge, MA: MIT Press.

Mervis, C. B. (1989). *Operating principles and early lexical development.* Paper presented at the biennial meeting of the Society for Research in Child Development, Kansas City, MO.

Mervis, C. B., & Rosch, E. (1981). Categorization of natural objects. *Annual Review of Psychology, 32,* 89–115.

Messer, D. J. (1980). The episodic structure of maternal speech to young children. *Journal of Child Language, 7,* 29–40.

Miller, J. F. (1981). *Assessing language production in children.* Baltimore: University Park Press.

Miller, J. F. (1983). Identifying children with language disorders and describing their language performance. In J. F. Miller, D. E. Yoder, & R. Schiefelbusch (Eds.), *Contemporary issues in language intervention* (pp. 61–74). Rockville, MD: ASHA.

Miller, J. F. (1987). Language and communication characteristics of children with Down syndrome. In S. M. Pueschel, C. Tingey, J. E. Rynders, A. C. Crocker, & D. M. Crutcher (Eds.), *New perspectives on Down syndrome*. Baltimore: Brookes Publishing.

Miller, J. F. (1988). The developmental asynchrony of language development in children with Down syndrome. In L. Nadel (Ed.), *The psychobiology of Down syndrome* (pp. 167–198). Cambridge, MA: MIT Press.

Miller, J. F., & Chapman, R. S. (1984). Disorders of communication: Investigating the development of language of mentally retarded children. *American Journal of Mental Deficiency, 88*, 536–545.

Miller, J. F., Chapman, R. S., Branston, M. B., & Reichle, J. (1980). Language comprehension in sensorimotor stages V and VI. *Journal of Speech and Hearing Research, 23*, 284–311.

Miller, J. F., Chapman, R. S., & MacKenzie, H. (1981, June). *Individual differences in the language acquisition of mentally retarded children.* Paper presented at the Second Annual Wisconsin Symposium on Research in Child Language Disorders, Madison, WI.

Miller, J. F., Chapman, R. S., & MacKenzie, H. (1981, August). *Individual differences in the language acquisition of mentally retarded children.* Paper presented at the Second International Congress for the Study of Child Language, University of British Columbia, Vancouver, BC, Canada.

Miller, J., & Yoder, D. (1974). An ontogenetic language teaching strategy for retarded children. In R. Schiefelbusch & L. Lloyd (Eds.), *Language perspectives: Acquisition, retardation, and intervention* (pp. 505–528). Baltimore: University Park Press.

Milosky, L. M. (1992). Children listening: The role of world knowledge in language comprehension. In R. S. Chapman (Ed.), *Processes in language acquisition and disorders* (pp. 20–44). Chicago: Mosby-Year Book.

Moran, M. J., Money, S. M., & Leonard, D. A. (1984). Phonological process analysis of the speech of mentally retarded adults. *American Journal of Mental Deficiency, 89*, 304–306.

Morgan, J. L., & Travis, L. L. (1989). Limits on negative information in language input. *Journal of Child Language, 16*, 531–552.

Mundy, P., Seibert, J. M., & Hogan, A. M. (1984). Relationship between sensorimotor and early communication abilities in developmentally delayed children. *Merrill-Palmer Quarterly, 30*, 33–48.

Mundy, P., Sigman, M., Kasari, C., & Yirmiya, N. (1988). Nonverbal communication skills in children with Down syndrome. *Child Development, 59*, 235–249.

Natsopoulos, D., & Xeromeritou, A. (1988). Comprehension of "before" and "after" by normal and educable mentally retarded children. *Journal of Applied Developmental Psychology, 9*, 181–199.

Neff, N. A., Walters, J., & Egel, A. L. (1984). Establishing generative yes/no responses in developmentally disabled children. *Journal of Applied Behavior Analysis, 17*, 453–460.

Nelson, K. (1973). Structure and strategy in learning to talk. *Monographs of the Society for Research in Child Development, 38*(Serial No. 149).

Nelson, K. (1975). The nominal shift in semantic–syntactic development. *Cognitive Psychology, 7*, 461–479.

Nelson, K. (1981). Individual differences in language development: Implications for development and language. *Developmental Psychology, 17*, 170–187.

Nelson, K. E. (1977). Facilitating children's syntax acquisition. *Developmental Psychology, 13*, 101–107.

Nelson, K. E., Carskaddon, G., & Bonvillian, J. D. (1973). Syntax acquisition: Impact of experimental variation in adult verbal interaction with the child. *Child Development, 44*, 497–504.

Nelson, K. E., Denninger, M. M., Bonvillian, J. D., Kaplan, B. J., & Baker, N. (1984). Maternal input adjustments and nonadjustments as related to children's linguistic advances and to language acquisition theories. In A. Pellegrini & T. Yawkey (Eds.), *The development of oral and written language in social contexts* (pp. 31–56). Norwood, NJ: Ablex.

Newfield, M. U., & Schlanger, B. B. (1968). The acquisition of English morphology by normal and educable retarded children. *Journal of Speech and Hearing Research, 11*, 693–706.

Newport, E. L. (1977). Motherese: The speech of mothers to young children. In N. Castellan, D. Pisoni, & G. Potts (Eds.), *Cognitive theory* (Vol. 2). Hillsdale, NJ: Lawrence Erlbaum Associates.

Newport, E. L., Gleitman, L. R., & Gleitman, H. (1977). Mother, I'd rather do it myself: Some effects and noneffects of maternal speech style. In C. E. Snow & C. A. Ferguson (Eds.), *Talking to children: Language input and acquisition* (pp. 109–149). New York: Cambridge University Press.

Newport, E. L., & Supalla, T. (1987). *A critical period effect in the acquisition of a primary language*. Unpublished manuscript, University of Illinois, Urbana.

Ninio, A., & Bruner, J. (1978). The achievements and antecedents of labeling. *Journal of Child Language, 5,* 1–15.

Nippold, M. A., Leonard, L. B., & Anastopoulos, A. (1982). Development in the use and understanding of polite forms in children. *Journal of Speech and Hearing Research, 25,* 193–202.

Nuccio, J. B., & Abbeduto, L. (1993). Dynamic contextual variables and the directives of persons with mental retardation. *American Journal on Mental Retardation, 97,* 547–558.

Nwokah, E. E. (1982). "Once upon a time"—Aspects of storytelling in normal and retarded children. *Language and Speech, 25,* 293–298.

Obrzut, J. E., Boliet, C. A., & Obrzut, A. (1986). The effect of stimulus type and directed attention on dichotic listening with children. *Journal of Experimental Child Psychology, 41,* 198–209.

Ochs, E., & Schieffelin, B. B. (1984). Language acquisition and socialization: Three developmental stories and their implications. In R. Shweder & R. LeVine (Eds.), *Culture theory: Essays on mind, self, and emotion* (pp. 276–319). New York: Cambridge University Press.

Oetting, J. B., & Rice, M. L. (1991). Influence of the social context on pragmatic skills of adults with mental retardation. *American Journal on Mental Retardation, 95,* 435–443.

Olenick, D. L., & Pear, J. J. (1980). Differential reinforcement of correct responses to prompts and probes in picture-naming training with retarded children. *Journal of Applied Behavior Analysis, 13,* 77–89.

Oliver, C. B., & Halle, J. W. (1982). Language training in the everyday environment: Teaching functional sign use to a retarded child. *Journal of the Association for the Severely Handicapped, 7,* 50–62.

Oller, D. K. (1980). The emergence of the sounds of speech in infancy. In G. Yeni-Komshian, J. Kavanagh, & C. Ferguson (Eds.), *Child phonology: Vol. 1. Production* (pp. 93–112). New York: Academic.

Oller, D. K., & Eilers, R. E. (1982). Similarity of babbling in Spanish- and English-learning babies. *Journal of Child Language, 9,* 565–577.

Oller, D. K., & Seibert, J. M. (1988). Babbling of prelinguistic mentally retarded children. *American Journal on Mental Retardation, 92,* 369–375.

Oller, D. K., Weiman, L. A., Doyle, W. J., & Ross, C. (1976). Infant babbling and speech. *Journal of Child Language, 3,* 1–11.

Olson-Fulero, L., & Conforti, J. (1983). Child responsiveness to mother questions of varying type and presentation. *Journal of Child Language, 10,* 495–520.

Olson, D. R., & Hildyard, A. (1981). Assent and compliance in children's language. In W. P. Dickson (Ed.), *Children's oral communication skills* (pp. 313–335). New York: Academic.

Olson, D. R., & Nickerson, N. (1978). Language development through the school years. In K. E. Nelson (Ed.), *Language development*. New York: Gardner Press.

Oshima-Takane, Y. (1988). Children learn from speech not addressed to them: The case of personal pronouns. *Journal of Child Language, 15,* 95–108.

Owens, R. E., Jr., & MacDonald, J. D. (1982). Communicative uses of the early speech of nondelayed and Down syndrome children. *American Journal of Mental Deficiency, 86,* 503–510.

Owings, N. O., & McManus, M. D. (1980). An analysis of communication functions in the speech of a deinstitutionalized adult mentally retarded client. *Mental Retardation, 18,* 309–314.

Owings, N. O., McManus, M. D., & Scherer, N. J.(1981). A deinstitutionalized retarded adult's use of communication functions in a natural setting. *British Journal of Disorders of Communication, 16,* 119–128.

Papania, N. (1954). A qualitative analysis of vocabulary responses of institutionalized mentally retarded children. *Journal of Clinical Psychology, 10*, 361–365.

Paris, S. G., Mahoney, G. J., & Buckholt, J. A. (1974). Facilitation of semantic integration in sentence memory of retarded children. *American Journal of Mental Deficiency, 78*, 714–720.

Patterson, C. J., Massad, C. M., & Cosgrove, J. M. (1978). Children's referential communication: Components of plans for effective listening. *Developmental Psychology, 14*, 401–406.

Paul, R., & Cohen, D. J. (1984). Responses to contingent queries in adults with mental retardation and pervasive developmental disorders. *Applied Psycholinguistics, 5*, 349–357.

Paul, R., & Cohen, D. J. (1985). Comprehension of indirect requests in adults with autistic disorders and mental retardation. *Journal of Speech and Hearing Research, 28*, 475–479.

Paul, R., Dykens, E., Lechman, J. F., Watson, M., Breg, W. R., & Cohen, D. J. (1987). A comparison of language characteristics of mentally retarded adults with fragile X syndrome and those with nonspecific mental retardation and autism. *Journal of Autism and Developmental Disorders, 17*, 457–468.

Pease, D. M., Gleason, J. B., & Pan, B. A. (1989). Gaining meaning: Semantic development. In J. B. Gleason (Ed.), *The development of language* (2nd ed., pp. 101–134). Columbus, OH: Merrill.

Pelligrini, A. D. (1984). A speech analysis of preschooler's dyadic interaction. *Communication and Cognition, 17*, 425–436.

Penner, S. (1987). Parental responses to grammatical and ungrammatical child utterances. *Child Development, 58*, 376–384.

Perez-Pereira, M. (1991). The acquisition of gender: What Spanish children tell us. *Journal of Child Language, 18*, 571–590.

Perner, J., & Leekam, S. R. (1986). Belief and quantity: Three year olds' adaptation to listener knowledge. *Journal of Child Language, 13*, 305–315.

Peters, A. M. (1977). Language learning strategies: Does the whole equal the sum of the parts? *Language, 53*, 560–573.

Peters, A. M. (1983). *The units of language acquisition*. New York: Cambridge University Press.

Peterson, C., & McCabe, A. (1983). *Developmental psycholinguistics: Three ways of looking at a child's narrative*. New York: Plenum.

Peterson, C. L., Danner, F. W., & Flavell, J. H. (1972). Developmental changes in children's responses to three indications of communicative failure. *Child Development, 43*, 1463–1468.

Petersen, G. A., & Sherrod, K. B. (1982). Relationship of maternal language to development and language delay of children. *American Journal of Mental Deficiency, 86*, 391–398.

Petitto, L. A. (1988). Language in the prelinguistic child. In F. S. Kessel (Ed.), *The development of language and language researchers* (pp. 187–221). Hillsdale, NJ: Lawrence Erlbaum Associates.

Petitto, L. A., & Marentette, P. F. (1991). Babbling in the manual mode: Evidence for the ontogeny of language. *Science, 25*, 1493–1496.

Piaget, J. (1952). *The origins of intelligence in children* (M. Cook, Trans.). New York: International Universities Press.

Piaget, J. (1980). Schemes of action and language learning. In P. Piatelli-Palmarini (Ed.), *Language and Learning* (pp. 163–183). Cambridge, MA: Harvard University Press.

Piaget, J., & Inhelder, B. (1969). *The psychology of the child*. New York: Basic.

Pine, J. M., & Lieven, E. V. M. (1990). Referential style at 13 months: Why age-defined cross-sectional measures are inappropriate for the study of strategy differences in early language development. *Journal of Child Language, 17*, 625–631.

Pinker, S. (1984). *Language learnability and language development*. Cambridge, MA: Harvard University Press.

Pinker, S. (1987). The bootstrapping problem in language acquisition. In B. MacWhinney (Ed.), *Mechanisms of language acquisition* (pp. 399–441). Hillsdale, NJ: Lawrence Erlbaum Associates.

Pinker, S. (1988). Learnability theory and the acquisition of a first language. In F. S. Kessel (Ed.), *The development of language and language researchers* (pp. 97–120). Hillsdale, NJ: Lawrence Erlbaum Associates.

Pinker, S. (1989). Language acquisition. In M. I. Posner (Ed.), *Foundations of cognitive science* (pp. 359–400). Cambridge, MA: MIT Press.

Pinker, S. (1990). Language acquisition. In D. N. Osherson & H. Lasnik (Eds.), *Language: An invitation to cognitive science* (Vol. 1, pp. 199–241). Cambridge, MA: MIT Press.

Pinker, S. (1991). Rules of language. *Science, 253*, 530–535.

Pipe, M. E. (1983). Dichotic listening performance following auditory discrimination training in Down's syndrome and developmentally retarded children. *Cortex, 19*, 481–491.

Pipe, M. E. (1985). Attenuation of dichotic-listening ear advantages by stimulus bias. *Neuropsychologia, 23*, 437–440.

Pipe, M. E. (1988). Atypical laterality and retardation. *Psychological Bulletin, 104*, 343–347.

Pisarchick, S. E. (1987). Down's syndrome. In C. R. Reynolds & L. Mann (Eds.), *Encyclopedia of special education* (Vol. 1, pp. 541–543). New York: Wiley.

Poizner, H., Klima, E. S., & Bellugi, U. (1987). *What the hands reveal about the brain.* Cambridge, MA: MIT Press.

Prater, R. J. (1982). Functions of consonant assimilation and re-duplication in early word productions of mentally retarded children. *American Journal of Mental Deficiency, 86*, 399–404.

Prelock, P. A., & Panagos, J. M. (1980). Mimicry versus imitative modeling: Facilitating sentence production in the speech of the retarded. *Journal of Psycholinguistic Research, 9*, 565–578.

Price-Williams, D., & Sabsay, S. (1979). Communicative competence among severely retarded persons. *Semiotica, 26*, 35–63.

Pueschel, S. M. (1988). Visual and auditory processing in children with Down syndrome. In L. Nadel (Ed.), *The psychobiology of Down syndrome* (pp. 199–216). Cambridge, MA: MIT Press.

Pye, C. (1986). Quiché Mayan speech of children. *Journal of Child Language, 13*, 85–100.

Quigley, S. P., & King, C. M. (1982). The language development of deaf children and youths. In S. Rosenberg (Ed.), *Handbook of applied psycholinguistics: Major thrusts of research and theory* (pp. 429–475). Hillsdale, NJ: Lawrence Erlbaum Associates.

Radford, A. (1990a). *Syntactic theory and the acquisition of English syntax: The nature of early child grammars of English.* Oxford, England: Blackwell.

Radford, A. (1990b). The syntax of nominal arguments in early child English. *Language Acquisition, 1*, 195–223.

Read, B., & Cherry, L. J. (1978). Preschool children's production of directive forms. *Discourse Processes, 1*, 233–245.

Reeder, K. (1980). The emergence of illocutionary skills. *Journal of Child Language, 7*, 13–28.

Reeder, K. (1983). Classifications of children's speech acts: A consumer's guide. *Journal of Pragmatics, 7*, 679–694.

Reeder, K. (1990). Text or context: The influence of early literate experience upon preschool children's speech act comprehension. In G. Conti-Ramsden & C. Snow (Eds.), *Children's language* (Vol. 7, pp. 305–326). Hillsdale, NJ: Lawrence Erlbaum Associates.

Reeder, K., & Wakefield, J. (1987). The development of young children's speech act comprehension: How much language is necessary? *Applied Psycholinguistics, 8*, 1–18.

Reeder, K., Wakefield, J., & Shapiro, J. (1988). Children's speech act comprehension strategies and early literacy experiences. *First Language, 8*, 29–48.

Reich, P. A. (1986). *Language development.* Englewood Cliffs, NJ: Prentice-Hall.

Reichle, J., Mirenda, P., Locke, P., Piche, L., & Johnston, S. (1992). Beginning augmentative communication systems. In S. F. Warren & J. Reichle (Eds.), *Causes and effects in communication and language intervention* (pp. 113–130). Baltimore, MD: Brookes.

Reichle, J., Rogers, N., & Barrett, C. (1984). Establishing pragmatic discriminations among the communicative functions of requesting, rejecting, and commenting in an adolescent. *Journal of the Association for Persons with Severe Handicaps, 9*, 31–36.

Revelle, G. L., Karabenick, J. D., & Wellman, H. M. (1981, April). *Comprehension monitoring in preschool children.* Paper presented at the meeting of the Society for Research in Child Development, Boston, MA.

Revelle, G. L., Wellman, H. M., & Karabenick, J. D. (1985). Comprehension monitoring in preschool children. *Child Development, 56,* 654–663.

Rice, M. (1983). Contemporary accounts of the cognitive/language relationship: Implications for speech-language clinicians. *Journal of Speech and Hearing Disorders, 48,* 347–359.

Rice, M. (1984). Cognitive aspects of communicative development. In R. L. Schiefelbusch & J. Pickar (Eds.), *The acquisition of communicative competence* (pp. 141–189). Baltimore: University Park Press.

Rice, M. (1986). Mismatched premises of the communicative competence model and language intervention. In R. Schiefelbusch (Ed.), *Language competence: Assessment and intervention* (pp. 261–280). San Diego, CA: College-Hill.

Roberts, R. J., Jr., & Patterson, C. J. (1983). Perspective taking and referential communication: The question of correspondence reconsidered. *Child Development, 54,* 1005–1014.

Robinson, E. J., & Robinson, W. P. (1976). The young child's understanding of communication. *Developmental Psychology, 12,* 328–333.

Robinson, E. J., & Robinson, W. P. (1977). Development in the understanding of causes of success and failure in verbal communication. *Cognition, 5,* 363–378.

Robinson, E. J., & Robinson, W. P. (1981). Ways of reacting to communicative failure in relation to the development of children's understanding about verbal communication. *European Journal of Social Psychology, 11,* 189–208.

Robinson, E. J., & Robinson, W. P. (1982). The advancement of children's verbal referential communication skills: The role of metacognitive guidance. *International Journal of Behavioural Development, 5,* 329–335.

Robinson, E. J., & Robinson, W. P. (1983). Communication and metacommunication: Quality of children's instructions in relation to judgments about the adequacy of instructions and the locus of responsibility for communication failure. *Journal of Experimental Child Psychology, 36,* 305–320.

Robinson, E. J., & Whittaker, S. J. (1986). Learning about verbal referential communication in the early school years. In K. Durkin (Ed.), *Language development during the school years* (pp. 155–171). London: Croom Helm.

Robinson, N., & Robinson, H. (1976). *The mentally retarded child* (2nd ed.). New York: McGraw-Hill.

Roeper, T. (1988). Grammatical principles of first language acquisition: Theory and evidence. In F. J. Newmeyer (Ed.), *Linguistics: The Cambridge survey* (Vol. 2, pp. 35–52). Cambridge, England: Cambridge University Press.

Rogers-Warren, A. K., & Warren, S. (1980). Mands for verbalization: Facilitating the generalization of newly trained language in children. *Behavior Modification, 4,* 230–245.

Rohr, A., & Burr, D. B. (1978). Etiological differences in patterns of psycholinguistic development of children of IQ 30–60. *American Journal of Mental Deficiency, 82,* 549–553.

Romski, M. A., & Sevcik, R. A. (1992). Developing augmented language in children with severe mental retardation. In S. F. Warren & J. Reichle (Eds.), *Causes and effects in communication and language intervention* (pp. 113–130). Baltimore, MD: Brookes.

Rondal, J. A. (1978a). Developmental sentence procedure and the delay-difference question in language development of Down's syndrome children. *Mental Retardation, 16,* 169–171.

Rondal, J. A. (1978b). Maternal speech to normal and Down's syndrome children matched for mean length of utterance. In C. E. Meyers (Ed.), *Quality of life in severely and profoundly mentally retarded people: Research foundations for improvements* (pp. 193–265). Washington, DC: American Association on Mental Deficiency.

Rondal, J. A. (1987). Language development in Down syndrome: A life-span approach. *International Journal of Behavioural Development* [special issue], 1–21.

Rondal, J. A. (1988). Down syndrome. In D. V. M. Bishop & K. Magford (Eds.), *Language development in exceptional circumstances.* Edinburgh: Churchill Livingstone.

Rondal, J. A. (in press). Parent-child interaction and the process of language acquisition in severe mental retardation: Beyond the obvious. In K. Marfo (Ed.), *Mental handicap and parent-child interaction.* New York: Praeger.

Rondal, J. A., & Cession, A. (1990). Input evidence regarding the semantic bootstrapping hypothesis. *Journal of Child Language, 17*, 711–722.

Rondal, J. A., Ghiotto, M., Brédart, S., & Bachelet, J. F. (1988). Mean length of utterance of children with Down syndrome. *American Journal of Mental Retardation, 93*, 64–66.

Rosch, E. (1975). Cognitive representation of semantic categories. *Journal of Experimental Psychology: General, 104*, 192–233.

Rosch, E. (1988). Coherences and categorization: A historical view. In F. S. Kessel (Ed.), *The development of language and language researchers* (pp. 373–391). Hillsdale, NJ: Lawrence Erlbaum Associates.

Rosch, E., & Mervis, C. B. (1975). Family resemblances: Studies in the internal structure of categories. *Cognitive Psychology, 7*, 573–605.

Rosenberg, S. (1982). The language of the mentally retarded: Development, processes, and intervention. In S. Rosenberg (Ed.), *Handbook of applied psycholinguistics: Major thrusts of research and theory* (pp. 329–392). Hillsdale, NJ: Lawrence Erlbaum Associates.

Rosenberg, S. (1984). Disorders of first-language development: Trends in research and theory. In E. S. Gollin (Ed.), *Malformations of development: Biological and psychological sources and consequences* (pp. 195–237). New York: Academic.

Rosenberg, S., & Abbeduto, L. (1987). Indicators of linguistic competence in the peer group conversational behavior of mildly retarded adults. *Applied Psycholinguistics, 8*, 19–32.

Rosenberg, S. A., & Robinson, C. C. (1985). Enhancement of mothers' interactional skills in an infant education program. *Education and Training of the Mentally Retarded, 20*, 163–169.

Rosin, M. M., Swift, E., Bless, D., & Vetter, D. (1985). *Communication profiles of adolescents with Down syndrome.* Unpublished manuscript, Waisman Center for Mental Retardation and Human Development, University of Wisconsin, Madison.

Roth, F. P., & Davidge, N. S. (1985). Are early verbal communicative intentions universal? A preliminary investigation. *Journal of Psycholinguistic Research, 14*, 351–363.

Rueda, R., & Chan, K. S. (1980). Referential communication skill levels of moderately mentally retarded adolescents. *American Journal of Mental Deficiency, 85*, 45–52.

Rusch, J. C., & Karlan, G. R. (1983). Language training. In J. L. Matson & J. A. Mulick (Eds.), *Handbook of mental retardation* (pp. 397–409). New York: Pergamon.

Ryan, J. (1975). Mental subnormality and language development. In E. H. Lenneberg & E. Lenneberg (Eds.), *Foundations of language development* (Vol. 2, pp. 269–277). New York: Academic.

Ryan, J. (1977). The silence of stupidity. In J. Morton & J. C. Marshall (Eds.), *Psycholinguistics: Developmental and pathological* (pp. 99–124). Ithaca, NY: Cornell University Press.

Sabo, H., Bellugi, U., & Vaid, J. (1986). *Selective sparing of grammatical functions in children with Williams syndrome.* Unpublished manuscript, The Salk Institute, San Diego.

Sachs, J. (1989). Communication development in infancy. In J. B. Gleason (Ed.), *The development of language* (2nd ed., pp. 35–57). Columbus, OH: Merrill.

Sachs, J., Bard, B., & Johnson, M. L. (1981). Language learning with restricted input: Case studies of two hearing children of deaf parents. *Applied Psycholinguistics, 2*, 33–54.

Sacks, H., Schegloff, E., & Jefferson, G. (1974). A simple systematics for the organization of turn-taking in conversation. *Language, 50*, 696–735.

Scarborough, H. S., Rescorla, L., Tager-Flusberg, H., Fowler, A. E., & Sudhalter, V. (1991). The relation of utterance length to grammatical complexity in normal and language-disordered groups. *Applied Psycholinguistics, 12*, 23–45.

Scarborough, H. S., & Wyckoff, J. (1986). Mother, I'd still rather do it myself: Some further non-effects of motherese. *Journal of Child Language, 13*, 431–437.

Schaffer, H. R., Collis, G. M., & Parsons, G. (1977). Vocal interchange and visual regard in verbal and preverbal children. In H. R. Schaffer (Ed.), *Studies in mother–infant interaction*. London: Academic.

Schaffer, H. R., Hepburn, A., & Collis, G. M. (1983). Verbal and nonverbal aspects of mother's directives. *Journal of Child Language, 10*, 337–355.

Scherer, N. J., & Owings, N. O. (1984). Learning to be contingent: Retarded children's responses to their mothers' requests. *Language and Speech, 27,* 255-267.

Schiefelbusch, R. L., & Pickar, J. (Eds.). (1984). *The acquisition of communicative competence.* Baltimore: University Park Press.

Schieffelin, B. B. (1979). Getting it together: An ethnographic approach to the study of the development of communicative competence. In E. Ochs & B. B. Schieffelin (Eds.), *Developmental pragmatics* (pp. 73-108). New York: Academic.

Schieffelin, B. B. (1986). *How Kaluli children learn what to say, what to do, and how to feel.* New York: Cambridge University Press.

Schlanger, B. B. (1973). *Mental retardation.* New York: Bobbs-Merrill.

Schloss, P. J., & Wood, C. E. (1990). Effect of self-monitoring on maintenance and generalization of conversational skills of persons with mental retardation. *Mental Retardation, 28,* 105-113.

Schneiderman, M. H. (1983). "Do what I mean, not what I say!" Changes in mothers' action-directives to young children. *Journal of Child Language, 10,* 337-356.

Schwartz, I. S. (1987). A review of techniques for naturalistic language training. *Child Language Teaching and Therapy, 3,* 267-276.

Schwartz, R. G., & Camarata, C. (1985). Examining relationships between input and language development: Some statistical issues. *Journal of Child Language, 12,* 199-207.

Scollon, R. (1976). *Conversations with a one year old: A case study of the developmental foundation of syntax.* Honolulu: University Press of Hawaii.

Seagoe, M. V. (1965). Verbal development in a mongoloid. *Exceptional Children, 21,* 269-273.

Searle, J. R. (1969). *Speech acts.* Cambridge, England: Cambridge University Press.

Searle, J. R. (1975). Indirect speech acts. In P. Cole & J. L. Morgan (Eds.), *Syntax and semantics* (Vol. 3, pp. 59-82). New York: Academic.

Searle, J. R. (1976). A classification of illocutionary acts. *Language in Society, 5,* 1-23.

Seibert, J. M., & Hogan, A. E. (1981). *Procedures manual for the Early Social-Communication scales.* Unpublished manuscript, Mailman Center for Child Development, University of Miami, FL.

Sells, P. (1985). *Lectures on contemporary syntactic theories.* Stanford: CSLI.

Shantz, C. U. (1981). The role of role-taking in children's referential communication. In W. P. Dickson (Ed.), *Children's oral communication skills* (pp. 85-102). New York: Academic.

Shantz, C. U. (1983). Social cognition. In P. H. Mussen (Ed.), *Handbook of child psychology* (Vol. 3, pp. 495-555). New York: Wiley.

Shatz, M. (1978). On the development of communicative understandings: An early strategy for interpreting and responding to messages. *Cognitive Psychology, 10,* 271-301.

Shatz, M. (1983). Communication. In P. Mussen (Ed.), *Handbook of child psychology* (Vol. 4, pp. 841-889). New York: Wiley.

Shatz, M., & Gelman, R. (1977). Beyond syntax: The influence of conversational constraints on speech modifications. In C. E. Snow & C. A. Ferguson (Eds.), *Talking to children* (pp. 189-198). Cambridge, England: Cambridge University Press.

Shatz, M., Hoff-Ginsberg, E., & MacIver, D. (1989). Induction and the acquisition of English auxiliaries: The effects of differentially enriched input. *Journal of Child Language, 16,* 121-140.

Shatz, M., & McCloskey, L. (1984). Answering appropriately: A developmental perspective on conversational knowledge. In S. Kuczaj II (Ed.), *Discourse development: Progress in cognitive development research* (pp. 20-36). New York: Springer-Verlag.

Shatz, M., & O'Reilly, A. W. (1990). Conversational or communicative skill? A reassessment of 2-year-olds' behavior in miscommunication episodes. *Journal of Child Language, 17,* 131-146.

Sigman, M., Mundy, P., Sherman, T., & Ungerer, J. (1986). Social interactions of autistic, mentally retarded, and normal children and their caregivers. *Journal of Child Psychology and Psychiatry, 27,* 647-656.

Silverman, K., Anderson, S. R., Marshall, A. M., & Baer, D. M. (1986). Establishing and generalizing audience control of new language repertoires. *Analysis and Intervention in Developmental Disabilities, 6,* 21-40.

Simeonsson, R. J., Monson, L. B., & Blacher, J. (1984). Social understanding and mental retardation. In P. Brooks, R. Sperber, & C. McCauley (Eds.), *Learning and cognition in the mentally retarded* (pp. 389–417). Hillsdale, NJ: Lawrence Erlbaum Associates.

Sinclair, H. (1975). Language and cognition in subnormals: A Piagetian view. In N. O'Connor (Ed.), *Language, cognitive deficits, and retardation* (pp. 155–168). London: Butterworths.

Siperstein, G. N. (1992). Social competence: An important construct in mental retardation. *American Journal on Mental Retardation, 96,* iii–vi.

Skinner, B. F. (1957). *Verbal behavior.* New York: Appleton-Century-Crofts.

Skinner, B. F. (1974). *About behaviorism.* New York: Knopf.

Slater, M. A. (1986). Modification of mother–child interaction in families with children at risk for mental retardation. *American Journal of Mental Deficiency, 91,* 257–267.

Slobin, D. I. (1982). Universal and particular in the acquisition of language. In E. Wanner & L. R. Gleitman (Eds.), *Language acquisition: The state of the art* (pp. 128–170). New York: Cambridge University Press.

Slobin, D. I. (1985). Crosslinguistic evidence for the language-making capacity. In D. I. Slobin (Ed.), *The crosslinguistic study of language acquisition: Vol. 2. Theoretical issues* (pp. 1157–1256). Hillsdale, NJ: Lawrence Erlbaum Associates.

Smeets, P., & Streifel, S. (1976). Training the generative usage of article-noun responses in severely retarded males. *Journal of Mental Deficiency Research, 20,* 121–127.

Smith, B. L. (1982). Some observations concerning premeaningful vocalizations of hearing-impaired infants. *Journal of Speech and Hearing Disorders, 47,* 439–442.

Smith, B. L. (1988). The emergent lexicon from a phonetic perspective. In M. D. Smith & J. L. Locke (Eds.), *The emergent lexicon* (pp. 75–106). San Diego, CA: Academic.

Smith, B. L., & Oller, D. K. (1981). A comparative study of premeaningful vocalizations produced by normally developing and Down's syndrome infants. *Journal of Speech and Hearing Disorders, 46,* 46–51.

Smith, B. L., & Stoel-Gammon, C. (1983). A longitudinal study of the development of stop consonant production in normal and Down's syndrome children. *Journal of Speech and Hearing Disorders, 48,* 114–118.

Smith, L., & von Tetzchner, S. (1986). Communicative, sensorimotor, and language skills of young children with Down syndrome. *American Journal of Mental Deficiency, 91,* 57–66.

Smith, L. B., Sera, M., Gattuso, B. (1988). The development of thinking. In R. J. Sternberg & E. E. Smith (Eds.), *The psychology of human thought* (pp. 366–391). New York: Cambridge University Press.

Smith, M. D., & Locke, J. L. (Eds.). (1988). *The emergent lexicon: The child's development of a linguistic vocabulary.* San Diego, CA: Academic.

Smolak, L. (1987). Child characteristics and maternal speech. *Journal of Child Language, 14,* 481–492.

Snart, F., O'Grady, M., & Das, J. P. (1982). Cognitive processing by subgroups of moderately mentally retarded children. *American Journal of Mental Deficiency, 86,* 465–472.

Snow, C. E. (1972). Mothers' speech to children learning language. *Child Development, 43,* 549–565.

Snow, C. E. (1977). The development of conversation between mothers and babies. *Journal of Child Language, 4,* 1–22.

Snow, C. E. (1984). Parent–child interaction and the development of communicative ability. In R. L. Schiefelbusch & J. Pickar (Eds.), *The acquisition of communicative competence* (pp. 69–108). Baltimore, MD: University Park Press.

Snow, C. E. (1986). Conversations with children. In P. Fletcher & M. Garman (Eds.), *Language acquisition* (2nd ed., pp. 69–89). Cambridge, England: Cambridge University Press.

Snow, C. E., & Ferguson, C. A. (Eds.). (1977). *Talking to children: Language input and language acquisition.* Cambridge, England: Cambridge University Press.

Snow, C. E., Perlmann, R. Y., Gleason, J. B., & Hooshyar, N. (1990). Developmental perspectives on politeness: Sources of children's knowledge. *Journal of Pragmatics, 14,* 289–305.

Snow, C. E., Perlmann, R., & Nathan, D. (1987). Why routines are different: Toward a multiple-factors model of the relation between input and language acquisition. In K. Nelson & A. van Kleeck (Eds.), *Children's language* (Vol. 6, pp. 65–98). Hillsdale, NJ: Lawrence Erlbaum Associates.

Snyder, L. S. (1978). Communicative and cognitive abilities and disabilities in the sensorimotor period. *Merrill-Palmer Quarterly, 24*, 161–180.

Sodian, B. (1988). Children's attributions of knowledge to the listener in a referential task. *Child Development, 59*, 378–385.

Sommers, R. K., & Starkey, K. L. (1977). Dichotic verbal processing in Down's syndrome children having qualitatively different speech and language skills. *American Journal of Mental Deficiency, 82*, 44–53.

Sonnenschein, S. (1984a). The effects of redundant communications on listeners: Why different types may have different effects. *Journal of Psycholinguistic Research, 13*, 147–166.

Sonnenschein, S. (1984b). Why young listeners do not benefit from differentiating verbal redundancy. *Child Development, 55*, 929–935.

Sonnenschein, S. (1986a). Development of referential communication: Deciding that a message is uninformative. *Developmental Psychology, 22*, 164–168.

Sonnenschein, S. (1986b). Development of referential communication skills: How familiarity with a listener affects a speaker's production of redundant messages. *Developmental Psychology, 22*, 549–552.

Sonnenschein, S. (1988). The development of referential communication: Speaking to different listeners. *Child Development, 59*, 694–702.

Sonnenschein, S., & Whitehurst, G. J. (1983). Training referential communication skills: The limits of success. *Journal of Experimental Child Psychology, 35*, 426–436.

Spearman, C. (1927). *The abilities of man.* New York: Macmillan.

Sperber, R. D., Davies, D., Merrill, E. C., & McCauley, C. (1982). Cross-category differences in the processing of subordinate–superordinate relationships. *Child Development, 53*, 1249–1253.

Sperber, R. D., Ragain, R. D., & McCauley, C. (1976). Reassessment of category knowledge in retarded individuals. *American Journal of Mental Deficiency, 81*, 227–234.

Spiegel, B. B. (1983). The effect of context on language learning by severely retarded young adults. *Language, Speech, and Hearing Services in Schools, 14*, 252–259.

Spradlin, J. E., & Siegel, G. (1982). Language training in natural and clinical environments. *Journal of Speech and Hearing Disorders, 47*, 2–6.

Stampe, D. L. (1969). The acquisition of phonetic representation. *Papers from the Fifth Regional Meeting of the Chicago Linguistic Society* (pp. 433–444).

Stark, R. E. (1980). Stages of speech development in the first year of life. In G. Yeni-Komshian, J. Kavanagh, & C. Ferguson (Eds.), *Child phonology: Vol. 1. Production* (pp. 73–90). New York: Academic.

Stark, R. E. (1986). Prespeech segmental feature development. In P. Fletcher & M. Garman (Eds.), *Language acquisition* (2nd ed., pp. 149–173). Cambridge, England: Cambridge University Press.

Steckol, K., & Leonard, L. (1981). Sensorimotor development and the use of prelinguistic performatives. *Journal of Speech and Hearing Research, 24*, 262–268.

Stephens, C. E., Pear, J. J., Wray, L. D., & Jackson, G. S. (1975). Some effects of reinforcement schedules in teaching picture names to retarded children. *Journal of Applied Behavior Analysis, 7*, 435–447.

Stern, D., Jaffe, J., Beebe, B., & Bennett, S. (1975). Vocalizing in unison and in alternation: Two modes of communication within the mother–infant dyad. In D. Aaronson & R. W. Rieber (Eds.), *Developmental psycholinguistics and communication disorders.* New York: New York Academy of Sciences.

Sternberg, R. J. (1988a). Intelligence. In R. J. Sternberg & E. E. Smith (Eds.), *The psychology of human thought* (pp. 267–308). New York: Cambridge University Press.

Sternberg, R. J. (1988b). *The triarchic mind: A new theory of human intelligence.* New York: Viking.

Stiles-Davis, M., Kritchevsky, M., & Bellugi, U. (Eds.). (in press). *Spatial cognition: Brain bases and development.* Chicago: University of Chicago Press.

Stoel-Gammon, C. (1980). Phonological analysis of four Down's syndrome children. *Applied Psycholinguistics, 1,* 31-48.

Stokes, T., & Baer, D. M. (1977). An implicit technology of generalization. *Journal of Applied Behavior Analysis, 10,* 349-367.

Stremel-Campbell, K., & Campbell, C. R. (1985). Training techniques that may facilitate generalization. In S. F. Warren & A. K. Rogers-Warren (Eds.), *Teaching functional language* (pp. 251-288). Austin, TX: Pro-Ed.

Sudhalter, V., Cohen, I. L., Silverman, W., & Wolf-Schein, E. G. (1990). Conversational analyses of males with fragile X, Down syndrome and autism: Comparison of the emergence of deviant language. *American Journal on Mental Retardation, 94,* 431-441.

Sugarman, S. (1984). The development of preverbal communication: Its contributions and limits in promoting the development of language. In R. L. Schiefelbusch & J. Pickar (Eds.), *The acquisition of communicative competence* (pp. 23-67). Baltimore, MD: University Park Press.

Surian, L. (1991). Do children exploit the maxim of antecedent in order to interpret ambiguous descriptions? *Journal of Child Language, 18,* 451-457.

Swinney, D. (1979). Lexical access during sentence comprehension: (Re)consideration of context effects. *Journal of Verbal Learning and Verbal Behavior, 18,* 645-660.

Tager-Flusberg, H. (1985a). Basic level and superordinate level categorization by autistic, mentally retarded, and normal children. *Journal of Experimental Child Psychology, 40,* 450-469.

Tager-Flusberg, H. (1985b). The conceptual basis for referential word meaning in children with autism. *Child Development, 56,* 1167-1178.

Tager-Flusberg, H. (1989). Putting words together: Morphology and syntax in the preschool years. In J. B. Gleason (Ed.), *The development of language* (2nd ed., pp. 135-165). Columbus, OH: Merrill.

Tannock, R. (1988). Mother directiveness in their interactions with their children with and without Down syndrome. *American Journal on Mental Retardation, 93,* 154-165.

Tannock, R., & Girolametto, L. (1992). Reassessing parent focused language intervention programs. In S. F. Warren & J. Reichle (Eds.), *Causes and effects in communication and language intervention* (pp. 49-79). Baltimore, MD: Brookes.

Tannock, R., Kershner, J. R., & Oliver, J. (1984). Do individuals with Down's syndrome possess right hemisphere language dominance? *Cortex, 20,* 221-231.

Thompson, M. M. (1963). Psychological characteristics relevant to the education of the pre-school mongoloid child. *Mental Retardation, 1,* 148-151.

Thurstone, L. L. (1938). *Primary mental abilities.* Chicago: University of Chicago Press.

Tomasello, M., Farrar, M., & Dines, J. (1984). Children's speech revisions for a familiar and unfamiliar adult. *Journal of Speech and Hearing Research, 27,* 359-363.

Tomasello, M., Mannle, S., & Kruger, A. C. (1986). Linguistic environment of 1- to 2-year-old twins. *Developmental Psychology, 22,* 169-176.

Tomasello, M., & Todd, J. (1983). Joint attention and lexical acquisition style. *First Language, 4,* 197-212.

Trehub, S. E. (1976). The discrimination of foreign speech contrasts by infants and children. *Child Development, 47,* 466-472.

Trevarthen, C. (1986). Facial, vocal, and gestural signs for motivation for speech in infants. In B. Lindblom & R. Zetterstrom (Eds.), *Precursors of early speech.* New York: Stockton Press.

Uzgiris, I. C., & Hunt, J. M. (1975). *Assessment in infancy: Ordinal scales of psychological development.* Urbana, IL: University of Illinois Press.

Valian, V. (1986). Syntactic categories in the speech of young children. *Developmental Psychology, 22,* 562-579.

van Kleeck, A., Maxwell, M., & Gunter, C. (1985). A methodological study of illocutionary coding in adult–child interaction. *Journal of Pragmatics, 9*, 659–681.

Vernon, P. E. (1971). *The structure of human abilities*. London: Methuen.

Vihman, M. M., Ferguson, C. A., & Elbert, M. (1986). Phonological development from babbling to speech: Common tendencies and individual differences. *Applied Psycholinguistics, 7*, 3–40.

Vihman, M. M., & Miller, R. (1988). Words and babble at the threshold of language acquisition. In M. D. Smith & J. L. Locke (Eds.), *The emergent lexicon* (pp. 151–183). San Diego: Academic.

Waldo, L., Guess, D., & Flanagan, B. (1982). Effects of concurrent and serial training on receptive labeling by severely retarded individuals. *Journal of the Association of Persons with Severe Handicaps, 7*, 56–66.

Warren, S. F. (1987, November). *Recent trends in language intervention research: Children and adolescents with mental retardation*. Paper presented at the American Speech and Hearing Association convention, New Orleans, LA.

Warren, S. F., & Kaiser, A. P. (1986). Incidental language teaching: A critical review. *Journal of Speech and Hearing Disorders, 51*, 291–299.

Warren, S. F., & Kaiser, A. P. (1988). Research in early language intervention. In S. L. Odom & M. B. Karnes (Eds.), *Research in early childhood special education* (pp. 89–108). Baltimore: Paul H. Brookes.

Warren, S. F., McQuarter, R. J., & Rogers-Warren, A. K. (1984). The effects of mands and models on the speech of unresponsive socially isolate children. *Journal of Speech and Hearing Disorders, 47*, 42–52.

Warren, S. F., & Rogers-Warren, A. K. (1983). A longitudinal analysis of language generalization among adolescents with severely handicapping conditions. *Journal of the Association for the Severely Handicapped, 8*, 18–31.

Waryas, C. L., & Stremel-Campbell, K. (1982). *Communication training program: Levels 1, 2, & 3*. Hingham, MA: Teaching Resources.

Waxman, S. R., & Kosowsky, T. D. (1990). Nouns mark category relations: Toddlers' and preschoolers' word-learning biases. *Child Development, 61*, 1461–1473.

Weeks, D. J., & Elliott, D. (1992). Atypical cerebral dominance in Down syndrome. *Bulletin of the Psychonomics Society, 30*, 23–25.

Weil, C., McCauley, C., & Sperber, R. D. (1978). Category structure and semantic priming in retarded adolescents. *American Journal of Mental Deficiency, 83*, 110–115.

Weiss, B., Weisz, J. R., & Bromfield, R. (1986). Performance of retarded and nonretarded persons on information-processing tasks: Further tests of the similar structure hypothesis. *Psychological Bulletin, 100*, 157–175.

Weisz, J. R., & Yeates, K. O. (1981). Cognitive development in retarded and nonretarded persons. Piagetian tests of the similar structure hypothesis. *Psychological Bulletin, 90*, 153–178.

Weisz, J. R., & Zigler, E. (1979). Cognitive development in retarded and nonretarded persons: Piagetian tests of the similar sequence hypothesis. *Psychological Bulletin, 86*, 831–851.

Welch, S. J., & Pear, J. J. (1980). Generalization of naming responses to objects in the natural environment as a function of training stimulus modality with retarded children. *Journal of Applied Behavior Analysis, 13*, 629–643.

Wellman, H. M., & Lempers, J. D. (1977). The naturalistic communicative abilities of 2-year-olds. *Child Development, 48*, 1052–1057.

Werker, J. F. (1980). Becoming a native listener. *American Scientist, 77*, 54–59.

Wexler, K. (1991). On the argument from the poverty of the stimulus. In A. Kasher (Ed.), *The Chomskyan turn* (pp. 252–269). Cambridge, MA: Blackwell.

Wexler, K., & Culicover, P. (1980). *Formal principles of language acquisition*. Cambridge, MA: MIT Press.

Wheldall, K. (1976). Receptive language development in the mentally handicapped. In P. Berry (Ed.), *Language and communication in the mentally handicapped* (pp. 36–55). London: Edward Arnold.

Whitehurst, G. J., & Sonnenschein, S. (1985). The development of communication: A functional analysis. In G. J. Whitehurst (Ed.), *Annals of child development* (Vol. 2, pp. 1–48). Greenwich, CT: JAI.

Wiegel-Crump, C. A. (1981). The development of grammar in Down's syndrome children between mental ages of 2-0 and 6-11 years. *Education and Training of the Mentally Retarded, 16*, 24–30.

Wildman, B. G., Wildman, H. E., & Kelly, W. J. (1986). Group conversational-skills training and social validation with mentally retarded adults. *Applied Research in Mental Retardation, 7*, 443–458.

Wilkinson, L. C. (Ed.). (1982). *Communicating in the classroom*. New York: Academic.

Wilkinson, L. C., & Calculator, S. (1982). Effective speakers: Students' use of language to request and obtain information and action in the classroom. In L. C. Wilkinson (Ed.), *Communicating in the classroom* (pp. 85–99). New York: Academic.

Wilkinson, L. C., & Spinelli, F. (1983). Using requests effectively in peer-directed instructional groups. *American Educational Research Journal, 20*, 479–501.

Wilkinson, L. C., Wilkinson, A. C., Spinelli, F., & Chiang, C. P. (1984). Metalinguistic knowledge of pragmatic rules in school-age children. *Child Development, 55*, 2130–2140.

Winner, E. (1988). *The point of words: Children's understanding of metaphors and irony*. Cambridge, MA: Harvard University Press.

Winters, J. J., & Brzoska, M. A. (1976). Development of formation of categories by normal and retarded persons. *Developmental Psychology, 12*, 125–131.

Winters, J. J., & Hoats, D. L. (1985). Comparison of verbal typicality judgments of mentally retarded and nonretarded persons. *American Journal of Mental Deficiency, 90*, 335–341.

Winters, J. J., & Hoats, D. L. (1986). Comparison of mentally retarded and nonretarded persons' organization of semantic memory. *American Journal of Mental Deficiency, 91*, 102–104.

Winters, J. J., Hoats, D. L., & Kahn, H. (1985). The relationship between typicality ratings and semantic characteristics as a function of intelligence level. *Bulletin of the Psychonomics Society, 23*, 195–198.

Witelson, S. F. (1988). Brain asymmetry, functional aspects. In J. A. Hobson (Ed.), *States of brain and mind* (pp. 13–16). Boston: Birkhauser.

Wright, R. E., & Rosenberg, S. (1993). Knowledge of text coherence and expository writing: A developmental study. *Journal of Educational Psychology*.

Yamada, J. E. (1990). *Laura: A case for the modularity of language*. Cambridge, MA: MIT Press.

Yoder, P. J., & Davies, B. (1990). Do parental questions and topic continuations elicit replies from developmentally delayed children?: A sequential analysis. *Journal of Speech and Hearing Research, 33*, 563–573.

Yoder, P. J., & Davies, B. (1992a). Do children with developmental delays use more frequent and diverse language in verbal routines? *American Journal on Mental Retardation, 97*, 197–208.

Yoder, P. J., & Davies, B. (1992b). Greater intelligibility in verbal routines with young children with developmental delays. *Applied Psycholinguistics, 13*, 77–91.

Yoder, P. J., & Feagans, L. (1988). Mothers' attributions of communication to prelinguistic behavior of developmentally delayed and mentally retarded infants. *American Journal on Mental Retardation, 93*, 36–43.

Yoder, P. J., & Kaiser, A. P. (1989). Alternative explanations for the relationship between maternal verbal interaction style and child language development. *Journal of Child Language, 16*, 141–160.

Yoder, P. J., Kaiser, A. P., & Alpert, C. L. (1989, March). *A comparison between didactic and milieu teaching in small groups of handicapped preschoolers of varying developmental levels*. Paper presented at American Speech and Hearing Association's Treatment Efficacy Conference in San Antonio, TX.

Zangwill, O. L. (1969). Intellectual status in aphasia. In P. J. Vinken & G. W. Bruyn (Eds.), *Disorders of speech perception and symbolic behavior*. Amsterdam: North-Holland.

Zekulin-Hartley, X. Y. (1981). Hemispheric asymmetry in Down's syndrome children. *Canadian Journal of Behavioral Science, 13*, 210–217.

Zekulin-Hartley, X. Y. (1983). Selective attention to dichotic input of retarded children. *Cortex*, *8*, 311–316.

Zetlin, A. G., & Sabsay, S. (1980, March). *Characteristics of verbal interaction among moderately retarded peers*. Paper presented at Gatlinburg Conference on Research in Mental Retardation, Gatlinburg, TN.

Zigler, E., & Hodapp, R. M. (1986). *Understanding mental retardation*. Cambridge, England: Cambridge University Press.

Zwitman, D., & Sonderman, J. (1979). A syntax program designed to present base linguistic structures to language-disordered children. *Journal of Communication Disorders*, *2*, 323–335.

Author Index

A

Abbeduto, L., 5, 6, 8, 27, 33, 34, 77, 80, 95, 96, 97, 99, 100, 106, 107, 110, 112, 117, 119, 120, 121, 129, 137, 139, 140, 141, 143, 144, 145, 146, 147, 148, 149, 150, 151, 152, 153, 154, 155, 156, 157, 158, 159, 160, 161, 162, 172, 182, 189, 213, *215, 216, 235, 239*
Ackerman, B. P., 109, 116, 120, 121, 140, *216*
Acunzo, M., 121, *216*
Adams, C., 140, *218*
Adamson, L. B., 174, 175, *230*
Adkins, J., 208, *232*
Aitchison, J., 173, 174, 181, *216*
Akhtar, N., 68, *216*
Allen, D. V., 95, *218*
Al-Mabuk, R., 120, *215*
Alpert, C. L., 193, 195, 202, 210, *216, 245*
Anastopoulos, A., 118, *235*
Anderson, B. J., 124, *216*
Anderson, S. R., 196, 205, 206, *216, 240*
Andrews, J. G., 90, *216*
Andrews, R. J., 90, *216*
Angelo, D., 197, 198, 199, *227*
Anisfeld, M., 85, *216*
Anselmi, D., 121, *216*

Applebaum, M. I., 141, *224*
Armstrong, V., 91, *232*
Ashman, A. F., 91, *216*
Aslin, R. N., 24, 40, *216, 222*
Astington, J., 117, 161, *216*
Astin-Smith, S., 209, *230*
Au, T. K. F., 69, *216*
August, D. L., 122, *225*
Austin, J. L., 110, 142, *216*
Axia, G., 118, 119, *216, 217*

B

Bach, K., 108, 110, 113, 142, 161, *216*
Bachelet, J. F., 88, *239*
Bacri, N., 25, *223*
Baer, D. M., 193, 199, 200, 203, 204, 205, 206, *228, 240, 243*
Baillargeon, R., 39, *226*
Baker, N., 44, *234*
Bambara, L. M., 202, 207, *221*
Bandura, A., 191, 196, 207, *216*
Bard, B., 41, 47, *239*
Barnes, S. B., 41, *216*
Barnett, J., 200, 202, 213, 214, *216*
Baroni, M. R., 118, 119, *216, 217*
Barrera, R. D., 132, *231*
Barrett, C., 200, 207, *237*
Barrett, M. D., 72, *217*

247

Subject Index

A

Adaptive behavior, 8-9
Adult-child interaction, 163-186
  child-directed adjustments, in Down syndrome
    children, 165-169
  lexical usage, 169
  following the child's lead, 172-174
    in Down syndrome children, 173-174
  parental directiveness, 174-181
    in Down syndrome children, 175-177, 178,
      179-180, 181
  parental speech acts, 181-183
    in Down syndrome children, 182-183
  prelinguistic intent, 170-171
  quantity of parental talk, 185
  social interactionist perspective, 163-165,
    171, 172, 173, 175, 183-184
  turn taking, in Down syndrome infants,
    171-172
  verbal routines, 183-184
Adults with mild mental retardation, 5-6
  grammatical morphemes, 6
  complex sentence structures, 6

C

Child-directed language, *see* Adult-child
  interaction

Cognition-language relationships, 2-5, 7-8,
  11-13, 13-14, 28-29, 33-39, 62-63,
  72, 73, 74-75, 75-77, 77-78, 86-87,
  90, 91, 93-94, 100-103
  cognition-first view, 33-39
  early grammatical development and, 2-5
  exceptional language development, 7-8, 77,
    78, 90, 100-103
  information processing deficits, 91
  MA-matching, 13-14
  modularity, 29
  morphosyntactic development, 86-87, 90
  phonological development, 62-63
  Piaget's theory, 11-13
  semantic development, 72, 73, 74-75,
    75-77
  Williams syndrome, 77-78

D

Down syndrome, 2-5, 55-59, 71-72, 76,
  89-92
  early grammatical development, 2-5
  exceptional language development, 90
  interaction with adults in, *see* Adult-child
    interaction
  morphosyntactic development, 89-92
  phonological development, 55-59
  semantic development, 71-72, 76

259

Printed and bound by CPI Group (UK) Ltd, Croydon, CR0 4YY

17/10/2024

01775685-0005